S0-AGU-063

An Irreverent
and Almost
Complete
Social History
of the
Bathroom

IN THE BATH

by Michael Flanders and Donald Swann

To be sung whilst taking a bath. Unaccompanied.

A percussion rhythm may be added with the aid of two toothbrushes and an empty glass.

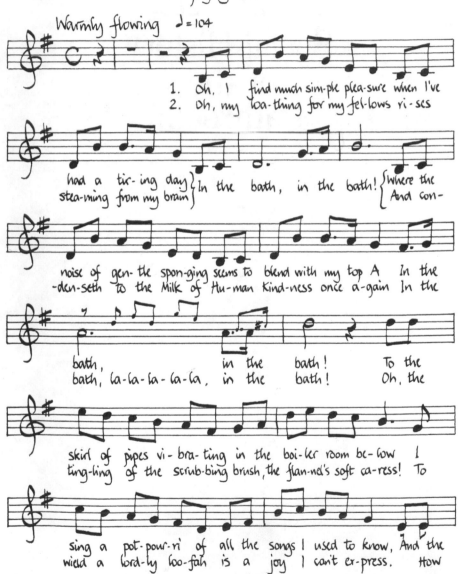

Warmly flowing ♩=104

1. Oh, I find much sim-ple plea-sure when I've had a tir-ing day
2. Oh, my loa-thing for my fel-lows ri-ses stea-ming from my brain

In the bath, in the bath!

Where the noise of gen-tle spon-ging seems to blend with my top A In the
And con-den-seth to the Milk of Hu-man Kind-ness once a-gain In the

bath, in the bath! To the
bath, la-la-la-la-la, in the bath! Oh, the

skirl of pipes vi-bra-ting in the boi-ler room be-low I
ting-ling of the scrub-bing brush, the flan-nel's soft ca-ress! To

sing a pot-pour-ri of all the songs I used to know, And the
wield a lord-ly loo-fah is a joy I can't ex-press. How

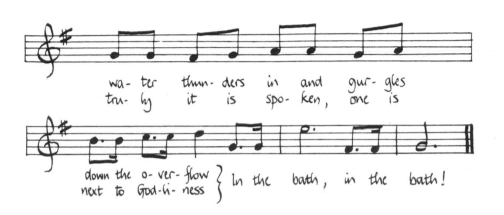

wa- ter thun- ders in and gur- gles
tru- ly it is spo- ken, one is

down the o- ver- flow } In the bath, in the bath!
next to God- li- ness }

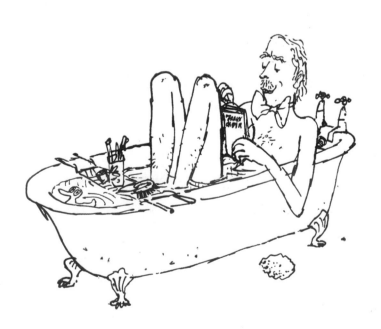

Also by FRANK MUIR

An Irreverent and Thoroughly
Incomplete Social History of
Almost Everything

With Denis Norden

The My Word! Stories

An Irreverent and Almost Complete Social History of the Bathroom

FRANK MUIR

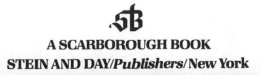

A SCARBOROUGH BOOK
STEIN AND DAY/*Publishers*/New York

First published in the United States of America in 1983
Copyright © 1982 by Frank Muir
All rights reserved
Printed in the United States of America

STEIN AND DAY/ *Publishers*
Scarborough House
Briarcliff Manor, N.Y. 10510

Library of Congress Cataloging in Publication Data

Muir, Frank.
    An irreverent and almost complete social history of the
bathroom.

    Originally published: A book at bathtime. London :
Heinemann, 1982.
    1. Bathing customs--History. 3. Bathrooms--History.
3. Baths--History. 4. Hygiene--History. 5. Toilets--
History. I. Title.
GT2845.M84 1983   391'.64   82-42838
ISBN 0-8128-2912-3
ISBN 0-8128-6186-8 (pbk.)

An Irreverent and Almost Complete Social History of the Bathroom

INTRODUCTION

A recent study of reading habits (*Book Industry Study Group Report No. 6*, 1978) revealed, without much pleasure, that as many readers do their reading in bathrooms as in libraries.

Many volumes have been written in the hope that they will be brooded upon in the dry silence of a library. In the light of the above statistic, it seemed high time that a modest volume was addressed specifically to the other half; to those who enjoy a read in the gurgling privacy of their bathroom.

It also seemed appropriate that as the impetus of this modest volume was the revelation that the bathroom is more than it seems in our social life, its subject should be an investigation into what part the bath, and the other facilities of a bathroom, played in the social life of our forefathers.

Letters, memoirs, poems, stories and gossip reveal that this social life was indeed 'social'. Only in comparatively recent years have we decided that we can only decently take a bath or perform our natural functions when we are alone. And only in even more recent years have we regularly smothered ourselves in lather, holding that Cleanliness is next to Godliness.

The concept of our modern bathroom as a hygienic, deodorized module with everything built-in is less than a hundred years old. As we glance round its constituent parts we can compare them with the facilities which our ancestors had to do battle with. How they coped is revealed in their writings. We learn of Disraeli, whose wife had to pull the string on his cold shower; of the Marquise who boiled her leg in the Seine; of Balzac whose ambition in life was to become so famous that he would be allowed to break wind in society;

of the lady in the public privy in Holland who kindly offered an English gentleman the loan of her mussel-shell scraper when she had finished with it. We also learn of the social dilemmas brought about by the W.C. (or whatever you call it) never having been given a simple, acceptable name, thus plunging posterity into the agony of having to sort out a mess of euphemisms; to separate, as it were, the U-bend words from the non-U-bend words.

For background information on the subject of bathrooms I am happily indebted to that Bible of Bathrooms, *Clean and Decent* by Lawrence Wright. Also to an odd volume of much charm and erudition, written it seems during the war whilst on Air Raid Precautions watch in Chelsea, *Cleanliness and Godliness*, by Reginald Reynolds.

> 'Go little book, on your chosen path
> To learning on the loo, laughter in the bath . . .'

Frank Muir
THORPE, 1982

P. S. Advances in modern science and technology have provided the solution to a problem which has bedevilled cleanly readers for centuries: how to read in a hot bath without your spectacles steaming up. You dip your spectacles into the hot bath for a moment and then polish them dry with a handy length of soft tissue.

There it rests, dominating the bathroom; a long rectangle of smooth porcelain falling into deep soft curves; unchanged in shape from the one into which King Midas of Knossos stepped some 3700 years ago.

Taking a bath is, to some people, a necessary chore to be got through as rapidly as possible, like cleaning one's shoes.

To a distinguished and immensely prolific modern author it was something else entirely:

> Lying in a hot bath, smoking a pipe. And Elagabalus himself, after driving his white horses through the gold-dusted streets of Rome, never knew anything better; nor indeed anything as good, not having either pipe or tobacco. People still say to me 'The way you work!', and behind the modest smirk I laugh secretly, knowing myself to be one of the laziest and most self-indulgent men alive. Long after they have caught the 8.20, opened the morning mail, telephoned to the managing director of the Cement Company, dictated yet another appeal to the Board of Trade, I am lying in my hot bath, smoking a pipe. I am not even soaping and scrubbing, but simply lying there, like a pink porpoise, puffing away. In a neighbouring room, thrown on the floor, are the morning papers, loud with more urgent demands for increased production, clamouring for every man and woman to save the country. And there I am,

lost in steam, the fumes of Latakia, and the vaguest dreams. Just beyond the bolted door, where the temperature drops nearly to freezing point, are delicate women, who have already been up for hours, toiling away. And do I care? Not a rap. Sometimes I pretend, just to test the credulity of the household, that I am planning my day's work; but I am doing nothing of the kind. Often I do not intend to do any work at all during the day; and even when I know I must do some, I could not possibly plan it, in or out of a bath. No, I am just lying there, a pampered slug, with my saurian little eyes half-closed, cancelling the Ice Ages, lolling again in the steamy hot morning of the world's time, wondering dimly what is happening to Sir Stafford Cripps. '. . . One of the most energetic and prolific of our authors. . . .' *Gertcha!*

J. B. Priestley (*1894–*)
DELIGHTS, 1949

Perhaps Mr. Priestley's pleasure was heightened by the knowledge that he was in no danger where he was:

'People born to be hanged are safe in water.'

Mark Twain's mother
Quoted in MARK TWAIN, A BIOGRAPHY, A. B. Paine

Young Master Robin, at prayers, remembered his romp in the bath with pleasure too:

God Bless Mummy. I know that's right.
Wasn't it fun in the bath to-night?
The cold's so cold, and the hot's so hot.
Oh! *God Bless Daddy* – I quite forgot.

A. A. Milne (*1882–1956*)
WHEN WE WERE VERY YOUNG

Getting up in the morning in the sixteenth century was rather different from today. A noted medical man of the time recommended it be accomplished with a light laugh and a prayer but not much in the way of ablutions:

> When you do rise in the morning, rise with
> mirth, and remember God. Let your hose be
> brushed within and without, and flavour the inside
> of them against the fire; use linen socks or linen
> hose next to your legs. When you be out of your
> bed, stretch forth your legs and your arms, and
> your body; cough and spit, and then go to your
> stool to make your egestion; and exonerate
> yourself at all times that nature would expel. After
> you have evacuated your body and trussed your
> points, comb your head oft; and so do divers times
> in the day. And wash your hands and wrists, your
> face and eyes, and your teeth, with cold water.

Andrew Boorde (*1490?–1549*)
DYETARY

When Lady Ruthven visited the young Pauline Borghese in Rome she found that personal cleanliness in 1862 among aristocrats was not vigorously pursued:

> When the guests arrived, they found the
> Princess – supremely lovely – with her beautiful
> little white feet exposed upon a velvet cushion.
> Then two or three maids came in, and touched the
> feet with a sponge and dusted them with a little
> powder – 'c'était la toilette des pieds.' The Duke
> of Hamilton used to take up one of the little feet
> and put it inside his waistcoat 'like a little bird'.

Augustus Hare (*1834–1903*)
THE STORY OF MY LIFE

The little Princess clearly did not have an English nanny to remind her of her obligations:

'We don't like that girl from Tooting Bec,
She washes her face and forgets her neck.'

Quoted in NANNY SAYS. (1972) Sir Hugh Casson and Joyce Grenfell

The Ancient Greeks and Romans had large and elaborate bath houses with water at varying temperatures. These became popular places to meet friends, cadge a free dinner, gossip. Slaves were on hand to anoint with oils, massage and generally mop up. But not everybody could be bothered with bathing. One mathematician, head full of isosceles triangles and acute angles, had to be forcibly cleansed:

Oftimes his [Archimedes'] servants got him
against his will to the baths, to wash and anoint
him: and yet being there, he would ever be
drawing out of the geometrical figures, even in the
very imbers of the chimney. And while they were
anointing of him with oils and sweet savours, with
his fingers he did draw lines upon his naked body:
so far was he taken from himself, and brought into
an extasy or trance, with the delight he had in the
study of geometry.

Plutarch (*1st. century A.D.*)
LIVES

The Ancients seemed to bath in considerable comfort. Even a Chinese Emperor's new concubine could count on a dip in a nice warm vase whilst on call:

Two days, two nights, and she was still in the
royal bed-chamber. Three times he slept and each
time she went to the door and beckoned to her
serving woman, and the woman came creeping
through the curtains to the boudoir beyond. There

the eunuchs had prepared a ready bath, a cauldron of water upon coals, so that the woman needed only to dip the water into the vast porcelain jar and make her mistress fresh again. She had brought clean garments and different robes and she brushed Yehonala's hair and coiled it smoothly. Not once did the young girl speak except to give direction and not once did the serving woman ask a question. Each time when her task was done Yehonala went in again to the imperial bedroom and the heavy doors were closed behind the yellow curtains.

Pearl S. Buck (*1892–1973*)
IMPERIAL WOMEN

In Turkey the ancient tradition of communal hot baths was maintained with such national enthusiasm that these steamy affairs became known to Europeans as 'Turkish Baths'. The first Englishwoman to penetrate one of these was Lady Mary Wortley Montagu, who wrote to a friend:

I won't trouble you with a relation of our tedious journey; but I must not omit what I saw remarkable at Sophia, one of the most beautiful towns in the Turkish empire, and famous for its hot baths, that are resorted to both for diversion and health. I stopped here one day on purpose to see them. Designing to go *incognita*, I hired a Turkish coach. These voitures are not at all like ours, but much more convenient for the country, the heat being so great that glasses would be very troublesome. They are made a good deal in the manner of the Dutch coaches, having wooden lattices painted and gilded; the inside being painted with baskets and nosegays of flowers, intermixed commonly with little poetical mottoes. They are covered all over with scarlet cloth, lined with silk, and very often richly embroidered and fringed. This covering entirely hides the persons in them, but may be thrown back at pleasure, and the ladies peep through the lattices. They hold four people very conveniently, seated on cushions, but not raised.

In one of these covered wagons, I went to the bagnio about ten o'clock. It was already full of women. It is built of stone, in the shape of a dome, with no windows but in the roof, which gives light enough. There were five of these domes joined together, the outmost being less than the rest, and serving only as a hall, where the portress stood at the door. Ladies of quality generally give this woman the value of a crown or ten shillings; and I did not forget that ceremony. The next room is a very large one paved with marble, and all round it, raised, two sofas of marble, one above another. There were four fountains of cold water in this room, falling first into marble basins, and then running on the floor in little channels made for that purpose, which carried the streams into the next room, something less than this, with the same sort of marble sofas, but so hot with steams of sulphur proceeding from the baths joining to it, it was impossible to stay there with one's clothes on. The two other domes were the hot baths, one of which had cocks of cold water turning into it, to temper it to what degree of warmth the bathers have a mind to.

I was in my travelling habit, which is a riding dress, and certainly appeared very extraordinary to them. Yet there was not one of them that shewed the least surprise or impertinent curiosity, but received me with all the obliging civility possible. I know no European court where the ladies would have behaved themselves in so polite a manner to a stranger. I believe in the whole, there were two hundred women, and yet none of those disdainful smiles, or satiric whispers, that never fail in our

8

assemblies when anybody appears that is not dressed exactly in the fashion. They repeated over and over to me, 'Uzelle, pék uzelle', which is nothing but Charming, very charming. The first sofas were covered with cushions and rich carpets, on which sat the ladies; and on the second, their slaves behind them, but without any distinction of rank by their dress, all being in the state of nature, that is, in plain English, stark naked, without any beauty or defect concealed. Yet there was not the least wanton smile or immodest gesture among them. They walked and moved with the same majestic grace which Milton describes of our general mother. There were many amongst them as exactly proportioned as ever any goddess was drawn by the pencil of Guido or Titian, – and most of their skins shiningly white, only adorned by their beautiful hair divided in many tresses, hanging on their shoulders, braided either with pearl or ribbon, perfectly representing the figures of the Graces.

I was here convinced of the truth of a reflection I had often made, that if it was the fashion to go naked, the face would be hardly observed. I perceived tha. the ladies with the finest skins and most delicate shapes had the greatest share of my admiration, though their faces were sometimes less beautiful than those of their companions. To tell you the truth, I had wickedness enough to wish secretly that Mr. Jervas could have been there invisible. I fancy it would have very much improved his art, to see so many fine women naked, in different postures, some in conversation, some working, others drinking coffee or sherbet, and many negligently lying on their cushions, while their slaves (generally pretty girls of seventeen or eighteen) were employed in braiding their hair in several pretty fancies. In short, it is the women's coffee-house, where all the news of the town is told, scandal invented, &c. – They generally take this diversion once a week, and stay there at least four or five hours, without getting cold by immediate coming out of the hot bath into the cold room, which was very surprising to me. The lady that seemed the most considerable among them, entreated me to sit by her, and would fain have undressed me for the bath. I excused myself with some difficulty. They being all so earnest in persuading me, I was at last forced to open my shirt, and shew them my stays; which satisfied them very well, for, I saw, they believed I was so locked up in that machine, that it was not in my own power to open it, which contrivance they attributed to my husband.

Lady Mary Wortley Montagu (1689–1762)
Letter to the Lady Rich, Adrianople, 1 April, 1717.

In more recent times a literary gentleman from America tried the baths and emerged unimpressed:

Here endeth my experience of the celebrated Turkish bath, and here also endeth my dream of the bliss the mortal revels in who passes through it. It is a malignant swindle. The man who enjoys it is qualified to enjoy anything that is repulsive to sight or sense . . .

Mark Twain (1835–1910)
THE INNOCENTS ABROAD

The sexes were usually segregated at these communal bath houses but a little mixed bathing was noticed by Pliny the Elder. According to first-hand reports from the poets Martial and Juvenal, ladies who dived in with the gentlemen were either whores or intellectuals (or both?). Mixed bathing was frowned upon but became prevalent in the Middle Ages when the baths were little more than brothels. Indeed the Italian word for bath *bagno*, and the English word *stews*, became synonyms for 'brothel'.

The nearest that the British got to the Roman/Turkish tradition of treating the bath house as the equivalent of a golf clubhouse or a W.I. Sewing Afternoon, or a house of assignation, was the development of Watering-Places, or Spas as they came to be called after the Belgian town of Spa where the whole thing started.

In 1606 it was discovered that a spring in the little town of Tunbridge, Kent, produced 'chalybeate waters' (chalybeate – not a word that drops from one's lips daily – means 'containing iron'). Citizens became convinced that if they forced some of this stuff down daily it would cure them of almost everything wrong with them so Tunbridge Wells – later Royal Tunbridge Wells – became a famous Watering-Place. A poet describes the elegant society to be met there in the seventeenth century:

At Five this Morn, when Phoebus rais'd his
    Head
From Thetis' Lap, I rais'd myself from Bed;
And mounting Steed, I trotted to the Waters,
The Rendezvous of Fools, Buffoons, and
    Praters,
Cuckolds, Whores, Citizens, their Wives and
    Daughters.
My squeamish Stomach I with Wine had
    brib'd,
To undertake the Dose that was prescrib'd;
But turning Head, a sudden cursed Crew
That innocent Provision overthrew,
Did, without drinking, make me purge and spew.

11

From Coach and Six a Thing unweildy roll'd,
Whom Lumber-Cart more decently would
   hold;
As wise as Calf it look'd, as big as Bully,
But handled, prov'd a mere Sir Nich'las
   Cully;
A bawling Fop, a *nat'ral* Nokes, and yet
He dar'd to *Censure*, to be thought a *Wit*.
To make him more ridiculous, in spight,
Nature contriv'd the Fool should be a Knight.
How wise is *Nature*, when she does dispense
A large Estate, to cover Want of Sense!
From hence unto the upper Walk I ran,
Where a new Scene of Foppery began;
A Tribe of Curates, Priests, Canonical Elves,
Fit Company for none beside themselves,
Were got together; each his Distemper told,
Scurvy, Stone, Strangury; some were so bold
To charge the Spleen to be their Misery,
And on that wise Disease lay Infamy.
But none had Modesty enough t'explain
His Want of Learning, Honesty, or Brain, . . .
Here, waiting for Gallant, young Damsel
   stood,
Leaning on Cane, and muffled up in Hood.
The Would-be-Wit, whose Bus'ness was to
   woe,

With Hat remov'd, and solemn Scrape of
    Shoe,
Advances bowing, then gentilely shrugs,
And ruffled Fore-Top into Order tugs;
And thus accosts her; *Madame, methinks the*
    Weather
Is grown much more serene since you came hither;
You influence the Heav'ns; but should the Sun
Withdraw himself, to see his Rays out-done
By your bright Eyes, They could supply the Morn,
And make a Day, before the Day be born.
With Mouth screw'd up, conceited winking
    Eyes,
And Breast thrust forward, *Lard, Sir,* (she
    replies,)
It is your goodness, and not my Deserts,
Which makes you shew this Learning, Wit, and
    Parts.
He, puzzled, bites his Nails, both to display
The sparkling Ring, and think what next to
    say,
And thus breaks forth afresh; *Madam, Egad,*
Your Luck at Cards Last Night was very bad;
At Cribbidge fifty nine —— and the next Shew,
To make the Game, —— and yet to want those two.
G—d D——, Madam, I'm the Son of a Whore,
If in my Life I saw the like before.

To Pedlar's Stall he drags her, and her Breast,
With Hearts and such like foolish Toys, he
    drest;
And then more smartly to expound the Riddle
Of all this Prattle, gives her a *Scotch* Fiddle.
Tir'd with this dismal Stuff, away I ran,
Faith, I was so asham'd, that with Remorse,
I us'd the Insolence to mount my *Horse*;
For *he*, doing only Things fit for his *Nature*,
Did seem to *me* by much the wiser *Creature*.

John Wilmot, Earl of Rochester (*1647–1680*)
TUNBRIDGE WELLS: A SATIRE

Townsfolk all over England dug furiously in the hope of locating a spring of foul-tasting water which would attract the fashionable world – the *ton* – and make everybody's fortune. An early, though fairly brief, success was made by Epsom, whose burghers located a spring so stiff with chemicals that they were able to produce not only a healing draught but also a crystallised version of the waters which proved to be a sure, rapid and explosive cure for constipation – Epsom Salts.

Tunbridge Wells was the upper-class Spa, much patronised by Nobility. At the other end of the social scale was Epsom, more convenient for London and a favourite haunt of London shopkeepers and their apprentices.

In between these two there were a number of other towns which had been lucky enough to tap a spring within their walls sufficiently sulphurous to attract the *beau monde*, e.g., Buxton, Malvern, Harrogate, Droitwich.

A slightly later but highly successful entry into the Spa racket (which it was) was Cheltenham. Set in a beautiful town the Spa became highly popular amongst the more elegant invalids and rose to even greater heights when it was Graced by the Condescension of a Visit from King George the Third and the Princesses.

What good its waters did was another matter:

> Here lie I and my four daughters,
> Killed by drinking Cheltenham waters.
> Had we but stuck to Epsom salts,
> We wouldn't have been in these here vaults.

Epitaph. Anon.

Cheltenham continued to flourish into the nineteenth century. The kind of people who foregathered there were not at all to the taste of a radical, four-square farmer/journalist/politician who saw it from the back of his horse:

> The Warwickshire Avon falls into the Severn here, and on the sides of both, for many miles back, there are the finest meadows that ever were seen. In looking over them, one wonders *what can become of all the meat?* By riding on about eight or nine miles further, however, this wonder is a little diminished; for here we come to one of the devouring WENS; namely CHELTENHAM, which is what they call a 'watering place'; that is to say, a place to which East India plunderers, West India floggers, English taxgorgers, together with gluttons, drunkards, and debauchees of all descriptions, *female* as well as male, resort, at the suggestion of silently laughing quacks, in the hope of getting rid of the bodily consequences of their manifold sins and iniquities. When I enter a place like this, I always feel disposed to squeeze up my nose with my fingers. It is nonsense, to be sure; but I conceit that every two-legged creature, that I see coming near me, is about to cover me with the poisonous proceeds of its impurities. To places like these come all that is knavish and all that is foolish and all that is base; gamesters, pick-

15

pockets, and harlots; young wife-hunters in search of rich and ugly and old women, and young husband-hunters in search of rich and wrinkled or half-rotten men, the former resolutely bent, be the means what they may, to give the latter heirs to their lands and tenements. These things are notorious.

William Cobbett (1763–1835)
RURAL RIDES

The Queen of English Spas, however, was Bath. It was the only city which could boast its own hot springs. There had been baths there since Roman times – hence its name – and during the Spa boom it had been put on the map by a visit from Queen Anne. It prospered. Elegant assembly rooms and terraces were built. Beau Nash was appointed the town's Master of Ceremonies and Bath settled down to its business of attracting the wealthy to wallow.

Taking the waters at Bath fell into a regular pattern. As soon as you arrived in town you were announced, in a kind of parody of death, by the tolling of a bell. Everybody who heard the bell knew that further gentry had joined them and quickly sent to know for whom the bell tolled.

The story is taken up by Oliver Goldsmith:

After the family is thus welcomed to *Bath*, it is the custom for the master of it to go to the public places, and subscribe two guineas at the assembly-houses towards the balls and music in the pump-house, for which he is entitled to three tickets every ball night. His next subscription is a crown, half a guinea, or a guinea, according to his rank and quality, for the liberty of walking in the private walks belonging to *Simpson's* assembly-house; a crown or half a guinea is also given to the booksellers, for which the gentleman is to have what books he pleases to read at his lodgings. And at the coffee-house another subscription is taken for pen, ink and paper, for such letters as the subscriber shall write at it during his stay. The ladies too may subscribe to the booksellers, and to an house by the pump-room, for the advantage of reading the news, and for enjoying each other's conversation.

Things being thus adjusted, the amusements of the day are generally begun by bathing, which is no unpleasing method of passing away an hour, or so.

The baths are five in number. On the south-west side of the abbey church is the King's Bath; which is an oblong square, the walls are full of niches, and at every corner are steps to descend into it: this bath is said to contain 427 tons and 50 gallons of water; and on its rising out of the ground over the springs, it is sometimes too hot to be endured by those who bathe therein. Adjoining to the King's Bath there is another, called the Queen's Bath; this is of more temperate warmth, as borrowing its water from the other.

In the south-west part of the city are three other baths, viz. The Hot Bath, which is not much inferior in heat to the King's Bath, and contains 53 tons 2 hogsheads, and 11 gallons of water. The Cross Bath, which contains 52 tons 3 hogsheads, and 11 gallons; and the Leper's Bath, which is not so much frequented as the rest.

The King's Bath (according to the best observations) will fill in about nine hours and a half; the Hot Bath in about eleven hours and a half; and the Cross Bath in about the same time.

The hours for bathing are commonly between six and nine in the morning; and the Baths are every morning supplied with fresh water; for when the people have done bathing, the sluices in each Bath are pulled up, and the water is carried off by drains into the river Avon.

In the morning the lady is brought in a close chair, dressed in her bathing cloaths, to the Bath; and, being in the water, the woman who attends, presents her with a little floating dish like a bason; into which the lady puts an handkerchief, a snuff-box, and a nosegay. She then traverses the Bath; if a novice with a guide, if otherwise by herself; and having amused herself thus while she thinks proper, calls for her chair, and returns to her lodgings.

The amusement of bathing is immediately succeeded by a general assembly of people at the pump-house, some for pleasure, and some to drink the hot waters. Three glasses, at three different times, is the usual portion for every drinker; and the intervals between every glass are enlivened by the harmony of a small band of music, as well as by the conversation of the gay, the witty, or the forward.

From the pump-house the ladies, from time to time, withdraw to a female coffee-house, and from thence return to their lodgings to breakfast. The gentlemen withdraw to their coffee-houses.

Oliver Goldsmith. (*1728–1774*)
THE LIFE OF RICHARD NASH, OF BATH, ESQ.

One of the publishing successes of the mid-eighteenth century was a poem, in a series of letters, describing a stay at Bath; Christopher Anstey's *The New Bath Guide*. It was issued in 1766 and went through ten editions before the end of the century. Horace Walpole wrote of it to his friend Montagu: 'What pleasure you have to come! There is a new thing published that will make you bepiss your cheeks with laughter.' That is, perhaps, rather too large a promise to make to modern readers but the verse gallops along and the author agreeably mocks the whole Taking the Cure charade.

Tabitha is the family's maid:

You cannot conceive what a number of ladies
Were wash'd in the water the same as our maid is:
Old Baron Vanteazer, a man of great wealth,
Brought his Lady, the Baroness, here for her
health;
The Baroness bathes, and she says that her case
Has been hit to a hair, and is mending apace;
And this is a point all the learned agree on,
The Baron has met with the fate of Acteon;
Who, while he peep'd into the bath, had the luck,
To find himself suddenly chang'd to a buck.
Miss Scratchit went in, and the Countess of Scales,
Both ladies of very great fashion in Wales:
Then all on a sudden two ladies of worth,
My Lady Pandora Macscurvy came forth,
With General Sulpher, arrived from the North.
So Tabby, you see, had the honour of washing
With folks of distinction, and very high fashion;
But in spite of good company, poor little soul,
She shook both her ears like a mouse in a bowl.
    Ods-bobs! how delighted I was unawares,
With the fiddles I heard in the room above stairs;
For music is wholesome, the doctors all think,
For ladies that bathe, and for ladies that drink:
And that's the opinion of Robin our driver,
Who whistles his nags while they stand at the river:
They say it is right that for every glass
A tune you should take that the water may pass.
So while little Tabby was washing her rump,
The ladies kept drinking it out of the pump.

Christopher Anstey. (*1724–1805*)
THE NEW BATH GUIDE

20

Those readers who are passionately devoted to limericks (if there can be any) might be interested to know that 'Roger the lodger', villain of the limerick which finishes 'It wasn't the Almighty Who lifted her nighty, but Roger the lodger the sod', seems to have been inspired by a poem in *The New Bath Guide*.

Miss Prudence informs Lady Betty that she has been elected to Methodism in a dream:

> Blessed I, tho' once rejected,
>   Like a little wand'ring sheep,
> Who this morning was elected
>   By a vision in my sleep.
>
> For I dream'd an apparition
>   Came, like Roger, from above;
> Saying, by divine commission,
>   I must fill you full of love.
>
> Just with Roger's head of hair on,
>   Roger's mouth and pious smile;
> Sweet, methinks, as beard of Aaron,
>   Dropping down with holy oil.
>
> I began to fall a-kicking,
>   Panted, struggled, strove, in vain;
> When the spirit whipt so quick in,
>   I was cur'd of all my pain.
>
> First I thought it was the night-mare
>   Lay so heavy on my breast;
> But I found new joy and light there,
>   When with heav'nly love possest.
>
> Come again then, apparition,
>   Finish what thou has begun;
> Roger, stay! thou soul's physician,
>   I with thee my race will run.

Ibid.

21

Innumerable authors took the waters at Bath and wrote about the experience, including Pope, Fielding, Sheridan, Fanny Burney, Jane Austen, Thackeray and Dickens. Tobias Smollett probably began his *The Expedition of Humphry Clinker* whilst staying there. The irascible Scottish doctor was highly critical of what he saw in the baths, even suggesting that the 'healing fluid' was foul to the taste because visitors were probably drinking the bath water:

I went into the King's Bath, by the advice of our friend Ch——, in order to clear the strainer of the skin, for the benefit of a free perspiration; and the first object that saluted my eye, was a child full of scrophulous ulcers, carried in the arms of one of the guides, under the very noses of the bathers. I was so shocked at the sight, that I retired immediately with indignation and disgust – Suppose the matter of those ulcers, floating on the water, comes in contact with my skin, when the pores are all open, I would ask you what must be the consequence? – Good Heaven, the very thought makes my blood run cold! we know not what sores may be running into the water while we are bathing, and what sort of matter we may thus imbibe; the king's-evil, the scurvy, the cancer, and the pox; and, no doubt, the heat will render the *virus* the more volatile and penetrating.

To purify myself from all such contamination, I went to the duke of Kingston's private Bath, and there I was almost suffocated for want of free air; the place was so small, and the steam so stifling.

After all, if the intention is no more than to wash the skin, I am convinced that simple element is more effectual than any water impregnated with salt and iron; which, being astringent, will certainly contract the pores, and leave a kind of crust upon the surface of the body. But I am now as much afraid of drinking, as of bathing; for, after a long conversation with the Doctor, about the construction of the pump and the cistern, it is very far from being clear with me, that the patients in the Pump-room don't swallow the scourings of the bathers. I can't help suspecting, that there is, or may be, some regurgitation from the bath into the cistern of the pump. In that case, what a delicate beveridge is every day quaffed by the drinkers; medicated with the sweat, and dirt, and dandriff; and the abominable discharges of various kinds, from twenty different diseased bodies, parboiling in the kettle below. In order to avoid this fithy composition, I had recourse to the spring that supplies the private baths on the Abbey-green; but I at once perceived something extraordinary in the taste and smell; and, upon inquiry, I find that the Roman baths in this quarter, were found covered by an old burying ground, belonging to the Abbey; thro' which, in all probability, the water drains in its passage: so that as we drink the decoction of living bodies at the Pump-room, we swallow the strainings of rotten bones and carcasses at the private bath – I vow to God, the very idea turns my stomach!

Tobias Smollett (*1721–1771*)
THE EXPEDITION OF HUMPHRY CLINKER

There is a modern anecdote which illustrates a more recent occasion when bathing and drinking became intertwined.

This story is absolutely true (or, if not true, a lie) and concerns a weekend when Lily Langtry was invited by an Earl to be a guest at his country houseparty. On Saturday morning milord took Miss Langtry aside and asked her whether she would be willing to sport in a bath in view of himself and the other male members of the houseparty, the bath to be filled with a light but sound hock.

Miss Langtry shyly agreed and the rendezvous was fixed at 11 p.m. that evening. At the given time the gentlemen filed solemnly into the mahogany bathroom in the guest wing and puffed silently at their cigars as Miss Langtry, with many a playful shriek, splashed and cavorted in the pale, transparent wine. They then filed out again, busy with their thoughts.

The Earl instructed the butler to rebottle the wine and serve it with the salmon mousse at Sunday luncheon as a fitting tribute to a beautiful and sporting lady. This was done, and the wine – and the gesture – was much appreciated by all.

But that afternoon the butler asked for a word with his master.

'Odd, milord' he said, 'Whereas I poured eight dozen bottles of the Esterhazy-Pierpont-Glückhauser '01 into Miss Langtry's bath – I re-bottled eight dozen bottles and one half'.

Probably the last examples of the large communal bath, endured for social and medicinal reasons for so many centuries, are municipal swimming-pools and a few institutional baths still used in some establishments as a cheap and simple method of getting batches of small boys, if not clean, at least wet:

> And there was the slimy water of the plunge
> bath – it was twelve or fifteen feet long, the whole
> school was supposed to go into it every morning,
> and I doubt whether the water was changed at all
> frequently – and the always-damp towels with
> their cheesy smell: and, on occasional visits in the
> winter, the murky sea-water of the local Baths,
> which came straight in from the beach and on
> which I once saw floating a human turd. And the
> sweaty smell of the changing-room with its greasy
> basins, and, giving on this, the row of filthy,
> dilapidated lavatories, which had no fastenings of
> any kind on the doors, so that whenever you were
> sitting there someone was sure to come crashing
> in. It is not easy for me to think of my schooldays
> without seeming to breathe in a whiff of something
> cold and evil-smelling – a sort of compound of
> sweaty stockings, dirty towels, faecal smells
> blowing along corridors, forks with old food
> between the prongs, neck-of-mutton stew, and the
> banging doors of the lavatories and the echoing
> chamber-pots in the dormitories.

George Orwell (*1903–1950*)
SUCH, SUCH WERE THE JOYS

Most hot-country religions laid down elaborate rules of hygiene. Ancient Eastern races and tribes, when they first came up against Western travellers, were horrified by their filthy habits: We did have *some* rules, of course:

> Wash your hands often, your feet seldom, your head never.
>
> English proverb. Sixteenth century.

And it was said, with considerable pride, that Queen Elizabeth I bathed once a month 'whether she needed it or no'.

Royalty and nobility frequently had elaborate baths constructed for their use but, of course, there was little or no plumbing to get the water in and take it away again. The water had to be warmed and poured in from jugs, like a marble version of a miner's galvanised iron tub. Bathing was a rare ritual event.

Some ladies preferred the simplicity of a dip in the river. One such dip inflamed a poet who wrote the lucky river a small ode:

> How fierce was I when I did see
> My Julia wash herself in thee!
> So lilies thorough crystal look,
> So purest pebbles in the brook,
> As in the river Julia did,
> Half with a lawn of water hid.
> Into thy stream myself I threw
> And struggling there I kissed thee too;
> And more had done, it is confessed,
> Had not the waves forbade the rest
>
> Robert Herrick (*1591–1674*)
> UPON JULIA'S WASHING HERSELF IN THE RIVER

The Marquise de Saint-Hérem, a slightly dotty French lady of the Court of Louis XIV, had an idea for making her dip in the river more agreeable. It was not a very good idea:

> She once succeeded in boiling her own leg in the
> middle of the River Seine, near Fontainebleau.
> The water had proved too cold for her liking when
> she was bathing, and she had had large quantities
> heated on the bank and poured around and over
> her, with the result that she was severely scalded
> and remained housebound for a week. In
> thunderstorms she had a habit of going down on all
> fours under her day-bed, and obliging her servants
> to lie piled on top of her, so that the thunder might
> lose its effect before it reached her.
>
> Duc de Saint-Simon (*1675–1755*)
> HISTORICAL MEMOIRS. Translated by Lucy Norton

What with one hazard and another, bathing seems to have been quite dangerous. The Dowager Duchess of Norfolk's great height almost provoked a catastrophe:

> The Dowager Duchess of Norfolk bathes, and
> being very tall she had like to have drowned a few
> women in the Cross Bath, for she ordered it to be
> filled till it reached to her chin, and so all those
> who were below her stature, as well as rank, were
> forced to come out or drown.
>
> Elizabeth Montagu (*1720–1800*)
> Letter to the Duchess of Portsmouth

A French Queen also got into difficulties:

> In this room there are several portraits of the
> French family, including pictures of the French
> Queen herself and of her husband Louis Philippe.
> Next door was her dressing room with a deep large
> bath, almost concealed, in which the old French

Queen was nearly drowned. Her attendant had left
her for a few minutes and when she returned the
old Queen was struggling and plunging about in
the bath almost at her last gasp.

Rev. Francis Kilvert (*1840–1879*)
DIARY Wed. 18 Jan. 1871

A bit of interest in bathing grew in the eighteenth century,
partly because people in the Age of Reason tended to be
enthusiastic about anything which could be called scientific,
and partly because they were obsessed with their health and
they came to believe that immersion in water was good for the
body. Cold baths, it seems, were a sovereign specific against
that widespread complaint – melancholia:

The cold Bath which I have gone into for three
weeks past have quite recovered my weak nerves
and restored me to good Spirits and the Blew
Devils are quite gone away, not, I suppose, very
well relishing the cold water.

Lord Dacre
Letter to Sanderson Miller, May 1745

They wrote poems and inscriptions about, and upon,
practically everything in that century. William Whitehead,
anxious to get the drooping patient into cold water once
med'cine had failed and balms and herbs essay'd their powers
in vain, wrote a poem to be inscribed on the side of the bath:

Whoe'er thou art, approach – Has med'cine
 fail'd?
 Have balms and herbs essay'd their powers
 in vain?
Nor the free air, nor fost'ring Sun prevail'd
 To raise thy drooping strength, or soothe
 thy pain?

Yet enter here. Nor doubt to trust thy frame
　To the cold bosom of this lucid lake.
Here Health may greet thee, and life's
　　languid flame,
　Ev'n from its icy grasp, new vigour take.

What soft Ausonia's genial shores deny,
　May Zembla give. Then boldly trust the
　　wave:
So shall thy grateful tablet hang on high,
　And frequent votaries bless this healing
　　cave.

William Whitehead (*1715–1785*)
INSCRIPTION FOR A COLD BATH

A superb example of an eighteenth-century didactic poem is *The Art of Preserving Health*, an extremely long, book-length poem telling the reader where it is healthiest to live, what to eat, etc., in blank verse so stately and rich that some passages have to be read many times with the help of a classical dictionary and the full-size O.E.D. before much of a message emerges.

In the following extract the poet, Dr. Armstrong, has something favourable to say about 'the gelid cistern' (the cold bath):

　　Against the rigours of a damp cold heav'n
　　To fortify our bodies, some frequent
　　The gelid cistern; and, where none forbids,
　　I praise their dauntless heart. A frame so steel'd
　　Dreads not the cough, nor those ungenial blasts,
　　That breathe the Tertian or fell Rheumatism;
　　The Nerves so temper'd never quit their tone,
　　No chronic langours haunt such hardy breasts...

29

Then he goes on a bit about 'the safe vicissitudes of life' which I do not wholly understand, and a passage 'ill-fitted he to want the known, or bear unusual things' which I do not understand at all. Then the mists clear and we find the poet advising global travellers to take three warm baths a day:

> Let those who from the frozen Arctos reach
> Parch'd Mauritania, or the sultry West,
> Or the wide flood that waters Indostan,
> Plunge thrice a day, and in the tepid wave
> Untwist their stubborn pores; that full and free
> Th' evaporation thro' the softened skin
> May bear proportion to the swelling blood.
> So shall they 'scape the fever's rapid flames;
> So feel untainted the hot breath of hell.
> With us, the man of no complaint demands
> The warm ablution, just enough to clear
> The sluices of the skin, enough to keep
> The body sacred from indecent soil.

John Armstrong M.D. (1769–1779)
THE ART OF PRESERVING HEALTH

It is no wonder that, apart from health cranks, hardly anybody at that time 'frequented the gelid cistern'. In his account of Samuel Johnson's middle years, James. L. Clifford describes what life was like without baths:

> But now back to Johnson's everyday life in the simple but commodious house in Gough Square. One may easily guess where Johnson and Tetty slept, but more perplexing problems have to do with sanitation and cleanliness. When Johnson wanted to wash his face, where did he find the water? And what happened to the dirty water after he was through? When he took a bath, if he ever did, where was the tub? In the bedroom? Or in the basement kitchen near one of the large fireplaces? And what happened to the contents of his chamber

pots? There are no references to such mundane matters in surviving diary entries or letters. All we can do is speculate, using such evidence as has come to light.

In 1749 in Gough Square there were certainly no bathrooms or running water. No ordinary London house at that time had bathrooms, and hardly any nobleman's. When Johnson and Tetty washed it was undoubtedly in a china bowl, with water from a nearby pitcher. By mid-century most houses on major streets did have leaden pipes bearing water from conduits coming into the basement or kitchen, but the water was turned on for short periods only three times a week. Thus the house-holder had to have a cistern or tank in the basement where water could be stored. For those without pipes the contents could be replenished by rain-water from gutters on the roof. And there were water carriers in most parts of London. Since Johnson did not live directly on a major street, it is unlikely that his house was supplied with pipes from the outside. In any case, water had to be carried upstairs by servants in pitchers or buckets, one explanation of the small size of portable tubs and the infrequency of bathing.

James L. Clifford (*1901–1979*)
DICTIONARY JOHNSON

It seems unlikely that the absence of washing facilities bothered Samuel Johnson. He did not regard personal cleanliness as being of much importance:

[of Kit Smart]
'He did not love clean linen, and I have no passion for it.'

Boswell's LIFE. 24 May, 1763

Boswell was more nattily dressed than Johnson but, it seems, was equally unwashed:

'James Boswell, the faithful biographer of Dr.
Johnson, meeting him in the pit of the Pantheon,
loudly exclaimed, "Why, Nollekens, how dirty
you go now! I recollect when you were the gayest
dressed of any in the house." To whom Nollekens
made, for once in his life, the retort-courteous of
"That's more than I could ever say of you!"
Boswell certainly looked very badly when dressed;
for, as he seldom washed himself, his clean ruffles
served as a striking contrast to his dirty flesh.'

J. T. Smith (*1766–1833*)
NOLLEKENS AND HIS TIME

For something like a hundred years after Johnson most baths were not plumbed in and those which were had only cold water on tap and usually had no waste-pipe. This dependence on a bath being filled from a hand-held jug tempted some eccentrics to bath in fluids other than water. Beau Brummel claimed that he bathed in milk but offered no proof. It is more readily believable of 'Old Q' the archetypal dissolute nobleman. Unfortunately for the dairy industry in London a rumour grew that the milk sold in the capital was recycled:

'There are many persons still living who
remember the almost universal prejudice against
drinking milk which prevailed in the metropolis, in
consequence of its being supposed that this
common necessary of life might have been retailed
from the daily lavations of the Duke of
Queensberry.'

J. H. Jesse (*1815–1874*)
GEORGE SELWYN AND HIS CONTEMPORARIES

Showers (cold-water only) came into use in the nineteenth century, although Dr. Routh could see little point in installing them in his Oxford college for, as he pointed out, undergraduates were only in residence for eight weeks at a stretch.

A shower took up much less room in a bedroom than did a bath and was cheaper. Servants would have to mop up a wider area of carpet but would have to carry down less volume of dirty water.

There was one snag, and that a nasty one – the shock to the nervous system when the cord was pulled and the icy needles hit warm flesh:

Trembling, as Father Adam stood
To pull the stalk, before the Fall,
So stand I here, before the Flood,
On my own head the shock to call:
How like our predecessor's luck!
'Tis but to pluck – but needs some pluck!

Still thoughts of gasping like a pup
Will paralyze the nervous pow'r;
Now hoping it will yet hold up,
Invoking now the tumbling show'r; –
But, ah! the shrinking body loathes,
Without a parapluie or clothes!

'Expect some rain about this time!'
My eyes are seal'd, my teeth are set –
But where's the Stoic so sublime
Can ring, unmov'd, for wringing wet?
Of going hogs some folks talk big –
Just let them try *the whole cold pig*!

Tom Hood (*1799–1845*)
STANZAS, COMPOSED IN A SHOWER-BATH

The nerve required for a person to turn on a cold shower proved too much for many people, including, it is shameful to relate, a pillar of Britain's political establishment. Mrs. Disraeli confided to friends:

'Dizzy has the most wonderful moral courage in
the world, but no physical courage. When he uses
his shower-bath, I always have to pull the string.'

G. W. E. Russell (<i>1853–1919</i>)
A POCKETFUL OF SIXPENCES

Of sterner stuff was a country parson. Unlike a cold shower, with its instant impact, a cold bath can be entered gingerly, a toe at a time, and withdrawn from instantly should gangrene or stoppage of the heart seem imminent.

All the same. Not much of a start to vicar's Christmas morning:

As I lay awake praying in the early morning I
thought I heard a sound of distant bells. It was an
intense frost. I sat down in my bath upon a sheet of
thick ice which broke in the middle into large
pieces whilst sharp points and jagged edges stuck
all round the sides of the tub like chevaux de frise,
not particularly comforting to the naked thighs and
loins, for the keen ice cut like broken glass. The
ice water stung and scorched like fire. I had to
collect the floating pieces of ice and pile them on a
chair before I could use the sponge and then I had
to thaw the sponge in my hands for it was a mass of
ice. The morning was most brilliant.

Rev. Francis Kilvert (<i>1840–1879</i>)
DIARY Sunday, December 25, 1870

A significant point which has probably already occurred to the reader is that nobody so far in their diaries and journals and poems has mentioned using the bath for the purpose of scrubbing the body.

The Romans used their baths mainly as social clubs, the cleaning process being a dubious system whereby they were massaged with oils which were squeegeed off by a slave with a *strigil*, a flesh-scraper.

During the dark centuries that followed perhaps the only people who bathed more than once or twice a year were monks in monasteries and, again, it was sitting in water which was the objective; there is little mention of scrubbing or indeed cleansing the sullied flesh.

The old Roman system of using oil – rather like cleaning a bicycle – was still current in the seventeenth century among the nobility, according to Francis Bacon. His instructions on how to take a bath read more like a course in Do-It-Yourself embalming:

First, before bathing, rub and anoint the Body with Oyle, and Salves, that the Bath's moistening heate and virtue may penetrate into the Body, and not the liquor's watery part: then sit 2 houres in the Bath; after Bathing wrap the Body in a seare-cloth made of Masticke, Myrrh, Pomander and Saffron, for staying the perspiration or breathing of the pores, until the softening of the Body, having layne thus in seare-cloth 24 houres, bee growne solid and hard. Lastly, with an oyntment of Oyle, Salt and Saffron, the seare-cloth being taken off, anoint the Body.

Francis Bacon, Baron Verulam (*1561–1626*)
SYLVA SYLVARUM

For the next two hundred years most citizens did not bath

at all. In hot Assembly Rooms and at the card tables this became something of a problem, which was solved by using scent, as did the Romans; 'a smell to cover a stink'.

The Age of Elegance, the eighteenth century, might have delighted the eye with its architecture and its fine fashions, and the ear with its music, but it must have been deeply offensive to the nose.

Then, early in the nineteenth century, a complete change came about. The middle-classes of the western world decided that washing was a good thing. And bathing was even better. Soap, used in previous centuries mainly for washing clothes and scrubbing the kitchen table, became heavily advertised and available commercially in a range of smells, from 'musk' to the hugely popular and reassuring odour of disinfectant, 'coal-tar'.

Ignoring the teachings of the early Christian leaders – St. Francis of Assisi taught that dirtiness was an indication of holiness, St. Jerome was ashamed of his followers for being too clean, St. Catherine of Siena gave up washing for good, St. Agnes died without ever having washed – the good people decided that washing was not only socially desirable but also highly pious. In support of this claim they made a line from one of John Wesley's sermons into a popular slogan: Cleanliness is next to Godliness:

> it is odd that the English
> > a rather dirty people
> should have invented the slogan
> *Cleanliness is next to Godliness*
> > meaning by that
> a gentleman smells faintly of tar
> persuaded themselves that constant cold
> hydropathy
> > would make the sons of gentlemen
> pure in heart
> > (not that papa or his chilblained offspring can
> > hope to be gentry)
> > still John Bull's

```
hip-bath it was
                    that made one carnal pleasure
lawful
        for the first time since we quarrelled
over Faith and Works
                    (Shakespeare probably stank
                            Le Grand
        Monarque certainly did)...
```

W. H. Auden (*1907–1973*)
ENCOMIUM BALNEI

John Wesley preached his sermon in the middle of the eighteenth century, perhaps the point when personal hygiene everywhere was at its lowest and parsons might be expected to scratch as they preached and dig around in their wigs with a quill to shift the lice about a bit. Why should he suddenly declare to his congregation that personal hygiene was a saintly virtue?

A glance at the text of Wesley's sermon reveals that he was not talking about personal cleanliness at all. He was warning his followers against wearing scruffy clothes:

Let it be observed, that slovenliness is no part of religion; that neither this, nor any text of Scripture, condemns neatness of apparel. Certainly this is a duty, not a sin. 'Cleanliness is, indeed, next to godliness'.

John Wesley (*1703–1791*)
SERMONS, No. xciii, ON DRESS

Wesley was clearly quoting an old saying. Brewer's Dictionary believes the phrase to have come from the writings of Phinehas ben Yair, an ancient Hebrew rabbi.

As the nineteenth century advanced, the new-found pleasure – now a duty – of soaping oneself and wallowing in a bath, or cringing under a shower, spread rapidly among those who could afford the soap and the ironmongery.

Leaps in technology brought water to increasing numbers of town houses and an urgent need to improve the drains meant that more baths and showers could be piped into the sewage system.

Manufacturers offered an increasingly bewildering range of reasonably priced baths in many materials, cast-iron, copper, papier-mâché, and in an assortment of designs; sponge baths, sitz baths, slipper baths, hip baths, and so on.

The British in their baths and the Americans under their showers had, at last, become wielders of soap and flannel.

Authorities on matters of health still urged caution, clinging to the old eighteenth-century attitude that baths were for therapeutic purposes only and should be on a doctor's prescription:

3523.   BATHS AND BATHING.
The frequency with which a bath should be repeated varies somewhat with different individuals. A safe rule, to which of course there are sundry exceptions, would be to bathe the body twice a week in winter and every other day in summer, gradually increasing the frequency to a tri-weekly washing in winter and a daily one in summer, if experience proves that better health is secured by such a habit.

3524.   HOT BATHS by which are meant those of a temperature of from 85° to 105° Fahrenheit, are chiefly used in the treatment of diseases as powerful stimulants. Every parent should remember that a hot bath, causing free perspiration, promoted by wrapping up warm in bed with blankets, will often save children and adults severe attacks of illness, if promptly resorted to after exposure to cold or wet.

3526. COLD BATHS are invaluable aids in promoting and preserving health, if properly used in suitable cases; but may become dangerous agents, causing even fatal results, if employed by the wrong individuals, at improper times, or with excessive frequency.

Baths should never be taken immediately after a meal, nor when the body is very much exhausted by fatigue or excitement of any kind, nor during nor just before menstruation; and they should be sparingly and guardedly used by pregnant women.

Mrs. Isabella Beeton (*1836–1865*)
HOUSEHOLD MANAGEMENT

Throughout the nineteenth century new comforts and facilities became available to the bather. Perhaps the most welcome was the happy combination of piped gas and piped water which made possible the invention of the geyser. At last it was no longer necessary to warm up the bath with jugs of hot water. The bather could have a bath at any temperature he or she desired:

> I test my bath before I sit,
> And I'm always moved to wonderment
> That what chills the finger not a bit
> Is so frigid upon the fundament.

Ogden Nash (*1902–1971*)

Unlike the old sitz and hip baths which were carried into the bedroom when needed and whisked away afterwards, the new baths were massive and permanent:

> The enormous mahogany-sided bath was approached by two steps, and had a sort of grotto containing a shower-bath at one end; this was lined with as many different stops as the organ in King's Chapel. And it was as difficult to control as it

would be for an amateur to play that organ.
Piercing jets of boiling, or ice-cold, water came
roaring at one from the most unexpected angles,
and hit one in the tenderest spots.

Gwen Raverat (*1885–1957*)
PERIOD PIECE: A CAMBRIDGE CHILDHOOD

In great houses a bedroom or dressing-room in the guest wing would be nominated the 'bathroom' and be suitably adapted.

When Charles revisited Brideshead he was always given the bedroom he had on his first visit:

It was next to Sebastian's, and we shared what had
once been a dressing-room and had been changed
to a bathroom twenty years back by the
substitution for the bed of a deep, copper,
mahogany-framed bath, that was filled by pulling a
brass lever heavy as a piece of marine engineering;
the rest of the room remained unchanged; a coal
fire always burned there in winter. I often think of
that bathroom – the water colours dimmed by
steam and the huge towel warming on the back of
the chintz armchair – and contrast it with the
uniform, clinical, little chambers, glittering with
chromium-plate and looking-glass, which pass for
luxury in the modern world.

Evelyn Waugh (*1903–1966*)
BRIDESHEAD REVISITED

The converted dressing-room or bedroom, with its fireplace and its chintz, would also have had plenty of cupboard space:

Miss Twye was soaping her breasts in her bath
When she heard behind her a meaning laugh
And to her amazement she discovered
A wicked man in the bathroom cupboard.

Gavin Ewart (*1916–*   )
MISS TWYE

The ex-bedroom would also have contained a mirror, probably a tall pier-glass large enough for the whole figure to be viewed and the dress or suit twitched and smoothed before going down to dinner.

As late as the 1950s a Bishop, staying as a guest in a large house, took a bath, skipped out of it and was appalled to see, in a large-pier glass which he had not noticed before, the reflection of his body stark naked.

He expressed his shock and dismay.

A poet replied:

> Beneath that Chasuble, my Lord, that holds
> You close (as Charity all men enfolds);
> Beneath that Cope that, opening before,
> Of Life Eternal signifies the Door,
> And (as Durandus taught) recalls the strength
> Of godly Perseverance by its length;
> Beneath that Rochet of pure lawn, and whiter
> Than Iceland's winter cap; beneath that Mitre;
> A body stands concealed, which God once chose
> The Spirits of his Children to enclose,
> And (as a Bishop surely must believe)
> His Very Self Incarnate to receive.
> Yet, through a mirror suddenly aware
> That 'Temples of the Spirit' can be bare,
> You shrink aghast, with pained and puzzled eyes,
> While God's great laughter peals about the skies.

Sir Lawrence Jones (*1885–1969*)
LINES TO A BISHOP WHO WAS SHOCKED (A.D. 1950)
AT SEEING A PIER-GLASS IN A BATHROOM

During the early years of the twentieth century a great many of the huge mansions in the inner suburbs of London were split up into flats to house the growing army of office workers. It was necessary to provide proper bathing facilities for the bed-sitters and flat-dwellers who now occupied the houses and so tiny bathrooms were built on each landing. Passengers on trains dawdling into the terminus can look up

at the back of these old mansions and see these bathrooms,
like little brick huts stuck to the wall:

From the geyser ventilators
    Autumn winds are blowing down
On a thousand business women
    Having baths in Camden Town.

Waste pipes chuckle into runnels,
    Steam's escaping here and there,
Morning trains through Camden cutting
    Shake the Crescent and the Square.

Early nip of changeful autumn,
    Dahlias glimpsed through garden doors,
At the back precarious bathrooms
    Jutting out from upper floors;

And behind their frail partitions
    Business women lie and soak,
Seeing through the draughty skylight
    Flying clouds and railway smoke.

Rest you there, poor unbelov'd ones,
    Lap your loneliness in heat.
All too soon the tiny breakfast,
    Trolley-bus and windy street!

John Betjeman (*1906–   *)
BUSINESS GIRLS

The notion of the modern bathroom, a small hygienic cell
into which was tightly packed the bath, wash-basin, bathroom
cabinet and mirror, and the W.C., an idea which Americans
pioneered, gradually became the accepted thing in Britain too.
    It was a triumph of ingenious and complicated plumbing.
And with complicated plumbing, and winter, came the
plumber:

Plumber is icumen in;
Bludie big tu-du.
Bloweth lampe, and showeth dampe,
And dripth the wud thru.
Bludie hel, boo-hoo!

Thawth drain, and runneth bath;
Saw sawth, and scruth scru;
Bull-kuk squirteth, leakë spurteth;
Wurry springeth up anew,
Boo-hoo, boo-hoo.

Tom Pugh, Tom Pugh, well plumbës thu, Tom
    Pugh;
Better job I naver nu.
Therefore will I cease boo-hoo,
Woorie not, but cry pooh-pooh,
Murie sing pooh-pooh, pooh-pooh,
Pooh-pooh!

A. Y. Campbell (1885–1958)
POEMS

This new network of up-pipes, down-pipes and assorted spouts on the exterior of buildings, according to a poet, proved a hazard to fauna:

We 'ad a bleed'n' sparrer wot
Lived up a bleed'n' spaht,
One day the bleed'n' rain came dahn
An' washed the bleeder aht.

An' as 'e layed 'arf drahnded
Dahn in the bleed'n street
'E begged that bleed'n' rainstorm
To bave 'is bleed'n' feet.

But then the bleed'n' sun came aht –
Dried up the bleed'n' rain –
So that bleed'n' little sparrer
'E climbed up 'is spaht again.

But, Oh! – the crewel sparrer'awk,
'E spies 'im in 'is snuggery,
'E sharpens up 'is bleed'n' claws
An' rips 'im aht by thuggery!

Jist then a bleed'n' sportin' type
Wot 'ad a bleed'n' gun
'E spots that bleed'n' sparrer'awk
An' blasts 'is bleed'n' fun.

The moral of this story
Is plain to everyone –
That them wot's up the bleed'n' spaht
Don't get no bleed'n' fun.

Anon

Perhaps the surest sign of the way that bathing had become a part of the daily domestic routine was the frequency with which it was mentioned in contemporary literature:

Mr. Salteena woke up rather early next day and was surprised and delighted to find Horace the footman entering with a cup of tea.

Oh thankyou my man said Mr. Salteena rolling over in the costly bed. Mr. Clark is nearly out of the bath sir anounced Horace I will have great plesure in turning it on for you if such is your desire. Well yes you might said Mr. Salteena seeing it was the idear and Horace gave a profound bow.

Ethel are you getting up shouted Mr. Salteena.

Very nearly replied Ethel faintly from the next room.

I say said Mr. Salteena excitedly I have had some tea in bed.

So have I replied Ethel.

Then Mr. Salteena got into a mouve dressing goun with yellaw tassles and siezing his soap he wandered off to the bath room which was most sumpshous. It had a lovly white shiny bath and sparkling taps and several towels arrayed in readiness by thourghtful Horace. It also had a step for climbing up the bath and other good dodges of a rich nature. Mr. Salteena washed himself well and felt very much better.

Daisy Ashford (*1881–1972*)
THE YOUNG VISITERS

However, even well into the twentieth century not everybody could afford to install bathrooms with dodges of a rich nature. To many people installing a bathroom with even modest dodges was a luxury:

Yesterday I heard from Harcourt Brace that Mrs. D. & C.R. are selling 148 and 73 weekly – Isn't that a surprising rate for the 4th month? Doesn't it portend a bathroom & w.c. either here or Southease? . . .

Virginia Woolf (*1882–1941*)
DIARY 22 Sept. 1925. ed: Anne Olivier Bell

In rural areas it was still unusual to find a bath in a cottage. The gentry may have had their bathrooms but the village folk made do:

Although only babies and very small children had baths, the hamlet folk were cleanly in their persons. The women would lock their doors for the whole afternoon once a week to have what they called 'a good clean-up'. This consisted of stripping to the waist and washing downward; then stepping into a footbath and washing upward. 'Well, I feels all the better for that,' some woman would say complacently. 'I've washed up as far as possible and down as far as possible,' and the

ribald would inquire what poor 'possible' had done
that it should not be included.

Flora Thompson (*1877–1947*)
LARK RISE TO CANDLEFORD, 1945.

Even the most genteel wash was accomplished with a huge
jug of water and a basin which usually sat upon the
'washstand' in the bedroom.

This had to suffice even for the lady's stripped-to-the-waist
ablution so happily painted by Degas and lovingly described
by D. H. Lawrence:

> When she rises in the morning
> I linger to watch her;
> She spreads the bath-cloth underneath the window
> And the sunbeams catch her
> Glistening white on the shoulders,
> While down her sides the mellow
> Golden shadow glows as
> She stoops to the sponge, and her swung breasts
> Sway like full-blown yellow
> Gloire de Dijon roses.

D. H. Lawrence (1885–1930)
GLOIRE DE DIJON

It was a less poetic and more difficult procedure for the
Rev. Wm. Archibald Spooner, Warden of New College,
Oxford, whose mind was habitually absent from what he was
doing at any given moment:

> Spooner was meditating ablution and had lifted a
> full jug of water from the wash-hand stand, where
> a basin also stood ready. Something that was
> passing through his mind caused him to walk, jug
> in hand, to the window. Then remembering his
> original purpose, he emptied the jug – but onto a
> passing undergraduate below.
> 'Warden, Warden!' the undergraduate cried out.

'Why did you do that?'
Spooner replied:
'Why are you in my basin?'

Quoted by T. F. Higham, M.A. (*1890–1975*)
A BOOK OF ANECDOTES

Among working folk in towns, too, baths were a novelty. Even when a landlord installed one it was seldom taken seriously:

'And a loovly bath where we can keep the coal . . .'

Will E. Haines and Jimmy Harper, 1928
IN MY LITTLE BOTTOM DRAWER
Performed by Gracie Fields

Miners, after their day's work at the coal face, traditionally soaped themselves clean in a tin bath in front of the kitchen fire:

With a look at the clock – the first thing Sammy had got out of pawn for her – she pulled the tin bath before the fire and began to fill it with hot water from the wash-house.

The clock struck five, and shortly after the tramp of feet echoed along the Terrace, the slow tramp of tired men. Nine hours from bank to bank and the Terraces to climb at the end of it. But it was good honest work, bred in their bones, and in her bones too. Her sons were young and strong. It was their work. She desired no other.

The door opened upon her thought and the three came in, Hughie first, then David, and finally Sammy with a sawn balk of timber tucked under his arm, for her kindling.

'How, mother,' Sammy smiled, his teeth showing white against the black coal dust that sweat had caked on him.

She loved the way he called her mother, not that 'mam' in common usage here; but she merely nodded towards the bath that was ready and turned back to set the table.

With their mother in the room the three lads took off their boots, jackets, their pit drawers and singlets, all sodden with water, sweat and pit dirt. Together, naked to the buff, they stood scouring themselves in the tiny steaming bath. There was never much room and it was always friendly. But there was not much joking to-night. Sam in a tentative way nudged Davey and grinned:

'Ower the bed a bit, ye elephant.' And again remarked: 'Whey, mon, have ye swallowed the soap?' But there was nothing genuine in the way of fun. The heaviness in the house, in Martha's face, precluded it. They dressed with no horse-play, sat in to their dinner almost in silence.

A. J. Cronin (1896–1980)
THE STARS LOOK DOWN

The miner in a novel by Emile Zola fared more happily. Well, he was married and what with all that soaping . . . They order, it seems, this matter better in France –

The tub was refilled with warm water and father was beginning to take off his jacket. A warning glance was the signal for Alzire to take Lénore and Henri to play outside. Dad did not like bathing in front of the family, as they did in many other homes in the village. Not that he was criticising anybody; he only meant that dabbling about together was all right for children.

'What are you doing up there?' Maheude called up the stairs.

'Mending my dress that I tore yesterday,' Catherine called back.

'All right, but don't come down; your father's washing.'

Maheu and his wife were alone. She had made

up her mind to put Estelle down in a chair as, for a wonder, she was not yelling, being near the fire. She gazed at her parents with the expressionless eyes of a tiny creature without intelligence. He crouched naked in front of the tub and began by dipping his head in, well lathered with soft soap. The use of this soap for generations past had discoloured the hair of all these people and turned it yellow. Then he stepped into the water, soaped his chest, belly, arms, and legs and rubbed them hard with his fists. His wife stood looking on.

'Well,' she began, 'I saw the look on your face when you came in. You were feeling pretty worried, weren't you? And the sight of the food cheered you up no end. Just fancy, those gentry up at La Piolaine never coughed up a sou. Of course, they were very nice – they gave the kids some clothes and I was ashamed to beg. It sticks in my throat when I have to cadge.'

She broke off to settle Estelle firmly in the chair, for fear she might topple over. Father went on pummelling his skin, without trying to hurry the story by asking questions. It interested him, but he patiently waited for things to be made plain.

'I must tell you that Maigrat had turned me down flat, like turning a dog out. You can imagine what a nice time I had. Woollen clothes may be all right for keeping you warm, but they don't fill your stomach, do they?'

He looked up, but still said nothing. Nothing from La Piolaine, nothing from Maigrat: well, what? But she was going on with the usual routine, having rolled her sleeves up so as to do his back and the places that are hard to get at. Anyway, he loved her to soap him and rub him all over fit to break her wrists. She took some soap and worked away at his shoulders, while he stiffened his body to withstand the attack.

'So back I went to Maigrat's and told him the tale. Oh, I didn't half tell him the tale! Said he couldn't have any heart, that he would come to a bad end if there was any justice in the world. He didn't like that at all, and he rolled his eyes round and would have liked to skedaddle. . . .'

She had gone down from his back to his buttocks and, warming up to the job, she pushed ahead into the cracks and did not leave a single part of his body untouched, making it shine like her three saucepans on spring-cleaning Saturdays. But the terrible arm-work made her sweat, shook her and took her breath away, so that her words came in gasps.

'Anyway, he called me an old limpet. . . . We've got enough bread till Saturday, and the best of it is that he lent me five francs. What's more, I got the butter, coffee, and chicory from him and was going to buy the meat and potatoes, but I saw he was beginning to jib. . . . Seven sous for the brawn, eighteen for the potatoes, that leaves me three francs seventy-five for a stew and some boiled beef. I haven't wasted my morning, have I, eh?'

She was now drying him, dabbing with a towel at the places that were difficult to dry. He, happy and carefree about the morrow's debts, laughed out loud and threw his arms round her.

'Don't be silly! You have made me all wet! Only. . . . I'm afraid Maigrat had got something in mind. . . .'

She was on the point of mentioning Catherine, but checked herself. Why upset father? It would start off an endless fuss.

'Got what in mind?'

'Oh, only how to swindle us. Catherine will have to go over the bill carefully.'

He seized her again, and this time did not leave

go. The bath always ended up like this – she made him excited by rubbing so hard and then towelling him everywhere, tickling the hairs on his arms and chest. It was the time when all the chaps in the village took their fun and more children were planted than anybody wanted. At night they had their families in the way. He pushed her to the table, cracking jokes to celebrate the one good moment a chap can enjoy during the whole day, calling it taking his dessert – and free of charge, what's more! She, with her flabby body and breasts hanging all over the place, put up a bit of resistance, just for fun.

'You silly, you! Oh, you are a one! And there's Estelle looking at us! Wait a minute while I turn her head the other way.'

'Oh, rubbish! What does she understand at three months?'

When it was over, he put on just a dry pair of trousers.

Emile Zola (1840–1902)
GERMINAL trans.: Leonard Tancock

To the inhabitants of hot and sunny Mediterranean islands the modern English preoccupation with personal hygiene was put down to diabolism or hypochondria:

English eccentricity remarked by the natives which the Count has missed; the English demand for houses with lavatories. An 'English' house in the island, has come to mean a house with a lavatory; and the landlord of such a house will charge almost double the ordinary rent for so remarkable an innovation. Bathrooms are even rarer and are considered a dangerous and rather satanic contrivance. For the peasants a bath is something you are sometimes forced to take by the doctor as a medicinal measure; the idea of

51

cleanliness does not enter into it. Theodore often quotes the old peasant who reverently crossed himself when shown the fine tiled bathroom at the Count's country house and said: 'Pray God, my Lord, that you will never need it.'

Lawrence Durrell (1912–)
PROSPERO'S CELL

It was only when bathrooms were present in almost all homes, ceased to be a novelty and were taken for granted, that there emerged the fact that mankind had created for itself a number of new dangers. Bathrooms, because of what they contained and what they were used for, presented a range of new ways in which the human species could do itself damage. There was the fearful danger of bathing a slender child in a bath with a wide plug-hole:

A muvver was barfin' 'er biby one night,
The youngest of ten and a tiny young mite,
The muvver was poor and the biby was thin,
Only a skelington covered in skin;
The muvver turned rahnd for the soap off the rack,
She was but a moment, but when she turned back,
The biby was gorn; and in anguish she cried,
'Oh, where is my biby?' – The angels replied:

'Your biby 'as fell dahn the plug-'ole,
Your biby 'as gorn dahn the plug;
The poor little thing was so skinny and thin
'E oughter been barfed in a jug;
Your biby is perfeckly 'appy,
'E won't need a barf any more,
Your biby 'as fell dahn the plug-'ole,
Not lorst, but gorn before.'

Anon.

And witness the disasters which befell Mr. Pooter when he decided to paint his bath:

APRIL 25. In consequence of Brickwell telling me his wife was working wonders with the new Pinkford's enamel paint, I determined to try it. I bought two tins of red on my way home. I hastened through tea, went into the garden and painted some flower-pots. I called out Carrie, who said: 'You've always got some new-fangled craze'; but she was obliged to admit that the flower-pots looked remarkably well. Went upstairs into the servant's bedroom and painted her washstand, towel-horse, and chest of drawers. To my mind it was an extraordinary improvement, but as an example of the ignorance of the lower classes in the matter of taste, our servant, Sarah, on seeing them, evinced no sign of pleasure, but merely said 'she thought they looked very well as they was before'.

APRIL 26. Got some more red enamel paint (red, to my mind, being the best colour), and painted the coal-scuttle, and the backs of our *Shakespeare*, the binding of which had almost worn out.

APRIL 27. Painted the bath red, and was delighted with the result. Sorry to say Carrie was not, in fact we had a few words about it. She said I ought to have consulted her, and she had never heard of such a thing as a bath being painted red. I replied: 'It's merely a matter of taste.'

APRIL 29, SUNDAY. Woke up with a fearful headache and strong symptoms of a cold. Carrie, with a perversity which is just like her, said it was 'painter's colic', and was the result of my having spent the last few days with my nose over a paint-pot. I told her firmly that I knew a great deal better what was the matter with me than she did. I had got a chill, and decided to have a bath as hot as I could bear it. Bath ready – could scarcely bear it so hot. I persevered, and got in; very hot, but very acceptable. I lay still for some time. On moving my hand above the surface of the water, I experienced the greatest fright I ever received in the whole course of my life; for imagine my horror on discovering my hand, as I thought, full of blood. My first thought was that I had ruptured an artery, and was bleeding to death, and should be discovered, later on, looking like a second Marat, as I remember seeing him in Madame Tussaud's. My second thought was to ring the bell, but remembered there was no bell to ring. My third was, that there was nothing but the enamel paint, which had dissolved with boiling water. I stepped out of the bath, perfectly red all over, resembling the Red Indians I have seen depicted at an East-End theatre. I determined not to say a word to Carrie, but to tell Farmerson to come on Monday and paint the bath white.

George and Weedon Grossmith
THE DIARY OF A NOBODY *1892*

The combination of warmth and smooth porcelain often tempted a most unwelcome visitor to call:

I have fought a grizzly bear,
Tracked a cobra to its lair,
Killed a crocodile who dared to cross my path;
But the thing I really dread
When I've just got out of bed
Is to find that there's a spider in the bath.

I've no fear of wasps or bees,
Mosquitoes only tease,

I rather like a cricket on the hearth;
But my blood runs cold to meet
In pyjamas and bare feet
With a great big hairy spider in the bath.

I have faced a charging bull in Barcelona,
I have dragged a mountain lioness from her cub,
I've restored a mad gorilla to its owner
But I don't dare to face that Tub...

What a frightful-looking beast –
Half an inch across at least –
It would frighten even Superman or Garth,
There's contempt it can't disguise
In the little beady eyes
Of the spider sitting glowering in the bath.

It ignores my every lunge
With the back-brush and the sponge;
I have bombed it with 'A Present from Penarth';
But it doesn't mind at all –
It just rolls into a ball
And simply goes on squatting in the bath...

For hours we have been locked in endless struggle;
I have lured it to the deep end, by the drain;
At last I think I've washed it down the plug-'ole
But here it comes a-crawling up the chain!

Now it's time for me to shave
Though my nerves will not behave,
And there's bound to be a fearful aftermath;
So before I cut my throat
I shall leave this final note:
DRIVEN TO IT –
   BY THE SPIDER IN THE BATH!

Michael Flanders and Donald Swann
THE SONGS OF MICHAEL FLANDERS AND DONALD SWANN

It seems that a huge percentage of all accidents occur in the home, so it is perhaps not surprising that the bathroom, the centre of family activity at least twice a day, has its share of jeopardies. The British Bathroom has been the stage for many a deeply harrowing drama:

The pub. Pub hubbub, over which:

LANDLORD: (*shouting*) Time, gentlemen, please! All your glasses please, gents. Come on, Mr. Glum, please let me get finished up early tonight. It's my bath-night, Mr. Glum, and you know how much I love a good old soak.

MR. GLUM: Yes, I've met her. But don't you talk to me about bath-nights, Ted. Not after what happened to *me* last week. Cor! That was something I shall remember till the day I die – if I'm spared that long. What happened was – (*changing to gently chiding tone*) – Ah, Ted, you weren't about to pour yet *another* brown ale in this glass, were you?

LANDLORD: No I wasn't, Mr. Glum.

MR. GLUM: (*grimly*) I thought you weren't! So shove one in there. No, reverting to last week, what happened was, I'd gone up to have a bath at my usual time – first of the month – and downstairs I'd left my son Ron – you know my boy Ron, don't you?

LANDLORD: He the one with the Tommy Steele haircut?

MR. GLUM: That's him. Except it's not a Tommy Steele haircut, it's a Davy Crockett hat gone mangy. Anyway, while I'm upstairs, he's on the sofa in our front room with his fiancée, Eth. And what *transpired* – as it transpires . . .

Music. The Glums' sitting-room,

ETH: Oh, Ron... Your father started having his bath at seven – it's now gone ten and he's still up there! That can't be good for an old man. Why should he be in that bath for three hours?

RON: Perhaps he's a *dirty* old man.

ETH: Even so, no one should stay in there all that time. I mean, I like my bath, but even allowing for a good old wallow – I'm in and out in twenty minutes. Oh, wouldn't you like to just pop your head round the bathroom door?

RON: (*eagerly*) Oh yes, Eth.

ETH: Your *father's* door! Please, Ron, please pop up and make sure nothing's happened to him.

RON: I'd rather not, Eth. I already popped up once – just after he got into the bath. He threw the dirty linen at me.

ETH: Whyever for?

RON: (*resentful*) Just 'cos I put Barbara Kelly in there with him.

ETH: Barbara Kelly?

RON: My goldfish. Poor little thing's got to stretch her fins somewhere.

ETH: But that's even more worrying, Ron. If Mr. Glum got into one of his *rages*...! A heavily built man like him all worked-up in a steamy little bathroom ...! Ron, he could go out just like *that*!

RON: Oh no, he couldn't go out like that, Eth. He'd be arrested.

ETH: What I meant, Ron –

RON: (*firmly*) Look, Eth, you're just making a mountain out of a mole-hole. Dad's all right. If anything had happened to him, we'd have heard.

From upstairs comes a muffled shout of infuriated frustration . . .

ETH: Ron, isn't that him? Listen.

From upstairs, more unintelligible shouting. This time, a muffled tirade of baffled profanity.

RON: (*triumphant*) There, Eth. See? (*fondly*) He's singing!

ETH: That was no singing, Ron, He's in difficulties! (*Shout*) Mr. Glum, are you feeling all right?

The bathroom. Mr. Glum is in the bath.

MR. GLUM: (*furious shout*) All right? No, I'm not all right. I can't get meself out of the *bath*!

Music and back to the pub.   *Pub hubbub.*

LANDLORD: Well, strike me rotten! Got your big toe jammed in the plug-hole? Dear oh dear. Must have been a bit unpleasant, I should think.

MR. GLUM: (*heavy sarcasm*) Oh no, Ted, it was delightful. If there's one thing I can thoroughly recommend, it's sitting for three hours in rapidly cooling water, with your toe stuck in the waste-pipe, and a flipping goldfish sporting round your southern hemisphere.

LANDLORD: Still you were lucky your Ron and Eth were there to lend a hand. Come to think of it, though, Eth couldn't have been that much help, really. Not in the circumstances.

MR. GLUM: Well, as it happens, we got *round* that

particular difficulty. I told Ron to empty a few packets of gravy browning into the bath water.

LANDLORD: Gravy browning...? Oh, that was shrewd, Mr. Glum. That really was shrewd.

MR. GLUM: Shrewd enough for *you* to think about pouring some brown in? (*As landlord pours –*) Yes, it worked a treat. By the time Ron had emptied the twelfth packet in, I'd have got a 'U' Certificate from any Watch Committee in the country. 'Course he had to stir it *round* a little...

Music and we're back in the bathroom.

MR. GLUM: That's it, Ron, give it a good swish round. Want to try one more packet for luck?

Knock on door.

ETH: (*Off*) All right for me to come in yet, Mr. Glum?

MR. GLUM: Hang on, Eth! How's it seem to *you*, Ron?

RON: Just a minute, Dad.

Ron licks his lips.

RON: Lovely.

MR. GLUM: I didn't mean *taste* it! Oh, it seems dark enough now. (*Calls*) Right ho, Eth, I'm decent.

The door opens and Eth enters.

ETH: Hallo, Mr. Glum.

MR. GLUM: (*weak voice*) Hallo, my dear. You'll pardon me not getting up. Well, Eth, this is a fine predicament for a man of my years to find himself in, eh? Sitting here like The Browning Version.

ETH: It's too awful, Mr. Glum. But what did you want to put your big toe in the plug-hole for in the first place?

MR. GLUM: (*irritable*) I didn't *want* to put it in. I had to put it in! There wasn't no plug.

ETH: No plug?

MR. GLUM: This afternoon, my son – your husband-to-be – he went round and collected the plug from the bath, the plug from the basin, the plug from the kitchen sink, both knobs off the telly and the check lino out the scullery.

ETH: Ron – whatever for?

RON: I'm teaching myself to play draughts.

MR. GLUM: Consequence was, when I turned on the tap this evening – what happened? The water runs straight out.

ETH: Yes, it would, wouldn't it?

MR. GLUM: Never mind it would, wouldn't it, it did, didn't it? The only thing I could do was get undressed, place myself in the *empty* bath and this time, prior to turning the taps on, stuff me big toe down the plug-hole. That part alone gave me a severe emotional shock.

ETH: Emotional shock?

MR. GLUM: You try sitting down naked on cold porcelain! But at least the bath filled up all right, so – after passing a lightly soaped flannel over my salient features, I lay me head back in the water, did my walrus impersonation – then went to get *out*. And what did I find? That toe was stuck fast! Wedged like a bung in a beer-barrel! Nothing'll shift it!

ETH: And that's how you've been for three hours? Oh, Ron, he hasn't even had any supper. Shouldn't you bring him up some?

RON: I think that might make him feel worse, Eth.

ETH: Why, Ron?

RON: It was toad in the hole.

MR. GLUM: Cor lummy, it's like Fate itself is perspiring against me.

ETH: Now, try not to get embittered, Mr. Glum. There must be *some* way of – look, how about this. Suppose we put a broomstick under your knee, wedge it against the side of the bath, then Ron and I throw all our weight on the other end. What would happen?

MR. GLUM: You'd break my ruddy *leg*, that's what would happen! Do you think I haven't been cudgelling my brains for a way out? There isn't one. I tell you, Ethel, I won't be shifted from this bathroom without major surgery! All because my dear son took it into his head to – (*emits a sudden, surprisingly maidenly shriek.*)

ETH: What is it?

MR. GLUM: That rotten *goldfish*! Keeps doing that when I least *expect* it. Where is it? (*Grabbing about in the dark water*) Just let me get my hands on it. I'll teach it to treat me like a subterranean grotto! (*Paddles his hand round.*)

RON: Watch it, Dad. You thrash around like that, you'll thin your gravy.

MR. GLUM: It's all so inexplainable. If the perishing toe went in, why won't it come out?

ETH: Oh, that's quite easily explainable, Mr. Glum. It was the heat of the hot water.

MR. GLUM: Eh?

ETH: It made your big toe swell. You see, heat always makes things get bigger.

RON: She's quite right, Dad. That's why days are longer in the summer than they are in the winter.

MR. GLUM: Thank you very much. So your suggestion is that I sit here till the winter?

ETH: Oh no, Mr. Glum. But we're on the right track.

MR. GLUM: How d'you mean?

ETH: Well, if we could – Ron, can you think of some way for your father to cool his big toe down?

RON: I think so, Eth.

MR. GLUM: How, Ron?

RON: Well, it seems obvious to me, Dad.

MR. GLUM: All right, don't keep it a secret. How can I cool that toe down?

RON: Take it out and blow on it.

MR. GLUM: (*containing his feelings*) Take it out and . . . Ron?

RON: Yes, Dad?

MR. GLUM: Once and for all, *admit* something to me. I just want the satisfaction of hearing you admit it.

RON: What, Dad?

MR. GLUM: Sometimes you're as dim as a sweep's ear-'ole! Aren't you?

RON: Yes, Dad.

MR. GLUM: Not just 'Yes, Dad'. Admit it.

RON: Sometimes I'm as dim as a sweep's ear-'ole.

MR. GLUM: Just plain honest-to-goodness gormless.

RON: Just plain honest-to-goodness gormless.

MR. GLUM: And stupid *with* it.

RON: And stupid *with* it.

MR. GLUM: Thank you, Ron. At least, that's made me feel a *little* better.

RON: I tell you one thing about me though, Dad.

MR. GLUM: What's that?

RON: I've never got my big toe stuck in a plug-hole.

MR. GLUM: (*to Eth, wildly*) Either take him away or – ! Look at me flesh – it's started going all *crinkly*. What with that and the gravy, I'll be like the edge of a steak-and-kidney pie. Please, Eth – think!

ETH: We are thinking, Mr. Glum. You really mustn't be so impatient.

MR. GLUM: Impatient? For heaven's sake, what am I asking? If they can raise ninety thousand tons of shipping out the Suez Canal, surely you two can get one old man's toe out a waste-pipe.

ETH: Waste-pipe! Yes, of course – that is a *pipe*, isn't it! I'd forgotten that. Ron – why don't we tackle the problem the other way about?

RON: You mean push his *head* in?

ETH: No, Ron. Get at the toe from the other end of the waste-pipe!

MR. GLUM: Ah! Now that's the first sensible suggestion yet. Yes – 'stead of *pulling* at the toe,

63

get to a position where you can *push* at it from beneath. Ron –

RON: Yes, Dad?

MR. GLUM: Bend down and have a look at the bottom of the bath.

Effect.   Bubbling.

MR. GLUM: Trouble is, you see, Eth – his mind has never really caught up with his body.

ETH: Mr. Glum, he'll drown!

Ron comes out of the water, gasping and spluttering.

RON: (*breathing hard*) Couldn't see *anything*, Dad. There was a toe in the way.

MR. GLUM: And the moment I get back the use of that toe, I know exactly where I'm going to place it. (*Patiently*) Ron, look *underneath* the bath. Down under the plug-hole. What you should find there is a waste-pipe coming out and forming a 'U'.

RON: A 'U'.

MR. GLUM: A 'U'. And at the base of that 'U' there is a nut.

RON: A nut.

MR. GLUM: A nut. Or, if you prefer – 'U' again. Now if you go and *undo* that nut, you will perceive a *hole* which, if you shove something up it, you can easily reach my ill-fated toe. Do you understand?

MR. GLUM AND RON: (*pause; then, together*) No, Dad.

ETH: I've got it, Ron. And it unscrews quite . . . (*grunt*) . . . Ah!   And there's the hole – oh, it can only be a couple of inches from the end of Mr.

64

Glum's toe.   Quick, Ron, get something out the bathroom cabinet you can shove up and push with.

RON: Right ho, Eth.

ETH: This'll do it, Mr. Glum. You're only a few seconds away from freedom now. See where you've got to push up, Ron?

RON: I see, Eth. Ready, Dad?

MR. GLUM: I been ready for three hours. A good hard push now, son.

RON: Right ho, Dad. (*Grunt of effort.*)

MR. GLUM: (*howl of agony*) Aagh! What did you –?

RON: You said find something to –

MR. GLUM: Not scissors! You great brainless –! That hole's only a couple of *inches* from where my toe is. You should be able to push it out with your finger.

RON: My finger. Ah! Question is . . . No, I've got a taller one somewhere. Ah, thought so. Stand by, Dad.

MR. GLUM: Feel me toe?

RON: Just a mo', just a mo' . . . Ah! Contact!

MR. GLUM: (*excited*) Now *push*, lad. *Hard*! All your weight behind it. I can feel it moving, moving – one more ought to . . . (*Triumph*) Aah! (*His foot pops out of water.*) I'm free! Free! Oh, the relief, the – Eth, I can't thank you enough for – (*his voice breaks.*)

ETH: Oh, that's all right.

MR. GLUM: And Ron – them remarks I made about you being dim and gormless and stupid . . . well, I apologize, son. It was just the heat of the moment. Will you – will you shake hands and say you forgive your nasty-tempered old Daddy?

RON: No, I won't, Dad.

MR. GLUM: Oh, no, Ron, don't bear grudges. Come on, stand up and shake hands.

RON: I just can't, Dad.

MR. GLUM: What do you mean 'can't'?

RON: It's my finger. Look – It seems to be stuck in the hole where . . .

MR. GLUM: Oh, gawd no! Oh, you dim, gormless, stupid, no-good –

BRING UP MUSIC AND FADE

Frank Muir and Denis Norden
From the radio programme TAKE IT FROM HERE, 1959

We leave the subject of baths as we began, with the musings of a writer immersed in his tub's comforting warmth.

But this time the writer is a little *triste*. He has noticed his toes and broods upon their loss of status:

> In the tub we soak our skin
> and drowse and meditate within.
>
> The mirror clouds, the vapors rise,
> We view our toes with sad surprise;
>
> The toes that mother kissed and counted,
> The since neglected and unwanted.

Edward Newman Horn (*1903?–1976*)

Next to the bath stands the washbasin. In a little hollow on its top there is a sliver of soap the size and thickness of an oval

66

postage stamp (how does a new cake of soap manage to reduce itself overnight to a barely visible sliver, which then lasts for three weeks?). There is also a pair of toothbrushes, colour-coded blue and pink, and a tube of toothpaste which has lost its cap.

Although in the past soap was mainly used for scrubbing and doing the laundry there was enough demand for it in Tudor times to support a Soapmakers' Guild, and Charles II farmed out the monopoly rights to manufacture it for a huge sum. The best soap, that is to say the slightly milder kind which did not immediately cause the user's skin to go scarlet and peel off, was imported from Castile in Spain.

But most households of any size boiled up their own. It was one of those domestic duties which fell to the womenfolk, like moulding the candles, brewing the beer, and preparing the medicines, cosmetics and herbal cure-alls which are sold nowadays under the horrid title of 'assorted toiletries'.

For those readers whose ambition to achieve self-sufficiency extends to assorted toiletries I give details of some old recipes. It is only fair to point out that when ordering some of the ingredients, e.g. dragon's-blood, japan-earth, virgin's wax, it might be as well to give your local drugstore a few days' notice:

How to make Ball Soap; of great Use in Families.

THIS soap is easily made, and goes much farther than any of the other soaps. You are to make a lee from ashes and tallow; then put the lees into a copper, and boil them till the watery part is quite gone, and there remains nothing in the copper but a sort of nitrous matter (the very strength and essence of the lee) to this the tallow is put, and the copper kept boiling and stirring for above half an hour, in which time the soap is made; it is then taken out of the copper, and put into tubs, or baskets, with sheets in them, and immediately (whilst warm) made into balls. You are to take notice, that it requires near 24 hours to boil away the watery part of the lee.

Peregrine Montague, Gent. (*mid-18th. century*)
THE FAMILY POCKET-BOOK
or, FOUNTAIN OF TRUE AND USEFUL KNOWLEDGE,
COMPILED AFTER THIRTY YEARS EXPERIENCE.

Factory-made toothbrushes are a product of our modern world and when they first appeared seemed a needless extravagance:

> Toothbrushes were not in general use; few
> could afford to buy such luxuries; but the women
> took a pride in their strong white teeth and cleaned
> them with a scrap of clean wet rag dipped in salt.
> Some of the men used soot as a sort of tooth-
> powder.

Flora Thompson.
LARK RISE TO CANDLEFORD.

Other tooth-powder substitutes used down the centuries besides soot, salt and perfumed water were pumicestone and – in Spain, according to Erasmus – human urine. Or you could put together a mixture of your own from one of the tried and true recipes published:

How to make the King of France's Teeth Powder, famous for making the Teeth white, and preserving them from the Scurvy.

Take of chalk and pebble-stones burnt, of each one oz. myrrh, bole-armoniac and dragon's-blood, of each half an ounce, of ammoniacum and cuttle-bones, of each 3 drachms, let them be all finely powder'd.

THE FAMILY INSTRUCTOR OF THE KNOWLEDGE OF MEDICINE. c. 1760.

Bad teeth were commonplace. Queen Elizabeth I had troublesome teeth; discoloured and green to begin with and finally, as gleefully reported back by foreign diplomats, virtually black, and there were recipes for keeping teeth steady and painless:

To fasten loose Teeth, and prevent the Tooth-ach.

Take myrrh and japan-earth, of each two drachms; bruise and boil them in a pint of claret, to the consumption of the third part, then strain it, and let it settle, wash your mouth with the clearest every morning. If your teeth are very foul, take a rag, and dip it in spirits of vitriol, and rub your teeth with it, washing your mouth with water after it.

Ibid.

The hint for cleaning foul teeth must have been effective as vitriol is used nowadays for cleaning badly stained baths.

A favoured form of primitive toothbrush was the end of a twig (hazel was favourite) but this ancient practice worried an eighteenth century gentleman who recommended that nothing more rigid than a sponge should be employed:

I hope you take great care of your mouth and teeth, and that you clean them well every morning with a ſpunge and tepid water, with a few drops of arquebuſade water dropped into it; beſides waſhing your mouth carefully after every meal. I do inſiſt upon your never uſing thoſe ſticks, or any hard ſubſtance whatſoever, which always rub away the gums, and deſtroy the varniſh of the teeth. I ſpeak this from woeful experience; for my negligence of my teeth, when I was younger than you are, made them bad; and afterwards, my deſire to have them look better, made me uſe ſticks, irons, &c. which totally deſtroyed them; ſo that I have not now above ſix or ſeven left. I loſt one this morning, which ſuggeſted this advice to you.

Lord Chesterfield's Letters to his son.
Letter LXXXV. London, 15 February, 1754.

'Arquebusade' was a lotion much valued for staunching gun-shot wounds.

The great medical school of Salernum took the view that toothache was caused by small worms burrowing into the tooth and setting up home there and that the cure was to smoke them out:

If in your teeth you hap to be tormented,
This means some little worms therein do breed:
Which pain (if heed be taken) may be prevented,
By keeping clean your teeth when as you feed.
Burn Frankincense (a gum not evil scented)
Put Henbane into this, and Onion seed,
And in a Tunnel to the Tooth that's hollow,
Convey the smoke thereof, and ease shall follow.

REGIMEN SANITATIS SALERNITANUM
English version by Sir John Harington, 1609

The science of dental care had made slow progress since Salernum. When the tooth had rotted irrevocably it had to be pulled out; a job for the barber or for a powerfully-shouldered quack at a Fair. But by the end of the eighteenth century a lot more was known about what caused teeth to go bad. And teeth became important enough to have a branch of medicine devoted to their study and care – dentistry:

> Whene'er along the ivory disks are seen
> The rapid traces of the dark gangrene,
> When caries comes, with stealthy pace, to throw
> Corrosive ink-spots on those banks of snow,
> Brook no delay, ye trembling, suffering Fair
> But fly for refuge to the Dentist's care.

> Solyman Brown (*1790–1865?*)
> THE DENTIAD

Up to the nineteenth century it was a widely held view in the Western world that washing the hair was an act of eccentricity and very dangerous to bodily health.

It took a poet of great courage (he personally founded Newfoundland) to advocate a washing of the head not just once a year but *quarterly*:

> *Is bathing of the head wholesome?*
> You shall find it wonderful expedient if you bathe
> your head four times in the year, and that with hot
> lye made of ashes. After which you must cause one
> presently to pour two or three gallons of cold
> fountain water upon your head. Then let your
> head be dried with cold towels. Which sudden
> pouring down of cold water, although it doth
> mightily terrify you, yet nevertheless it is very
> good, for thereby the natural heat is stirred within
> the body, baldness is kept back, and the memory
> is quickened.

> William Vaughan (*1557–1641*)
> NATURALL AND ARTIFICIAL DIRECTIONS FOR HEALTH

> The poet also recommended eating young ducks which had
> been stifled in borage smoke to 'increase natural seed'.

71

More typical was an eighteenth century reaction to a recipe for an oatmeal-and-egg shampoo:

> The Method is this, Let a Woman wash her Hair
> with a Mixture of beaten Eggs and Oatmeal, and
> go afterwards into a warm Bath, and she will poison
> the Water to such a Degree, that there will be a
> stinking noisome Smell communicated to it, and a
> great Quantity of a light and frothy Sea Green
> Matter will swim in it; the whole Body of the
> Water will also partake of this Colour, and it will
> taint the very Walls, tinging them green and
> making them stink.

'Sir' John Hill (*1716?–1775*)
A REVIEW OF THE ROYAL SOCIETY

Most of the recipes which our fore-parents used for their cosmetics were cheerfully medieval, relying heavily on blind trust in mumbo-jumbo and the belief that something with a long name must be beneficial:

> To clere, to clense, and to mundifie the face use
> stufes and bathes, and euery mornyne after
> keymyng of the head, wype the face with a Skarlet
> cloth, and washe not the face ofte, but ones a weke
> anoynt the face a lytle ouer with the oyle of
> Costine, and vse to eat *Electuary de aromatibus*, or
> the confection of Anacardine, or the syrupe of
> Fumitery, or confection of Manna . . .

Andrew Boorde (*1490?–1549*)
BREUYARY OF HEALTH

The head anointed with the juice of leeks preserveth the hair from falling. A mouse roasted and given to children to eat remedieth pissing the bed.

THE WIDDOWES TREASURE 1595

To preserve the Face from being deform'd by the Small-pox.

Take an ounce and a half of pomatum; of oil of almonds one ounce; of spermaceti and virgin's wax, of each three drachms; of damask rose-water one ounce, set them all together over the fire, and as soon as they are melted take them off, let them stand then till they are cold, then make a hole, and drain out the water, and with a feather anoint the patient's face.

THE FAMILY INSTRUCTOR IN THE KNOWLEDGE OF MEDICINE C. 1760

One of the remedies makes one feel that one would prefer to keep the sore lip, unsightly though it might be:

For a Bruise, occasion'd by a Cold.

Take horse-dung and sheep's suet, of each equal parts, boil them well together, and apply warm to the part affected, like a poultice.   Ibid.

Our last recipe seems to require the user to slap on a mixture of calvesfoot-jelly and bread-and-butter pudding:

A Very Good Water to Make the Face Appear of the Age of 25 year

Take a couple of calves' feet and seethe them in seven pound of river water until half be consumed; then put in a pound of rice, and let it seethe with crumbs of fine manchet bread steeped in milk, two pounds of fresh butter and seven new laid eggs with their shells and all: set those all things to distil, and into the water that shall come of it out a little camphor and saccharine alum, and you shall have an excellent noble thing of it.

THE SECRETS OF THE REVEREND MAISTER ALEXIS OF PIEMINT 1558
trans.: William Warde

Bizarre and revolting though most of the early cures appear to modern eyes it is reasonable to suppose that some of them must have done *some* good because they appeared over a period of many centuries and were reprinted endlessly. Take a scientifically-minded gentleman's recipe for eye-lotion:

Take *Paracelsus's Zebethum Occidentale*, (*viz.* Human Dung) of a good Colour and Consistence, dry it slowly till it be pulverable: Then reduce it into an impalpable Powder; which is to be blown once, twice or thrice a Day, as occasion shall require, into the Patient's Eyes.

The Hon. Robert Boyle (*1627–1691*)
MEDICINAL EXPERIMENTS

This was the Boyle who propounded 'Boyle's Law'.

In previous centuries a household's medical and cosmetic needs required a large room to themselves. Herbs had to be hung to dry; pestles and mortars, jars and bottles, drying cabinets, scales, tubs of ingredients, all had to be stored, and a fair amount of space had to be allocated to the various vigorous processes which were necessary, e.g., distillation, seething, beating, grinding, pulverizing.

Nowadays our remedies are prepared for us, and they come in pleasant little bottles which we can arrange neatly in a box on the wall specially designed for our modern bathrooms – the Medicine Cabinet:

I am sure that many a husband has wanted to wrench the family medicine cabinet off the wall and throw it out of the window, if only because the average medicine cabinet is so filled with mysterious bottles and unidentifiable objects of all kinds that it is a source of constant bewilderment and exasperation to the American male. Surely the British medicine cabinet and the French medicine cabinet and all the other medicine cabinets must be simpler and better ordered than ours. It may be that the American habit of saving everything and never throwing anything away, even empty bottles, causes the domestic medicine cabinet to become as cluttered in its small way as the American attic becomes cluttered in a major way. I have encountered few medicine cabinets in this country which were not pack-jammed with something between a hundred and fifty and two hundred different items, from dental floss to boracic acid, from razor blades to sodium perborate, from adhesive tape to coconut oil. Even the neatest wife will put off clearing out the medicine cabinet on the ground that she has something else to do that is more important at the moment, or more diverting. It was in the apartment of such a wife and her husband that I became enormously involved with a medicine cabinet one morning not long ago.

I had spent the week-end with this couple –
they live on East Tenth Street near Fifth Avenue –
such a week-end as left me reluctant to rise up on
Monday morning with bright and shining face and
go to work. They got up and went to work, but I
didn't. I didn't get up until about two-thirty in the
afternoon. I had my face all lathered for shaving
and the wash-bowl was full of hot water when
suddenly I cut myself with the razor. I cut my ear.
Very few men cut their ears with razors, but I do,
possibly because I was taught the old Spencerian
free-wrist movement by my writing teacher in the
grammar grades. The ear bleeds rather profusely
when cut with a razor and is difficult to get at.
More angry than hurt, I jerked open the door of
the medicine cabinet to see if I could see a styptic
pencil, and out fell, from the top shelf, a little
black paper packet containing nine needles. It
seems that this wife kept a little packet containing
nine needles on the top shelf of the medicine
cabinet. The packet fell into the soapy water of the
wash-bowl, where the paper rapidly disintegrated,
leaving nine needles at large in the bowl. I was,
naturally enough, not in the best condition, either
physical or mental, to recover nine needles from a
wash-bowl. No gentleman who has lather on his
face and whose ear is bleeding is in the best
condition for anything, even something involving
the handling of nine large blunt objects.

It did not seem wise to me to pull the plug out of
the wash-bowl and let the needles go down the
drain. I had visions of clogging up the plumbing
system of the house, and also a vague fear of
causing short circuits somehow or other (I know
very little about electricity and I don't want to have
it explained to me). Finally I groped very gently
around the bowl and eventually had four of the
needles in the palm of one hand and three in the

palm of the other – two I couldn't find. If I thought quickly and clearly I wouldn't have done that. A lathered man whose ear is bleeding and who has four wet needles in one hand and three in the other may be said to have reached the lowest known point of human efficiency. There is nothing he can do but stand there. I tried transferring the needles in my left hand to the palm of my right hand, but I couldn't get them off my left hand. Wet needles cling to you. In the end I wiped the needles off on to a bath-towel which was hanging on a rod above the bath-tub. It was the only towel that I could find. I had to dry my hands afterwards on the bath-mat. Then I tried to find the needles in the towel. Hunting for seven needles in a bath-towel is the most tedious occupation I have ever engaged in. I could find only five of them. With the two that had been left in the bowl, that meant there were four needles in all missing – two in the wash-bowl and two others lurking in the towel or lying in the bath-tub under the towel. Frightful thoughts came to me of what might happen to anyone who used that towel or washed his face in the bowl or got into the tub, if I didn't find the missing needles. Well, I didn't find them. I sat down on the edge of the tub to think, and I decided finally that the only thing to do was wrap up the towel in a newspaper and take it away with me. I also decided to leave a note for my friends explaining as clearly as I could that I was afraid there were two needles in the bath-tub and two needles in the wash-bowl, and that they better be careful.

I looked everywhere in the apartment, but I could not find a pencil, or a pen, or a typewriter. I could find pieces of paper, but nothing with which to write on them. I don't know what gave me the idea – a movie I had seen, perhaps, or a story I had read – but I suddenly thought of writing a message with a lipstick. The wife might have an extra lipstick lying around and, if so, I concluded it would be in the medicine cabinet. I went back to the medicine cabinet and began poking around in it for a lipstick. I saw what I thought looked like the metal tip of one, and I got two fingers around it and began to pull gently – it was under a lot of things. Every object in the medicine cabinet began to slide. Bottles broke in the wash-bowl and on the floor; red, brown, and white liquids spurted; nail files, scissors, razor blades, and miscellaneous objects sang and clattered and tinkled. I was covered with perfume, peroxide, and cold cream.

It took me half an hour to get the debris all together in the middle of the bathroom floor. I made no attempt to put anything back in the medicine cabinet. I knew it would take a steadier hand than mine and a less shattered spirit. Before I went away (only partly shaved) and abandoned the shambles, I left a note saying that I was afraid there were needles in the bath-tub and the wash-bowl and that I had taken their towel and that I would call up and tell them everything – I wrote it in iodine with the end of a toothbrush. I have not called up yet, I am sorry to say. I have neither found the courage nor thought up the words to explain what happened. I suppose my friends believe that I deliberately smashed up their bathroom and stole their towel. I don't know for sure, because they have not yet called me up, either.

James Thurber (*1894–1961*)
NINE NEEDLES

'Toilet paper' – as it is described in the trade – is a modern invention dating back only as far as the 1880s, when it became available from the British Perforated Paper Company; an excellent example of a go-ahead company creating public demand for a product for which there was no need.

Our ancestors would have laughed themselves silly at the notion of us paying good money to buy rolls of plain paper when our houses are full of old magazines and newsprint.

In ancient times, before the invention of paper, the cleaning-off problem was solved in a number of ways. Water was the answer where water existed. Failing that it was a matter of using a scraper or an abrasive.

The Romans favoured a kind of miniature hockey-stick (in wood or precious metal according to the user's status), or a sponge on the end of a stick (origin of the phrase 'to get hold of the wrong end of the stick'?).

In desert areas it was normal to use sand, powdered brick, or earth. A book on Muslim law published as late as 1882, *Manuel de Jurisprudence Musulman selon le Rite de Chafi*, recommends using stones: 'There shall be three stones employed or three sides of the same stone'.

A favourite scraper throughout the ages, probably because of its convenient shape and easy availability, was a mussel shell. A writer in the eighteenth century recalls a charming incident involving its use:

'Whereas I have known an old woman in Holland set herself on the next hole to a gentleman, and civilly offer him her muscle shell by way of scraper after she had done with it herself.'

PHILOSOPHICAL DIALOGUE CONCERNING DECENCY 1751

Perhaps a similar encounter in a two-seater inspired the poet to write:

Then her cheek was pale and thinner than should
   be for one so young,
And her eye on all my motions with a mute
   observance hung.

Alfred Lord Tennyson (*1809–1892*)
LOCKSLEY HALL

A form of scraper which lingered on and perhaps is still in use in rural America is the corncob, a box of which would be to hand in all well-appointed privies:

'Now, about her furnishin's. I can give you a nail
or hook for the catalogue, and besides, a box for
cobs. You take your pa, for instance; he's of the old
school and naturally he'd prefer the box; so put
'em both in, Elmer.

Charles Sale
THE SPECIALIST. 1930

Charles (Chick) Sale's tiny best-seller, *The Specialist,* is a publishing phenomenon. Sale was not an author or a journalist but a character comedian whose best-known act was to play the part of an old craftsman, Lem Putt, whose speciality, and love, was building privies. Piracy and plagiarism was a great problem to comedians in the early years of this century and Sale was persuaded to establish his copyright on the character by putting him into print. In 1929 he set up a little publishing company for the sole purpose of printing *The Specialist.*

It has never since been out of print. Its sales exceed a million, in ten languages. It is thirty pages long and has about 3000 words. George Bernard Shaw wrote – on one of his famous postcards – 'The illustrations are excellent; but the frontispiece fails in courage. Clearly it should represent the Elmer family *in situ.* G.B.S.'

A rural American privy in the heat of summer, cool beneath a leafy tree, a box of soft, fresh cobs waiting, sounds tolerable enough. However, the seasons changed. And some parents practised thrift:

But when the crust was on the snow and the sullen
    skies were gray,
In sooth the building was no place where one could
    wish to stay.
We did our duties promptly, there one purpose
    swayed the mind;

We tarried not, nor lingered long on what we left
    behind.
The torture of that icy seat would make a Spartan
    sob,
For needs must scrape the goose flesh with a
    lacerating cob,
That from a frost-encrusted nail, was suspended
    by a string –
For Father was a frugal man and wasted not a
    thing.

James Whitcomb Riley (*1849–1916*)
THE OLD BACKHOUSE

A soft alternative to those of tender skin who had to ply the mussel shell or lacerating cob came in the late fifteenth century when the development of printing brought about a massive increase in the manufacture of paper. From the days of Queen Elizabeth I it became the custom to retire to stool with a book, ripping out pages as they were called for.

This use to which their work was put did not please authors. Robert Herrick wrote a little cautionary verse in his book to give it protection:

Who with thy leaves shall wipe (at need)
The place, where swelling *Piles* do breed:
May every ill, that bites, or smarts,
Perplex him in his hinder-parts.

Robert Herrick (*1591–1674*)
TO HIS BOOKE

Correspondence also came in handy:

> I am seated in the necessary house. I have your letter before me. Soon it will be behind me.
>
> Anon.

By the eighteenth century the use of books in the privy was so commonplace that a poem was published with the title:

BUM-FODDER
for the
LADIES
a
POEM
(Upon Soft PAPER)
1753

The poem itself turned out to be a deeply boring political satire. 'Bum-fodder' is, of course, the origin of the modern word 'bumph'.

The good point about taking a book into the privy with you was that the time spent in there was not wasted but spent on self-improvement.

Samuel Johnson, musing on the fact that as flogging decreased in the great schools so did learning, commented 'What the boys get at one end they lose at the other.' One could say about someone sitting in the privy reading and tearing out pages 'What they lose at one end they gain at the other.'

Reading and tearing out the pages was highly recommended by many eminent men, including Lord Chesterfield, who wrote to his son:

I knew a gentleman, who was fo good a manager of his time, that he would not even lofe that fmall portion of it, which the calls of nature obliged him to pafs in the neceffary-houfe ; but gradually went through all the Latin Poets, in thofe moments. He bought, for example, a common edition of Horace, of which he tore off gradually a couple of pages, carried them with him to that neceffary place, read them firft, and then fent them down as a facrifice to Cloacina : this was fo much time fairly gained ; and I recommend to you to follow his example. It is better than only doing what you cannot help doing at thofe moments; and it will make any book, which you fhall read in that manner, very prefent in your mind. Books of fcience, and of a grave fort, muft be read with continuity; but there are very many, and even very ufeful ones, which may be read with advantage by fnatches, and unconnectedly; fuch are all the good Latin poets, except Virgil in his Æneid: and fuch are moft of the modern poets, in which you will find many pieces worth reading, that will not take up above feven or eight minutes. Bayle's, Moreri's, and other dictionaries, are proper books to take and fhut up for the little intervals of (otherwife) idle time, that every body has in the courfe of the day, between either their ftudies or their pleafures. Good night.

Lord Chesterfield. Letters to his Son.
Letter C1, London, December the 11th. O.S. 1747.

The noble Lord Chesterfield would hardly have been pleased had he known that his advice was to be encapsulated for all time in a humble limerick:

> There was a young fellow named Chivy
> Who, whenever he went to the privy,
> First solaced his mind,
> Then wiped his behind,
> With some well-chosen pages of Livy.

Anon.
QUOTED IN THE LIMERICK ed.: G. Legman

Books are rarely torn up for lavatorial purposes these days; they are too valuable and there are many cheaper sources of waste paper. But they are still read there (John Cowper Powys revealed that he had read his way, seated, through *The Anatomy of Melancholy*, *Tristram Shandy*, half of *Don Quixote*, all of Rabelais and two volumes of the works of Montaigne). Further evidence came in *The Bookseller* of Dec. 19 and 26, 1981 which reported that Crown Paint's Gallup survey into what people would choose to have as 'fantasy extras' in their 'dream loo' produced the following list:

1. A musical toilet-paper holder.
2. Gold taps.
3. Built-in stereo.
4. A heated seat.
5. A copy of *Jane's Fighting Ships*.

One of the traditional American sources of suitable paper in farming areas was the enormously thick mail-order catalogue which was sent seemingly to everybody by the firm of Sears Roebuck. This massive work, normally printed on reasonably flexible paper, was pierced in its top lefthand corner, threaded with string and hung in the privy on a nail:

I'll tell you about a technical point that was put to me the other day. The question was this: 'What is the life, or how long will the average mail order catalogue last, in just the plain, ordinary eight family three holer?' It stumped me for a spell; but this bein' a reasonable question I checked up, and found that by placin' the catalogue in there, say in January – when you get your new one – you should be into the harness section by June; but, of course, that ain't through apple time, and not countin' on too many city visitors, either.

An' another thing – they've been puttin' so many of those stiff-coloured sheets in the catalogue here lately that it makes it hard to figger. Somethin' really ought to done about this, and I've thought about takin' it up with Mr. Sears Roebuck hisself.

Charles Sale
THE SPECIALIST 1930

It seems that the older generation of farmer preferred using a corncob and it was the young folk who took to the catalogue but both were part of the U.S rural tradition, hence the phrase used to describe the farmlands: 'the cob and catalogue belt'

84

Town dwellers did their shopping in person so were not usually sent mail-order catalogues. It was their custom, until quite recent years, to collect old paper-bags, circulars, used envelopes and so on and put them away for a later session of cutting-up. This little task, as Diana Holman-Hunt remembers, was the sort of employment given to a young girl on a visit to her granny:

'Now my dear, you can make yourself useful; there are many circulars, envelopes and paper bags ready on the Moorish throne.'

'Which do you need most, spills or lavatory paper?'

'Let me see – the latter I think, as none has been made for so long. Here is your knife.' It was engraved with the name Helen Faucit. 'You will find the stiletto, the template and string in the Indian box over there.' She settled at the writing-table, and with a pin-like nib, scratched away at her letters.

I ripped the blade through the stiff paper folded round the template. 'Some of these bags from Palmer's Stores are very thick and covered with writing.'

'Print is all right on one side you know. Try not to talk.'

When I had cut a hundred sheets, I pierced their corners and threaded them with a string; I tied this in a loop to hang on a nail by the 'convenience'. I made a mental note of the softer pieces and put them together in the middle, between the back of a calendar from Barkers and an advertisement for night-lights.

Diana Holman-Hunt
MY GRANDMOTHERS AND I

When the company first put their 'toilet tissue' on the market, in the 1880s, they hit a considerable snag. Shoppers were to embarrassed to ask for it. The company overcame the problem by using an almost plain wrapper which merely gave a trade name and did not reveal what the wrapper contained. A well brought-up shopper could then, cheeks flaming, mutter 'Two, please' to the shop assistant and with a bit of luck none of her neighbours would know that she was buying a couple of rolls of That Which Must Not Be Mentioned.

Perhaps at no time was the practice of prudery brought to such a high form of art as during the reign of Queen Victoria. We all know splendid examples of this: the invention of the expression 'white meat' so that when stipulating which bit of chicken was preferred it was not necessary to say the dread word 'breast'; the titled lady who recommended that books by male and female authors should be kept on separate shelves; the hiding of lushly rounded piano legs beneath frilly drapery. The general feeling was that these were sensible precautions designed to protect the innocent and that breaking the taboos would only result in social oblivion, dizzy spells and an early death.

These taboos were at their strongest in anything to do with the natural functions performed in the bathroom (with the functions performed naturally in the bedroom a close second). In order to avoid using those words which had such earthy, beastly connotations, euphemism was piled upon euphemism. Ladies and gentlemen bent over backwards until their foreheads were (metaphorically) touching the carpet behind them to avoid mentioning, say, the china chamber pot which ladies sat upon and gentlemen stood before nightly.

Victorian delicacy of this order was the subject of a short story, rather surprisingly by an author better known for his sea-stories:

THE BEDCHAMBER MYSTERY

Now that a hundred years have passed, one of the scandals in my family can be told. It is very doubtful if in 1843 Miss Forester (she was Eulalie, but being the eldest daughter unmarried, she of

86

course was Miss Forester) and Miss Emily Forester and Miss Eunice Forester ever foresaw the world of 1943 to which their story would be told; in fact it is inconceivable that they could have believed that there ever would be a world in which their story could be told blatantly in public print. At that time it was the sort of thing that could only be hinted at in whispers during confidential moments in feminine drawings rooms; but it was whispered about enough to reach in the end the ears of my grandfather, who was their nephew, and my grandfather told it to me.

In 1843 Miss Forester and Miss Emily and Miss Eunice Forester were already maiden ladies of a certain age. The old-fashioned Georgian house in which they lived kept itself modestly retired, just like its inhabitants, from what there was of bustle and excitement in the High Street of the market town. The ladies indeed led a retired life; they went to church a little, they visited those of the sick whom it was decent and proper for maiden ladies to visit, they read the more colourless of the novels in the circulating library, and sometimes they entertained other ladies at tea.

And once a week they entertained a man. It might almost be said that they went from week to week looking forward to those evenings. Dr. Acheson was (not one of the old ladies would have been heartless enough to say 'fortunately', but each of them felt it) a widower, and several years older even than my great-great-aunt Eulalie. Moreover, he was a keen whist player and a brilliant one, but in no way keener or more brilliant than were Eulalie, Emily, and Eunice. For years now the three nice old ladies had looked forward to their weekly evening of whist – all the ritual of setting out the green table, the two hours of silent cut-and-thrust play, and the final twenty minutes of conversation with Dr. Acheson as he drank a glass of old madeira before bidding them good night.

The late Mrs. Acheson had passed to her Maker somewhere about 1830, so that it was for thirteen years they had played their weekly game of whist before the terrible thing happened. To this day we do not know whether it happened to Eulalie or Emily or Eunice, but it happened to one of them. The three of them had retired for the night, each to her separate room, and had progressed far toward the final stage of getting into bed. They were not dried-up old spinsters; on the contrary, they were women of weight and substance, with the buxom contours even married women might have been proud of. It was her weight which was the undoing of one of them, Eulalie, Emily, or Eunice.

Through the quiet house that bedtime there sounded the crash of china and a cry of pain, and two of the sisters – which two we do not know – hurried in their dressing gowns to the bedroom of the third – her identity is uncertain – to find her bleeding profusely from severe cuts in the lower part of the back. The jagged china fragments had inflicted severe wounds, and, most unfortunately, just in those parts where the injured sister could not attend to them herself. Under the urgings of the other two she fought down her modesty sufficiently to let them attempt to deal with them, but the bleeding was profuse, and the blood of the Foresters streamed from the prone figure face downward on the bed in terrifying quantity.

'We shall have to send for the doctor,' said one of the ministering sisters; it was a shocking thing to contemplate.

'Oh, but we cannot!' said the other ministering sister.

'We must,' said the first.

'How terrible!' said the second.

And with that the injured sister twisted her neck and joined in the conversation. 'I will not have the doctor,' she said. 'I would die of shame.'

'Think of the disgrace of it!' said the second sister. 'We might even have to explain to him how it happened!'

'But she's bleeding to death,' protested the first sister.

'I'd rather die!' said the injured one, and then, as a fresh appalling thought struck her, she twisted her neck even further. 'I could never face him again. And what would happen to our whist?'

That was an aspect of the case which until then had occurred to neither of the other sisters, and it was enough to make them blench. But they were of stern stuff. Just as we do not know which was the injured one, we do not know which one thought of a way out of the difficulty, and we shall never know. We know that it was Miss Eulalie, as befitted her rank as eldest sister, who called to Deborah, the maid, to go and fetch Dr. Acheson at once, but that does not mean to say that it was not Miss Eulalie who was the injured sister – injured or not, Miss Eulalie was quite capable of calling to Deborah and telling her what to do.

As she was bid, Deborah went and fetched Dr. Acheson and conducted him to Miss Eunice's bedroom, but of course the fact that it was Miss Eunice's bedroom is really no indication that it was Miss Eunice who was in there. Dr. Acheson had no means of knowing. All he saw was a recumbent form covered by a sheet. In the center of the sheet a round hole a foot in diameter had been cut, and through the hole the seat of the injury was visible.

Dr. Acheson needed no explanations. He took his needles and his thread from his little black bag and set to work and sewed up the worst of the cuts and attended to the minor ones. Finally he straightened up and eased his aching back.

'I shall have to take those stitches out,' he explained to the still and silent figure which had borne the stitching stoically without a murmur. 'I shall come next Wednesday and do that.'

Until next Wednesday the three Misses Forester kept to their rooms. Not one of them was seen in the streets of the market town, and when on Wednesday Dr. Acheson knocked at the door Deborah conducted him once more to Miss Eunice's bedoom. There was the recumbent form, and there was the sheet with the hole in it. Dr. Acheson took out the stitches.

'It has healed very nicely,' said Dr. Acheson. 'I don't think any further attention from me will be necessary.'

The figure under the sheet said nothing, nor did Dr. Acheson expect it. He gave some concluding advice and went his way. He was glad later to receive a note penned in Miss Forester's Italian hand:

Dear Dr. Acheson,
We will all be delighted if you will come to whist this week as usual.

When Dr. Acheson arrived he found that the 'as usual' applied only to his coming, for there was a slight but subtle change in the furnishings of the drawing room. The stiff, high-backed chairs on which the three Misses Forester sat bore, each of them, a thick and comfortable cushion upon the seat. There was no knowing which of the sisters needed it.

C. S. Forester (*1899–1966*)
COSMOPOLITAN MAGAZINE, 1943

Distaste for talking about bodily functions seems to have been mainly confined to the middle-aged, and to the middle-class. Generalising wildly, it could be said that those who toil with their hands live a physical life and are not ashamed of the physics of the body, and aristocrats are above bourgeois social taboos. Similarly old folk cannot be bothered with social niceties, and children – well, children find all bodily functions fascinating and hilarious. Children have a seemingly endless repertoire of gleeful jokes, about everything that the body can get up to and should not in polite company:

> He who farts in church
> Sits in his own pew.

Schoolboy joke of great age.

That particular bodily action was so natural to young children that it took years of patient persuasion to get them to stop. It seems that Nannies used a code phrase to remind the expellent that his breach of manners had been audible:

> 'Master Robert is talking German.'

Quoted in NANNY SAYS.
Sir Hugh Casson and Joyce Grenfell.

'Talking German' is perhaps the one activity of those we are considering that has always been looked upon as a private rather than a social pleasure:

> Every man likes the smell of his own farts.

Icelandic Proverb.
Quoted in THE FABER BOOK OF APHORISMS, 1962
ed.: W. H. Auden and Louis Kronenberger.

I once accused Mr. Auden of making this up. He strongly denied it and assured me that he had come across the proverb during his tour of Iceland with Louis MacNeice in the thirties.

History records that a gentle antiquarian and writer not only enjoyed his own emanations but believed that he was giving pleasure to others:

91

Sir Henry Englefield had a fancy (which some greater men have had) that there was about his person a natural odour of roses and violets. Lady Grenville, hearing of this, and loving a joke, exclaimed, one day when Sir Henry was present, 'Bless me, what a smell of violets!' – 'Yes,' said he with great simplicity; 'it comes from me.'

TABLE-TALK OF SAMUEL ROGERS, 1856

The idea of achieving artificially what Sir Henry seemed to have achieved naturally had already occurred to a writer, who went on to become 'the world's most respected American'. Benjamin Franklin, infuriated by the way the Royal Academy of Brussels had belittled his discoveries, wrote a satirical letter to them (which for some reason he did not send):

A LETTER TO THE ROYAL ACADEMY OF BRUSSELS

Gentlemen:

It is universally well known that, in digesting our common food, there is created or produced in the bowels of human creatures a great quantity of wind.

That the permitting this air to escape and mix with the atmosphere is usually offensive to the company, from the fetid smell that accompanies it.

That all well-bred people, therefore, to avoid giving such offense, forcibly restrain the efforts of nature to discharge that wind.

That so retained contrary to nature it not only gives frequently great present pain, but occasions future diseases such as habitual cholics, ruptures, tympanies, etc., often destructive of the constitution, and sometimes of life itself.

Were it not for the odiously offensive smell accompanying such escapes, polite people would probably be under no more restraint in discharging such wind in company than they are in spitting or blowing their noses.

My prize question therefore should be: To discover some drug, wholesome and not disagreeable, to be mixed with our common food, or sauces, that shall render the natural discharge of wind from our bodies not only inoffensive, but agreeable as perfumes.

That this is not a chimerical project and altogether impossible, may appear from these considerations. That we already have some knowledge of means capable of *varying* that smell. He that dines on stale flesh, especially with much addition of onions, shall be able to afford a stink that no company can tolerate; while he that has lived for some time on vegetables only, shall have that breath so pure as to be insensible to the most delicate noses; and if he can manage so as to avoid the report, he may anywhere give vent to his griefs, unnoticed. But as there are many to whom an entire vegetable diet would be inconvenient, and as a little quicklime thrown into a jakes will correct the amazing quantity of fetid air arising from the vast mass of putrid matter contained in such places, and render it rather pleasing to the smell, who knows but that a little powder of lime (or some other thing equivalent), taken in our food, or perhaps a glass of limewater drunk at dinner, may have the same effect on the air produced in and issuing from our bowels? This is worth the experiment. Certain it is also that we have the power of changing by slight means the smell of another discharge, that of our water. A few stems of asparagus eaten shall give our urine a disagreeable odor; and a pill of turpentine no bigger than a pea shall bestow on it the pleasing smell of violets. And why should it be thought more impossible in nature to find means of making perfume of our wind than of our water?

For the encouragement of this inquiry (from the immortal honor to be reasonably expected by the inventor), let it be considered of how small importance to mankind, or to how small a part of mankind have been useful those discoveries in science that have heretofore made philosophers famous. Are there twenty men in Europe this day the happier, or even the easier, for any knowledge they have picked out of Aristotle? What comfort can the vortices of Descartes give to a man who has whirlwinds in his bowels! The knowledge of Newton's mutual *attraction* of the particles of matter, can it afford ease to him who is racked by their mutual *repulsion*, and the cruel distensions it occasions? The pleasure arising to a few philosophers, from seeing, a few times in their lives, the threads of light untwisted, and separated by the Newtonian prism into seven colors, can it be compared with the ease and comfort every man living might feel seven times a day, by discharging freely the wind from his bowels? Especially if it be converted into a perfume; for the pleasures of one sense being little inferior to those of another, instead of pleasing the *sight*, he might delight the *smell* of those about him, and make numbers happy, which to a benevolent mind must afford infinite satisfaction. The generous soul, who now endeavors to find out whether the friends he entertains like best claret or Burgundy, champagne or Madeira, would then inquire also whether they chose musk or lily, rose or bergamot, and provide according-ly. And surely such a liberty of *ex-pressing one's scentiments, and pleasing one another*, is of in-finitely more importance to human happiness than that liberty of the *press*, or of *abusing one another*, which the English are so ready to fight and die for.

In short, this invention, if completed, would be, as Bacon expresses it, *bringing philosophy home to men's business and bosoms*. And I cannot but conclude that in comparison therewith for *universal* and *continual utility*, the science of the philosophers abovementioned, even with the addition, gentlemen, of your *'figure quelconque,'* and the figures inscribed in it, are all together, scarcely worth a

Fart-hing

Benjamin Franklin (*1706–1790*)
Stevens Collection of Franklin Manuscripts,
State Department, Washington, D.C.

Some hundred years later, in 1882, another American wrote on the subject, but this time a piece of fiction, an imagined conversation at the court of Queen Elizabeth I. In 1870 Mark Twain had married a conservative and somewhat puritanical lady and it has been suggested that this drove underground a natural talent for satire and revolt. At any rate in 1882 he wrote what in those days was regarded as a 'vile' and 'unutterably coarse' story, which he managed to get printed secretly at West Point Military Academy, to amuse his friend the Rev. Joseph Twichell. There were originally fifty copies. Here are the opening pages:

Conversation, as it was by the Social Fireside in the time of the Tudors

Yesterday took Her Majesty ye Queen a fantasy such as she sometimes hath, and had to her closet certain that do write plays, books, and such like, these being my Lord Bacon, his worship Sir Walter Raleigh, Mr. Ben Jonson, and ye child Francis Beaumont, which being but sixteen, hath yet turned his hand to ye doing of ye Latin masters into our English tongue, with great discretion and much applause. Also came with these ye famous Shakespeare. A right strange mixing truly of mighty blood with mean, ye more in especial since ye Queen's Grace was present, as likewise these following, *to wit*, ye Duchess of Bilgewater, twenty-two years of age; ye Countess of Granby, twenty-six; her daughter, ye Lady Helen, fifteen; (sic) as also these two maids of honour, *to wit:* ye Lady Margery Boothy, sixty-five, and ye Lady Alice Dilberry, turned seventy, she being two years ye Queen's Grace's elder.

I being Her Majesty's cup-bearer, had no choice but to remain and behold rank forgotten, and ye high hold converse with ye low as upon equal terms, a great scandal did ye world hear thereof.

In ye heat of ye talk it befell that one did break wind, yielding an exceeding mighty and distressful stink, whereat all did laugh full sore, and then:

Ye Queen. Verily in mine eight and sixty years have I not heard ye fellow to this fart. Meseemeth, by ye great sound and clamour of it, it was male; yet ye belly it did lurk behind should now fall lean and flat against ye spine of him that hath been delivered of so stately and so vast a bulk, whereas ye guts of them that do quiff-splitters bear, stand comely still and round. Prithee, let ye author confess ye offspring. Will my Lady Alice testify?

Lady Alice. Good your Grace, an' I had room for such a thundergust within mine ancient bowls, 'tis not in reason I could discharge ye same and live to thank God for that He did choose handmaid so humble whereby to shew his power. Nay, 'tis not I that have brought forth this rich o'ermastering fog, this fragrant gloom, so pray you seek ye further.

Ye Queen. Maybe ye Lady Margery hath done ye company this favour?

Lady Margery. So please you Madam, my limbs are feeble with ye weight and drought of five and sixty winters, and it behoveth that I be tender unto them. In ye good providence of God, an' I had contained this wonder, forsooth would I have given ye whole evening of my sinking life to ye dribbling of it forth, with trembling and uneasy soul, not launched it sudden in its matchless might, taking mine own life with violence, rending my weak frame like rotten rags. It was not I, your Majesty:

Ye Queen. In God's name, who hath favoured us? Hath it come to pass that a fart shall fart *itself?* Not such a one as this, I trow. Young Master Beaumont; but no, 'twould have wafted him to Heaven like down of goose's body. 'Twas not ye little Lady Helen – nay, ne'er blush, my child; thou wilt tickle thy tender maidenhead with many a mousie-sqeak before thou learnest to blow a hurricane like to this. Wast you, my learned and ingenious Jonson?

Jonson. So fell a blast hath ne'er mine ears saluted, nor yet a stench so all-pervading and immortal. 'Twas not a novice did it, good Your Majesty, but one of veteran experience –

else had he failed of confidence. In sooth it was not I.

Ye Queen.   My Lord Bacon?

Lord Bacon.   Not from my lean entrails hath this prodigy burst forth, so please Your Grace. Naught so doth befit ye great as great performance; and haply shall ye find that 'tis not from mediocrity this miracle hath issued.

(Though ye subject be but a fart, yet will this tedious sink of learning ponderously philosophize. Meantime did ye foul and deadly stink pervade all places to that degree, that never smelt I ye like, yet dared I not to leave ye presence, albeit I was like to suffocate.)

Ye Queen.   What saith ye worshipful Master Shakespeare?

Shakespeare.   In ye great hand of God I stand, and so proclaim my innocence. Though ye sinless hosts of Heaven had foretold ye coming of this most desolating breath, proclaiming it the work of uninspired man, its quaking thunders, its firmament clogging rottenness his own achievement in due course of nature, yet had I not believed it; but had said ye pit itself hath furnished forth ye stink, and Heaven's artillery hath shook ye globe in admiration of it.

(Then was there a silence, and each did turn himself toward ye worshipful Sir Walter Raleigh, that browned embattled, bloody swashbuckler, who rising up did smile, and simpering, say:)

Sir Walter.   Most Gracious Majesty, 'twas I that did it, but indeed it was so poor and frail a note, compared with such as I am wont to furnish, that in sooth I was ashamed to call ye weakling mine in so august a presence. It was nothing – less than nothing, Madam, I did it but to clear my nether throat; but had I come prepared then had I delivered something worthy. Bear with me, please Your Grace, till I can make amends.

Mark Twain *(1835–1910)*

Mark Twain's fiction does not do justice to Queen Elizabeth. History reveals that when the same situation actually occurred the Queen managed matters with exquisite tact:

> This Earle of Oxford, making of his low obeisance to Queen Elizabeth, happened to let a Fart, at which he was so abashed and ashamed that he went to Travell, 7 yeares. On his return the Queen welcomed him home, and sayd, My Lord, I had forgott the Fart.

John Aubrey *(1626–1697)*
BRIEF LIVES. ed.: Oliver Lawson Dick

Victorians were by no means the only people to find the practice repugnant. In the early travel book *Purchas, His*

Pilgrims (II, vii, 936), 1619, there is a description of the negroes of Guinea, who were happy to wander about naked, being most upset by Netherland sailors 'who could not (or would not) hold their wind, which the natives held to be a shame and contempt done to them.'

European 'courtesy books' of the Middle Ages gave clear instructions to would-be courtiers:

> Beware of thy hinder parts from gun-blasting.
>
> BOKE OF CURTASYE, 14th. c.

But others thought differently. The Roman Emperor Claudius is reported to have considered making it socially acceptable on humanitarian grounds:

> He is reported to have had some thoughts of
> making a decree that it might be lawful for any
> man to break wind at the table, being told of a
> person whose modest retention had like to have
> cost him his life.
>
> Suetonius. (*c.A.D. 70–c. 160*)
> DE VITA CAESARUM

The great medical school of the eleventh century at Salerno agreed with Claudius that retention could be a serious hazard to health:

> *To release certain winds is considered almost a*
> *   crime.*
> *Yet those who suppress them risk dropsy, convulsions,*
> *Vertigo and frightful colics.*
> *These are too often the unhappy outcome*
> *Of a sad discretion.*
>
> REGIMEN SANITATIS SALERNITATUM

Montaigne, in the sixteenth century, devoted one of his essays to contemplating his inner workings. He seems to have believed that Claudius actually did make it all legal because he wrote:

'**G**od alone knows how many times our bellies, by the refusal of one single fart, have brought us to the door of an agonising death. May the Emperor who gave us the freedom to fart where we like, also give us the power to do so.'

Michel Eyquem Montaigne (*1533–1592*)
ESSAIS. I.XXI.

This, perhaps ultimate, freedom was also the concern of the great French writer, Honoré de Balzac:

'I should like one of these days to be so well known, so popular, so celebrated, so famous, that it would permit me. . . .' Try to imagine the most enormous ambition that has entered the head of man since time began; the most impossible, the most unattainable, the most monstrous, the most Olympian, ambition; an ambition that neither Louis XIV nor Napoleon had; an ambition Alexander the Great would not have been able to satisfy in Babylon; an ambition forbidden to a dictator, to a nation's saviour, to a pope, to a master of the world. He, Balzac, said simply, '. . . so celebrated, so famous, that it would permit me to break wind in society and society would think it a most natural thing.'

JOURNAL DES GONCOURTS trans: Lewis Galantière
18 October, 1855.

Freedom was in fact spectacularly, though temporarily, achieved in France at the end of the nineteenth century. Not 'in society' or on medical grounds but on a public stage.

Oddly, a sentence in Montaigne's Essay adumbrates the whole strange phenomenon:

103

'That staunch upholder of will-power Saint Augustine (*Cite de Dieu* Book XIV, Chapter XXIV) claims to have seen someone in such control of his backside that he could break wind at will and follow the tone of verses spoken to him.

Michel Eyquem Montaigne (*1533–1592*)
ESSAIS, I.XXI

Modern churchmen have also held liberal views on this issue. In April 1982, the *Standard* newspaper reported that in a sermon, televised throughout the U.S.A. from the small town of Muncie, Indiana, the preacher assured his flock that 'the escape of any gas from the body is a sign that the devil is making his exit'.

In 1892 a Frenchman who billed himself as 'Le Petomane' (*péter*: to break wind) could not only follow the tone of verses with the control of his backside but perform a range of virtuoso tricks. His music-hall act was described by his son:

Before presenting the star of this story to the reader, it is important to remember the extraordinary, extravagant place which Le Petomane held in Parisian life between 1892 and 1900. 'At this time,' writes Marcel Pagnol, 'Sarah Bernhardt, Rejane, Lucien Guitry dominated the Paris stage along with the splendid Variety company the mere memory of which still makes actors who saw it when they were young feel modest and immature. These were some of the box office receipts of the time: Sarah Bernhardt 8,000 F, Lucien Guitry 6,500 F, Rejane 7,000 F, Variety 6,000 F. There was also a comic artist making himself heard at the Moulin Rouge. He seemed to be alone on the stage and his backside had more to say than his face. He called himself Le Petomane and in a single Sunday he took 20,000 F at the box office . . .'

104

My father was sure of himself. He had worked up his act very carefully. He would present himself in an elegant costume. Red coat with a red silk collar, breeches in black satin ruched at the knee. Black stockings and Richelieu patent leather pumps, white butterfly tie and white gloves held in the hand.

My father was never tired of telling us that he had bought this magnificent rig out of his own money and was proud of it. Contrary to what has often been said or implied, the Moulin Rouge paid not a penny towards this splendid attire, worthy of a great star.

'My children,' our father would tell us often, 'I never had stage fright before going on – not even on my opening night at the Moulin Rouge.'

The hour struck. When the compère announced 'a sensational act never before seen or heard' there was a long silence in the auditorium until the artist appeared. Then as soon as he was on, he explained what he was going to do. But, in order to get them laughing with him, he had prepared a funny little speech which I can remember word for word, having heard it so often.

This is how Le Petomane presented himself with an ease and good humour which worked beautifully on the public.

'Ladies and Gentlemen, I have the honour to present a session of Petomanie. The word Petomanie means someone who can break wind at will but don't let your nose worry you. My parents ruined themselves scenting my rectum.'

During the initial silence my father coolly began a series of small farts, naming each one 'This is a little girl, this the mother-in-law, this the bride on her wedding night (very little) and the morning after (very loud), this the mason (dry – no cement) this the dressmaker tearing two yards of calico (this one lasted at least ten seconds and imitated to perfection the sound of material being torn) then a cannon (Gunners stand by your guns! Ready – fire!) the noise of thunder, etc., etc.

Then my father would disappear for a moment behind the scenes to insert the end of a rubber tube, such as are used for enemas. It was about a yard long and he would take the other end in his fingers and in it place a cigarette which he lit. He would then smoke the cigarette as if it were in his mouth the contraction of his muscles causing the cigarette to be drawn in and then the smoke blown out. Finally my father removed the cigarette and blew out the smoke he had taken in. He then placed a little flute with six stops in the end of the tube and played one or two little tunes such as 'Le Roi Dagobert' and, of course, 'Au clair de la lune'. To end the act he removed the flute and then blew out several gas jets in the footlights with some force. Then he invited the audience to sing in chorus with him.

From the beginning of the 'audition' mad laughter had come. This soon built up into general applause. The public and especially women fell about laughing. They would cry from laughing. Many fainted and fell down and had to be resuscitated.

'This was all splendid for me,' my father said, 'the whole of my act went across without a hitch and full steam ahead.'

The director enthusiastically offered my father a month's contract renewable. And since his triumph grew all the time, neither side delayed signing a contract which bound them for several years with the right for Le Petomane to play abroad or elsewhere in France.

My father installed his family in a turreted chalet in Saint Maur des Fosses. There we had servants,

106

who became at the same time friends, and in particular a coachman-cum-valet, Pitalugue, who also acted as my father's manager.

He had a pretty little English carriage, a cabriolet drawn by a mare called Aida and when he drove it himself all dressed up in his best, with Le Petomane in the driver's seat, he was recognised and saluted affectionately as an important personage wherever he went:

'That's Le Petomane who went past then...!'
He was the talk of the town.

Jean Nohain and F. Caradec
LE PETOMANE. 1967. trans.: Warren Tute.

Proceeding on our tour of the bathroom, we have examined the bath and ruminated on the washbasin and its Assorted Toiletries. We should now be faced with the bidet but this is highly unlikely. For some reason the Anglo-Saxon races have never been able to take seriously this useful and efficient adjunct to personal hygiene. Instead, when met with on European holidays it gives rise either to a shudder of distaste at the strange practices which foreigners get up to or thigh-slapping jokes about 'the doll's bath' and 'so that's where we're supposed to wash our feet'.

Suffice it to say that the first mention of a bidet was made in 1710, in France of course, when it was reported that Marc René de Voyer, Marquis d'Argenson, lieutenant of the Paris police, was graciously received by Madame de Prie whilst she was astride her bidet. Though how he knew what she was astride considering the voluminous skirts of the period raises doubts. She might just as well have been astride a unicycle.

So leaping lightly over the bidet, or where it would have been had there been one, we arrive at what the French sometimes call *le petit coin*. There in the corner It stands. The porcelain bowl with its seat and lid.

The lavatory/loo/bog/john/can/dunny/W.C./*le double*/toilet/comfort-station/doings/gents/penny-house/carsey.

The modern domestic Thing is, as it were, dual purpose

and normally is happy to accept the products of both the minor and the major natural functions.

I say 'normally' because local customs can vary. The actress Gretchen Franklyn recalls arriving at a Theatrical boarding-house in the North-East of England which boasted a 'toilet' downstairs and another on the top landing. Anxious to make herself comfortable after her journey she tactfully made for the one at the top of the stairs. As she mounted the stairs there came a pounding on the banisters and the voice of the landlady rose up the stairwell 'We doan't use that toilet for solids, dear'.

Performance of the minor – or non-solids – natural function crops up frequently in tribal myth and legend. It is recorded that the Ancient Celts elected Maeve as their queen because she won a contest to see which of the tribal maidens could squat down and make the biggest hole in the snow. They later murdered her but perhaps for another reason.

The contest was echoed in modern times during the last war. Professor R. V. Jones, the scientist who 'bent the beam', reveals in his book *Most Secret War* that he won a male version of the Celts' competition by peeing over a six-foot wall.

Tribes living in warm climates formulated sensible rules of personal hygiene. In the old Testament, in Deuteronomy, it is recommended that a spot be chosen well away from the tents, a hole be dug with a mattock and filled in again afterwards – a routine still practised by army patrols and cats.

A Greek didactic poet penned some helpful hints for gentlemen:

> *When you would have your urine pass away,*
> *Stand not upright before the eye of day;*
> *And scatter not your water as you go*
> *Nor let it, when you're naked, from you flow:*
> *In either case 'tis an unseemly sight:*
> The gods observe alike by day and night:
> *The man whom we devout and wise may call*
> *Sits in that act, or streams against a wall.*

Hesiod (c. 8th century B.C.)
WORKS AND DAYS. trans.: Thomas Cooke

108

Pliny, in *Naturalis Historia*, quoted Ostanes as saying that to allow a little urine to fall upon the foot in the morning was beneficial to health. So according to Hesiod and Ostanes the old Corsican I once saw turning away from the wall of a church buttoning his flies, his left boot damp and shiny, was both devout and healthy. But not law-abiding. Above his head on the wall of the church a large notice said *Défense d'uriner contre le mur de l'église.*

Instructions as to where to dig and where to stand are all very well but they presuppose that there is plenty of time in hand and everything is under control, which is not always so:

Adrian Mitchell's Famous Weak Bladder Blues

Now some praise God because he gave us the
    bomb to drop in 1945
But I thank the Lord for equipping me with the
    fastest cock alive.

You may think a sten-gun's frequent, you can call
    greased lightning fast,
But race them down to the Piccadilly bog and
    watch me zooming past.

Well it's excuse me,
And I'll be back.
Door locked so rat-a-tat-tat.
You mind if I go first?
I'm holding this cloudburst.
I'll be out in 3·7 seconds flat.

I've got the Adamant Trophy, the Niagara Cup,
    you should see me on the M.1 run,
For at every comfort station I've got a reputation
    for – doing the ton.

Once I met that Speedy Gonzales and he was first
    through the door.
But I was unzipped, let rip, zipped again and out
    before he could even draw.

Now God killed Vicky and he let Harold Wilson
    survive,
But the good Lord blessed little Adrian Mitchell
    with the fastest cock alive.

Adrian Mitchell
OUT LOUD, 1968

Others who are not able to choose either the time or place
are young children Going Through a Phase:

A dry bed deserves a boiled sweet.

NANNY SAYS, Hugh Casson and Joyce Grenfell

Sleeping next to a child who is soaking wet and steaming
seems an odd thing to be nostalgic about but an American
poet and journalist managed it:

When Willie was a little boy,
    Not more than five or six,
Right constantly he did annoy
    His mother with his tricks.
Yet not a picayune cared I
    For what he did or said
Unless, as happened frequently,
    The rascal wet the bed.

Closely he cuddled up to me
    And put his hand in mine,
Till all at once I seemed to be
    Afloat in seas of brine.
Sabean odors clogged the air
    And filled my soul with dread,
Yet I could only grin and bear
    When Willie wet the bed.

'Tis many times that rascal has
    Soaked all the bedclothes through,
Whereat I'd feebly light the gas
    And wonder what to do.

110

Yet there he lay, so peaceful-like,
    God bless his curly head!
I quite forgave the little tyke
    For wetting of the bed.

Ah, me! those happy days have flown,
    My boy's a father too,
And little Willies of his own
    Do what he used to do.
And I, ah! all that's left for me
    Are dreams of pleasure fled;
My life's not what it used to be
    When Willie wet the bed!

Eugene Field (1850–1895)

It was Eugene Field, reviewing a production of *King Lear*, who wrote of Creston Clarke: 'He played the King as though under momentary apprehension that someone else was about to play the ace.'

The indiscriminate showering of the natural blessings was not confined to Corsicans, incontinent poets and small children but popped up throughout history, in fact and in fiction.

There was the giant Gargantua, whose mighty effusion resulted in a noble city being renamed:

Some few days after that they had refreshed themselves, he went to see the city, and was beheld of everybody there with great admiration: for the people of Paris are such fools, such puppies, and naturals, that a juggler, a carrier of indulgencies, a sumpter-horse, a mule with his bells, a blind fiddler in the middle of a cross lane, shall draw a greater confluence of people together than an evangelical preacher. And they pressed so hard upon him, that he was constrained to rest himself upon the steeple of our Lady's church; at which place, seeing so many about him, he said with a loud voice, 'I believe that these buzzards will have me to pay them here my welcome hither, and my beverage: it is but good reason. I will now give them their wine, but it shall be only a *par ris*, that is, in sport.' Then smiling, he untied his goodly codpiece, and lugging out his Roger into the open air, he so bitterly all-to-be-pissed them, that he drowned two hundred and sixty thousand four hundred and eighteen, besides the women and little children.

Some, nevertheless, of the company escaped this piss-flood by mere speed of foot, who when they were at the higher end of the university, sweating, coughing, spitting, and out of breath, they began to swear and curse, some in good hot earnest, and others *par ris*, *carimari*, *carimara*; *golynoly*, *golynolo*; 'ods-bodkins, we are washed *par ris*,' from whence the city hath been ever since called Paris.

François Rabelais (*1495?–1553*)
THE BOOK OF GARGANTUA. trans.: Sir Thomas Urquhart
and Peter Motteux

Perhaps it was this story which put an Italian gentleman off:

The pleasantest dotage that ever I read, saith *Laurentius*, was of a Gentleman at *Senes* in *Italy* who was afraid to pisse, lest all the towne should bee drowned; the Physicians caused the bells to be rung backward, and told him the towne was on fire, whereupon he made water, and was immediately cured.

Robert Burton (*1577–1640*)
ANATOMY OF MELANCHOLY

And perhaps reading Burton gave Dean Swift an idea for a way in which Lemuel Gulliver could render the King of Lilliput a most signal service:

I was alarmed at Midnight with the Cries of many Hundred People at my Door; by which being suddenly awaked, I was in some Kind of Terror. I heard the Word *Burglum* repeated incessantly; several of the Emperor's Court making their Way through the Croud, intreated me to come immediately to the Palace, where her Imperial Majesty's Apartment was on fire, by the Carelessness of a Maid of Honour, who fell asleep while she was reading a Romance. I got up in an Instant; and Orders being given to clear the Way before me; and it being likewise a Moonshine Night, I made a shift to get to the Palace without trampling on any of the People. I found they had already applied Ladders to the Walls of the Apartment, and were well provided with Buckets, but the Water was at some Distance. These Buckets were about the Size of a large Thimble, and the poor People supplied me with them as fast as they could; but the Flame was so violent, that they did little Good. I might easily have stifled it with my Coat, which I unfortunately left behind me for haste, and came away only in my Leather Jerkin. The Case seemed wholly desperate and deplorable; and this magnificent Palace would have infallibly been burnt down to the Ground, if, by a Presence of Mind, unusual to me, I had not suddenly thought of an Expedient. I had the Evening before drank plentifully of a most delicious Wine, called *Glimigrim*, (the *Blefuscudians* called it *Flunec*, but ours is esteemed the better Sort) which is very diuretick. By the luckiest Chance in the World, I had not discharged myself of any Part of it. The Heat I had contracted by coming very near the Flames, and by my labouring to quench them, made the Wine begin to operate by Urine; which I voided in such a Quantity, and applied so well to the proper Places, that in three Minutes the Fire was wholly extinguished; and the

rest of that noble Pile, which had cost so many
Ages in erecting, preserved from Destruction.

Jonathan Swift *(1667–1745)*
GULLIVER'S TRAVELS

These passages would hardly have surprised or shocked most eighteenth-century readers. Ladies were accustomed to relieving themselves discreetly almost anywhere. Until the early nineteenth century they wore long dresses and no drawers so it was simply a matter of standing astride some sort of gutter and gazing dreamily about for a minute or so. In extremely cold climates where gutters were frozen more sophisticated measures were called for. Marco Polo writes that in Siberia it became fashionable for a lady's serving-maid to follow her mistress carrying a large sponge which she could, without indelicacy, insert beneath her lady's dress to absorb the effluent.

Gentlemen did the best they could in the circumstances. For instance, during troop manoeuvres:

> M. de Vendôme (I report only the bare,
> unvarnished facts) arrived independently at Ghent
> between seven and eight o'clock in the morning,
> as troops were entering the town. He stopped with
> the remnant of his suite still accompanying him,
> dismounted, let down his breeches, and there and
> then planted his stools quite close to the troops as
> he watched them go by.

Duc de Saint-Simon *(1675–1755)*
HISTORICAL MEMOIRS, trans. Lucy Norton

After a jolly party:

> Sir Charles Sedley, Bart., sometimes of Wadham
> coll., Charles lord Buckhurst (afterwards earl of
> Middlesex), Sir Thom Ogle, &c. were at a cook's
> house, at the signe of the cock in Bow-street neare
> Covent-garden, within the libertie of Westminster;

and being all inflamed with strong liquors, they
went into the balcony, joyning to their chamber-
window, and putting downe their breeches, they
excrementized in the street.

Anthony Wood (*1632–1695*)
LIFE AND TIMES

A noted Puritan divine in skittish mood became quite
inventive:

Of Dr. Thomas Goodwin, when ffelow of
Catherine Hall. – He was somewhat whimsycall, in
a frolic pist once in old Mr. Lothian's pocket.

Thomas Woodcock (*fl. 1695*)
PAPERS

While an aristocratic lady at the Court of Louis XIV at
Versailles must have been less than a social asset at dinner
parties:

The Princesse d'Harcourt ... was a glutton, and so eager to relieve herself that she drove her hostesses to desperation, for although she never denied herself the use of the convenience on leaving table, she sometimes allowed herself no time to reach it at leisure, leaving a dreadful trail behind her that made the servants of M. du Maine and M. le Grand wish her to the devil. As for her, she was never in the least embarrassed, but lifted her skirts and went her way, saying on her return that she had felt a little faint.

Duc de Saint-Simon (*1675–1755*)
HISTORICAL MEMOIRS, trans.: Lucy Norton

The French Court was notorious for this kind of behaviour:

Mademoiselle de Montpensier, and the Palatine Duchess of Orléans, though women of the highest birth and rank, as well as of unimpeached conduct, conceal nothing on these points, in their writings. The former, speaking of the Duchess of Orléans, her step-mother, second wife of Gaston, brother of Louis the Thirteenth, says, 'She had contracted a singular habit of always running into another room, *pour se placer sur la Chaise percée*, when dinner was announced. As she never failed in this particular, the Grand Maître, or Lord Steward of Gaston's Household, who performed the ceremony of summoning their Royal Highnesses to table; observed, smelling to his Baton of office, that there must certainly be either Senna or Rhubarb in its composition, as it invariably produced the effect of sending the Duchess to the Garderobe.' I have, myself, seen the late Electress Dowager of Saxony, daughter of the Emperor Charles the Seventh, at her own palace, in the suburbs of Dresden, rise from the table where she was playing, when the room has been full of company of both sexes; lay down her cards, retire for a few minutes, during which time the game was suspended, and then return, observing to those near her, '*J'ai pris Médecine aujourd'huy.*'

Sir Nathaniel Wraxall (*1751–1831*)
HISTORICAL MEMOIRS

Other memoirs and diaries give similar accounts of courtiers using the walls of the Hall of Mirrors, corners of staircases, in fact any part of the building where they were unobserved by the King. The custom at Fontainebleau was to wait until dusk and then make for a lawn outside. Here lords, ladies and the Swiss Guard would assemble, each trying to ignore the other and get on with his or her business. The pretty walks became unwalkable.

The English Court was almost as bad in its habits. When the plague slackened its grip and the Court of King Charles II gave up living in Oxford and returned to London, a university diarist recorded:

> To give a further character of the court, they,
> though they were neat and gay in their apparell,
> yet they were very nasty and beastly, leaving at
> their departure their excrements in every corner,
> in chimneys, studies, colehouses, cellers.

Anthony Wood (*1632–1695*)
LIFE AND TIMES

Not all recorded examples of this sort of thing show gross slovenliness of manners or drunken caperings. There was the episode concerning a Lady and the minister of Thames Ditton, the Rev. George Harvest. Mr. Harvest was in every way well-mannered and gentlemanly. But he was extremely absent minded:

> One day Lady Onslow, being desirous of knowing
> the most remarkable planets and constellations,

requested Mr. Harvest, on a fine starlight night, to
point them out to her, which he undertook to do;
but in the midst of his lecture, having occasion to
make water, thought that need not interrupt it,
and accordingly directing that operation with one
hand, went on in his explanation, pointing out the
constellations with the other.

Francis Grose (<i>1731–1791</i>)
THE OLIO

It was not that our male ancestors had no place to Go.
There had always been areas and rooms allocated for their
relief; the Palace of Versailles had many, as had the colleges of
Oxford. The problem was to get gentlemen to use them.
Gentlemen, endowed by nature with directional control, had
developed over the centuries a tradition of using whatever was
at hand rather than what was especially provided for the
purpose. In the early years of the last century Lord Byron was
banned from Long's Hotel in Bond Street for peeing in a
corner of the entrance hall rather than going to the bother of
seeking out a necessary house.

It is recorded that at a meeting of clergy in the 1920s at an
Oxford college a rather hearty young vicar asked whether it
was permitted to pee in the bedroom basin. 'Certainly not!'
said the Dean. Adding, after thought, 'Unless the window is
closed.'

It seems that this male privilege is tolerated, under certain
conditions, in the clubland of St. James's where one gentle-
man's club has a notice, I am told, reading DURING THE
ASPARAGUS SEASON MEMBERS ARE REQUESTED
NOT TO RELIEVE THEMSELVES IN THE HAT-
STAND.

It was a simple matter for people who lived in the country
to allocate a special place; they had plenty of room. Like the
biblical hole in the ground which was well away from the
tents, the hole they dug was well away, and down wind, from
their dwelling. The next development was to put a hut round
the hole, partly to stop the pig falling in but also for protection
against the weather. It came to be called the 'privy' (or in

Tudor times, the 'jakes', probably from 'Jack's place', Jack being the nickname for a simple countryman). The countryman's privy was not only a convenient and fairly hygienic answer to the problem but was also a considerable asset to his kitchen garden:

> The privy had from time immemorial been an important source of soil fertility. By the mid-nineteenth century human urine and excrement had been subjected to scientific analysis. *The Cottage Gardener* published the fascinating fact that 'the annual urine of two men is said to contain sufficient mineral food for an acre of land, and mixed with ashes will produce a fair crop of turnips'. When the shed at the bottom of the garden was supplanted by indoor plumbing the cottage garden was the poorer. I myself often stayed as a child in a cottage with an outdoor privy where squares cut from the *Daily Mail* and a bucket of ashes were placed beside the seat. All was used on the garden which grew, I remember, spectacularly good runner beans.
>
> Anne Scott-James (*1913–*)
> THE COTTAGE GARDEN

It was usual for the cottager to shift his privy from time to time so that the whole of his garden enjoyed the benefit. When the structure had to be permanent the resultant soil could become very rich indeed:

> In [New] Colledge, the house of office or Bog-house is a famous pile of building, the dung of it computed by old Jacob Bobart to be worth a great deal of money, who said this Compost when rotton was an excellent soil to fill deep holes to plant young vines.
>
> Thomas Baskerville (*c. 1675*)

119

A drawback to the privy was that not only the domestic pig was in danger of falling in. The principle was that the occupier was suspended above the hole in the ground on a wooden pole, or plank, or a seat with a hole cut in it. And wood rots. Or is not strong enough to support the weight suddenly applied to it:

> 'And when it comes to construction,' I sez, 'I can
> give you joists or beams. Joists make a good job.
> Beams cost a bit more, but they're worth it.
> Beams, you might say, will last forever. 'Course, I
> could give you joists, but take your Aunt Emmy,
> she ain't gettin' a mite lighter. Some day she might
> be out there when them joists give away and there
> she'd be – catched. Another thing you've got to
> figger on, Elmer,' I sez, 'is that Odd Fellows picnic
> in the fall. Them boys is goin' to get in there in
> fours and sixes, singin' and drinkin', and the like,
> and I want to tell you there's nothin' breaks up an
> Odd Fellows picnic quicker than a diggin' party.'

> Charles Sale
> THE SPECIALIST

Records show that diggin' parties were required fairly frequently. A famous royal catastrophe occurred in 1184 when the Emperor Frederick I summoned a group of notables, including eight ruling princes, to a Diet in the Great Hall at Erfurt:

> The Emperor . . . had occasion to go to the
> privy, whither he was followed by some of the
> nobles, when suddenly the floor that was under
> them began to sink; the emperor immediately took
> hold of the iron grates of a window, whereat he
> hung by the hands till some came and succoured
> him. Some gentlemen fell to the bottom where
> they perished. And it is most observable, that
> amongst those who died was Henry earl of

Schwartzenburg, who carried the presage of his death in a common imprecation of his, which was this, *If I do it not, I wish I may sink in a privy.*

Rev. Nathaniel Wanley *(1634–1680)*
THE WONDERS OF THE LITTLE WORLD

One sad incident concerned a gentleman who fell in on an inappropriate day:

A Jewe at Tewkesbury fell into a Privie on the Saturday and would not that day bee taken out for reverence of his sabbath, wherefore Richard Clare Earle of Glocester kepte him there till Munday that he was dead.

John Stowe *(1525?–1605)*
A SURVEY OF LONDON, 1603.

Reverence for the sabbath was still strong in the 1890s but the threat to life and limb was much smaller and awkward dilemmas could be dealt with tactfully:

A lady got locked into the lavatory on a Sunday morning; so her brother-in-law, a clergyman, sat on a chair up against the door and read the morning service aloud to her from outside.

Gwen Raverat *(1885–1957)*
PERIOD PIECE: A CAMBRIDGE CHILDHOOD

It is encouraging to learn that a nasty experience in a House of Office resulted in at least one spiritual awakening:

WILLIAM TWISSE

His sonne Dr. Twisse, Minister of the New-church neer Tothill-street Westminster, told me, that he had heard his father say, that when he was a schoole-boy at Winton-college, that he was a rakell; and that one of his Schoolefellowes and camerades (as wild as himselfe) dyed there; and

121

that, his father goeing in the night to the House of
office, the phantome or Ghost of his dead
schoolefellow appeared to him, and told him *I am
damn'd*: and that this was the Beginning of his
Conversion.

John Aubrey (*1626–1697*)
BRIEF LIVES, ed. Oliver Lawson Dick

The misfortune of falling into the privy – or perhaps the
fear of it happening – was so prevalent that it gave rise to a
popular limerick:

There was a young man from Kilbride
Who fell in a privy and died.
His broken-hearted brother
Fell into another,
And now they're interred side by side.

Anon.
Quoted in THE LIMERICK, ed. G. Legman

The backyard privy has by no means disappeared, particularly in rural areas, but it is no longer such a cornerstone of
family life as it once was. Poets, especially American poets,
sigh for the memory of those dear, dead days with –
considering sentiments like 'I ween the old familiar smell will
sooth my jaded soul' – what might be called *nostalgie de la ph-
e-e-e-w:*

When memory keeps me company and moves to
   smiles or tears,
A weather-beaten object looms through the mist of
   years.
Behind the house and barn it stood, a hundred
   yards or more,
And hurrying feet a path had made, straight to its
   swinging door.
Its architecture was a type of simple classic art,
But in the tragedy of life it played a leading part.

And oft the passing traveller drove slow, and
    heaved a sigh,
To see the modest hired girl slip out with glances
    shy.

We had our posey garden that the women loved so
    well,
I loved it, too, but better still I loved the stronger
    smell
That filled the evening breezes so full of homely
    cheer,
And told the night-o'ertaken tramp that human life
    was near.
On lazy August afternoons, it made a little bower
Delightful, where my grandsire sat and whiled
    away an hour.
For there the morning-glory its very eaves
    entwined,
And berry bushes reddened in the steaming soil
    behind.

All day fat spiders spun their webs to catch the
    buzzing flies
That flitted to and from the house, where Ma was
    baking pies.
And once a swarm of hornets bold, had built a
    palace there,
And stung my unsuspecting aunt – I must not tell
    you where.
Then Father took a flaming pole – that was a
    happy day –
He nearly burned the building up, but the hornets
    left to stay.
When summer bloom began to fade and winter to
    carouse
We banked the little building with a heap of
    hemlock boughs.

But when the crust was on the snow and the sullen
    skies were gray,
In sooth the building was no place where one could
    wish to stay.
We did our duties promptly, there one purpose
    swayed the mind;
We tarried not, nor lingered long on what we left
    behind.
The torture of that icy seat would make a Spartan
    sob,
For needs must scrape the goose flesh with a
    lacerating cob,
That from a frost-encrusted nail, was suspended
    by a string –
For Father was a frugal man and wasted not a
    thing.

When Grandpa had to 'go out back' and make his
    morning call,
We'd bundle up the dear old man with a muffler
    and a shawl,
I knew the hole on which he sat – 'twas padded all
    around,
And once I dared to sit there – 'twas all too wide I
    found.
My loins were all too little, and I jackknifed there
    to stay,
They had to come and get me out, or I'd have
    passed away.
Then Father said ambition was a thing that boys
    should shun,
And I just used the children's hole 'till childhood
    days were done.

And still I marvel at the craft that cut those holes so
    true,
The baby hole, and the slender hole that fitted
    Sister Sue;

That dear old country landmark! I've tramped
   around a bit,
And in the lap of luxury my lot has been to sit,
But ere I die I'll eat the fruit of trees I robbed of
   yore,
Then seek the shanty where my name is carved
   upon the door.
I ween the old familiar smell will sooth my jaded
   soul,
I'm now a man, but none the less, I'll try the
   children's hole.

James Whitcomb Riley (*1849–1916*)
THE OLD BACKHOUSE

Vastly more complicated sewage-disposal problems arose for town dwellers. The rich and the mighty had little trouble, of course, with an army of servants and plenty of space. Monasteries, invariably sited near running water, sat their monks in rows above a conduit. Castles had privies built into the thickness of the walls, with a channel to lead the effluent down the outside of the wall and into the moat. But as the water in moats was usually static this could produce problems. Owners of yachts still have the same problem today when they are tied up alongside each other in harbour or in a marina, all pumping their sewage overboard. Noël Coward defined the problem when he reappeared on the deck of a friend's boat after a visit to the ship's 'toilet' and said 'Not so much "good-bye" as "au revoir"'.

Many owners of great mansions had huge drains dug which led the waste well away from the house and into a stream (some of these were discovered later and were claimed to be secret passages). Other noble houses had little rooms specially built behind fire-places for warmth or tucked away where they would avoid embarrassment (to be claimed later as priest-holes and secret rooms). Almost all of them were unventilated and must have been appalling to use.

Even today, in the hot climate of a Greek island a privy represents a considerable health hazard:

Nimiec . . . arrived at a fishing village in Merlera on one of his fishing jaunts, and was housed in a small cottage with an earth lavatory, primitive and so full of flies that he drew the attention of his host to its condition. His host said briskly, 'Flies? Of course there are flies. If you could do as we all do and wait until just before the midday meal you would not find a fly in the lavatory. They all come round to the kitchen.'

Lawrence Durrell
PROSPERO'S CELL

Monarchs and the Gentry got round the problem of having to sit in a reeking privy by having the privy brought to their chamber in portable form and then having it smartly taken away again after use. These portable privies were called 'close stools' (In France, *'chaise percée'*, i.e. chair with a hole in it), and royal close stools were sumptuously decorated. Samuel Johnson did not approve of an elegant stool which Boswell had seen at an Embassy in Paris:

'Sir, that is Dutch; quilted seats retain a bad smell.
No Sir, there is nothing so good as the plain board.'

BOSWELL'S JOURNAL OF A TOUR TO THE HEBRIDES WITH SAMUEL JOHNSON, ed. F. A. Pottle and C. H. Bennett

A simpler, even more portable, version of the close stool was the chamber-pot, which could be kept handy in the dining-room or salon and used almost anywhere, frequently behind a screen so that conversation need not be interrupted.

The British used them widely. Judges often kept a porcelain pot below their bench. Travellers took their own pot for use during long journeys by coach.

A noble gentleman once sent a china chamber-pot as a gift to the Countess of Hillsborough. Attached was a short explanatory poem:

Too proud, too delicate to tell her wants
Her lover guesses them, and gladly grants;

The wish that he still trembles to explain
She long has known but bids him wish in vain;
With tears incessant he laments his case,
And can have small occasion for this vase.
Go then beneath her bed or toilet stand,
But chiefly after tea be near at hand;
Sure of her notice then, then take your fill,
Nor fear one drop her tidy hand should spill,
Though Cyder or Champagne supply the source,
And laughter hurry forth the rapid course.
Who talks of the Pierian spring or stream?
But stop dear Muse, lest on th'enchanting theme
My warm imagination should proceed
To what you must not write, she must not read.

Henry Fox, Lord Holland (*1705–1774*)
Kings-gate, 1764

The chamber-pot no longer exists but Lord Holland's house at Kingsgate, Kent, or what is left of the house, still stands. It lies back from the road opposite Joss Bay.

The use of some sort of small portable receptacle goes back many centuries. The Unspeakable Trimalchio in ancient Rome used one at the public baths:

Suddenly we saw a bald old man in a reddish shirt, playing ball with some long-haired boys. It was not so much the boys that made us watch, although they alone were worth the trouble, but the old gentleman himself. He was taking his exercise in slippers and throwing a green ball around. But he didn't pick it up if it touched the ground; instead there was a slave holding a bagful, and he supplied them to the players. We noticed other novelties. Two eunuchs stood around at different points: one of them carried a silver chamber pot, the other counted the balls, not those flying from hand to hand according to the rules, but those that fell to the ground. We were still admiring these elegant arrangements when

Menelaus hurried up to us.

'This is the man you'll be dining with,' he said. 'In fact, you are now watching the beginning of the dinner.'

No sooner had Menelaus spoken than Trimalchio snapped his fingers. At the signal the eunuch brought up the chamber pot for him, while he went on playing. With the weight off his bladder, he demanded water for his hands, splashed a few drops on his fingers and wiped them on a boy's head.

Petronius (*fl. 1st century A.D.*)
THE SATYRICON, trans.: John Sullivan

Inhabitants of hot climes had little interest in chamber-pots but those who dwelt midst ice and snow and could not nip out in the night to a convenient patch of *maquis* or rain-forest knew their worth. As a writer found when he bedded down with some Eskimos in their igloo:

I slipped into my fur bag. The children squeezed themselves under the skins, and the wrinkled granny, grumbling and complaining like any old lady, squatted on her heels and stripped off all her clothes. She got into bed, muttering to herself and grunting, tossing about for a while before she fell asleep. Ayallik, meanwhile, had stripped to the nude. With a cheerful 'Alapa!' . . . 'Cold!' he vanished under his covers. Ongirlak was the last to go to bed. She plugged the door-hole with a snow block and fixed her lamps for the night, beating out all of the flame except for a tiny glow in the corner, a night-light. Then she distributed small empty tins, improvised chamber-pots, placing one at each of our heads.

Roger P. Buliard
INUK

128

The French had always used chamber-pots and had even invented a special female version. At the time of Louis XIV there was a Jesuit preacher at Versailles whose sermons were of such an inordinate length that ladies could not last the course, so someone invented a china container, shaped like a large sauce-boat without a lip, which they could secrete beneath their skirts (dexterity must have been needed when leaving the church). The famous Jesuit preacher was Louis Bourdaloue and it seems only proper that the pot, which brought comfort and ease to many of the ladies of his congregation, should have been named a *bourdaloue*. Examples can still be found in junk shops, cottage hospitals and homes, usually filled with flowers or gravy.

It seems that coping with nature's needs was not all that difficult for countrymen, Kings, Eskimos, and anybody who was rich. Privacy was not a major problem because very few sought it. Communal privies, family privies and two and three seaters were normal and the 'house of necessity', or whatever it was called at the time, was a convivial place where husband and wife went together and strangers exchanged gossip; you were not expected to be in there alone:

> *You may, as your great French lord doth, invite some special friend of yours from the table, to hold discourse with you as you sit in that with-drawing-chamber.*

> Thomas Dekker (*c. 1570–c. 1641*)
> GULL'S HORNBOOK

The French were noted for their gregariousness whilst on stool. The novelist Smollett was most alarmed at the practice and its implications:

I have known a lady handed to the house of office by her admirer, who stood at the door, and entertained her with *bons mots* all the time she was within. But I should be

129

glad to know, whether it is possible for a fine lady to speak and act in this manner, without exciting ideas to her own disadvantage in the mind of every man who has any imagination left, and enjoys the intire use of his senses, howsoever she may be authorised by the customs of her country?

Tobias Smollett (1721–1771)
TRAVELS THROUGH FRANCE AND ITALY

Although our Kings and Princes received guests while they were at stool, the practice was particularly widespread at the French court:

> The Duc d'Humières asked if I would take him one morning to Versailles, as he wished to thank M. le Duc D'Orléans. The Regent was not dressed when we arrived, but still in the cupboard under the stairs, which he had made his privy. I found him there, sitting on his *chaise percée*, surrounded by two or three of his gentlemen and valets.

Duc de Saint-Simon (1675–1755)
HISTORICAL MEMOIRS, trans. Lucy Norton

Being in company with a Great Man in such intimate circumstances was most useful in the elaborate game of gaining preferment at Versailles:

> The Abbé Jules, later Cardinal, Alberoni wormed himself into Vendôme's confidence by making delicious cheese soup and pandering to his revolting habits. Saint-Simon says that he once exclaimed, 'Oh! Angelic bottom!', when Vendôme rose from his *chaise-percée*.

Duc de Saint-Simon (1675–1755)
HISTORICAL MEMOIRS, trans. Lucy Norton
Note by Lucy Norton, Chap. XVIII

Gregariousness at stool was also the custom in Italy, as a young English traveller noted when staying in Naples with Sir William and Lady Hamilton. Acts and functions which were studiously concealed in England he found openly performed at the court of Ferdinand IV of Naples:

> When the King has made a hearty meal, and feels an inclination to retire, he commonly communicates that intention to the Noblemen around him in waiting, and selects the favoured individuals, whom, as a mark of predilection, he chooses shall attend him. *'Sono ben pransato,'* says he, laying his hand on his belly, *'Adesso bisogna un buona panchiata.'* The persons thus preferred, then accompany his Majesty, stand respectfully round him, and amuse him by their conversation, during the performance.
>
> Sir Nathaniel Wraxall (*1751–1831*)
> HISTORICAL MEMOIRS

The young Sir Nathaniel, fired by these discoveries of continental practices hitherto unmentionable in polite society, went on to make a little list of sordid behaviour in French royalist circles:

> Henry the Third, it is well known, was stabbed in the belly, of which wound he died, in 1589, while sitting on the *Chaise percée*; in which indecorous situation he did not scruple to give audience to Clement, the regicide Monk, who assassinated him. Marshal Suarrow, in our own time, received his Aides du Camp and his General Officers, precisely in a similar manner. Madame de Maintenon, as the Duke de St. Simon informs us, thought those moments so precious, that she commonly accompanied Louis the Fourteenth to the 'Garderobe'. So did Louvois, when Minister of State. The Duke de Vendôme, while commanding the

Armies of France in Spain and Italy, at the commencement of the last Century, was accustomed to receive the greatest personages, on public business, in the same situation. We have Cardinal Alberoni's authority for this fact. If we read the account written by Du Bois, of the last illness of Louis the Thirteenth, we may there see what humiliating functions Anne of Austria performed for that Prince in the course of his malady; over which an English writer, more fastidious, would have drawn a veil.

Ibid.

The real sufferers from the problem of where to Go were poor people who increasingly began to congregate in towns. Here there were no fields or bushes to disappear into, no running water to dispose of the end product. Everybody had a fairly noisome time of it in towns but at least the wealthier had their close-stools and their privies (into which the close-stools and the chamber-pots were emptied) but, as in Pepys' house, these were usually in the basement or under the stairs and had to be dug out and carried through the house at night by 'dung-farmers'.

The poor, living in rookeries of lodgings, usually had no facilities at all within the house. There were public 'necessary houses' but the nearest might be a mile away. It was customary to use chamber-pots and just empty them into the roadway.

In Edinburgh, where there were no public and very few private privies, most of the population lived in tall tenement buildings and a special tradition of pot-emptying evolved:

On six evenings of the week the taverns were filled with men of all classes at their ale and claret, till the ten o'clock drum, beaten at the order of the magistrates, warned every man that he must be off home. Then were the High Street and Canongate filled with parties of every description, hurrying

132

unsteadily along, High Court Judges striving to walk straight as became their dignity, rough Highland porters swearing in Gaelic as they forced a passage for their sedan-chairs, while far overhead the windows opened, five, six, or ten storeys in the air, and the close stools of Edinburgh discharged the collected filth of the last twenty-four hours into the street. It was good manners for those above to cry 'Gardy-loo' (*gardez l'eau*) before throwing. The returning roysterer cried back 'Haud yer han',' and ran with humped shoulders, lucky if his vast and expensive full-bottomed wig was not put out of action by a cataract of filth. The ordure thus sent down lay in the broad High Street and in the deep, well-like closes and wynds around it making the night air horrible, until early in the morning it was perfunctorily cleared away by the City Guard. Only on Sabbath morn it might not be touched, but lay there all day long, filling Scotland's capital with the savour of a mistaken piety.

G. M. Trevelyan, O.M. (*1876–1962*)
ENGLISH SOCIAL HISTORY: 'The Eighteenth Century'

Perhaps the first civic father to provide some sort of relief to his citizens was the Roman Emperor Vespasian (A.D. 9–79) who built a number of handsome urinals (gentlemen only). The chronicler tells us that he 'of his princely bounty and magnificence erected diverse places of fair polished marble, for this special purpose, requiring and no less straightly charging all persons, as well citizens as strangers, to refrain from all other places, saving these specially appointed'.

Making the use of the urinals compulsory gives a clue that Vespasian's action was not wholy benevolent. In true Roman style he also made a handsome profit by collecting the effluent in tanks and selling it to dyers.

Suetonius tells us that Vespasian's son Titus complained that the urinals and their tanks smelt. To which the father replied '*sed non olet denarius*'. 'But the money doesn't smell'.

133

Madrid is reported to have instituted portable privies on the back of carts. These toured the streets, heralded by a crier (what would he have cried?).

Even in Edinburgh there is record of an entrepreneur trying to provide some sort of relief:

> The streets of Edinburgh were perambulated by a
> man carrying a bucket and a great cloak, with the
> cry 'Wha wants me for a bawbee?' meaning 'Who
> wishes to hire the services of my bucket and
> shielding cloak for a halfpenny?'

Lawrence Wright
CLEAN AND DECENT

What the town-dwellers of the western world badly needed was the device that we now have; a hygienic container, washed with running water, with a valve system so that the effluent is borne away, odour-free, through a ventilated pipe.

Surprisingly, such devices have popped up throughout history. When Sir Arthur Evans excavated King Midas's Palace of Knossos in Minoan Crete he found it elaborately plumbed with a latrine complete with marble pan (which probably had a wooden seat) and a removable plug with a cistern of water above it to flush it clean. (It is said that when Sir Arthur was asked by somebody what the clay thing was which he was holding in his hand, he replied 'Tis an ill-favoured thing, sir, but Minoan'). King Midas's Palace was dated as about 2,000 years B.C.

In Elizabethan times a tremendous leap forward was made by Sir John Harington, Queen Elizabeth's godson. In 1596 he published a book which he called *Metamorphosis of Ajax* (in reference books the title is followed by the note – A pun on 'A jakes' – as inevitably as any reference to the writer 'Saki' is followed by – H. H. Munro).

In the book the author describes, and gives the plans of, a water closet which he has invented:

To. M.E.S., Esquire.

Sir,

My master having expressly commanded me to finish a strange discourse that he had written to you, called the Metamorpho-sis of Ajax, by setting certain pictures thereto... Wherefore now, seriously and in good sadness, to instruct you and all gentlemen of worship, how to reform all unsavoury places, whether they be caused by privies or sinks, or such like (for the annoyance coming all of like causes, the remedies need not be much unlike) this shall you do.

AN ANATOMY.

In the privy that annoys you, first cause a cistern, containing a barrel, or upward, to be placed either in the room or above it, from whence the water may, by a small pipe of lead of an inch be conveyed under the seat in the hinder part thereof (but quite out of sight); to which pipe you must have a cock or a washer, to yield water with some pretty strength when you would let it in.

If that which follows offend the reader, he may turn over a leaf or two, or but smell to his sweet gloves, and then the savour will never offend him. The cistern in the first plot is figured at the letter A; and so likewise in the second plot. The small pipe in the first plot at D, in the second E; but it ought to lie out of sight.

Next make a vessel of an oval form, as broad at the bottom as at the top; two feet deep, one foot broad, sixteen

The vessel is expressed in the first

This is Don A JAX house, of the new fashion, all in sunder, that a workeman may see what he hath to do.

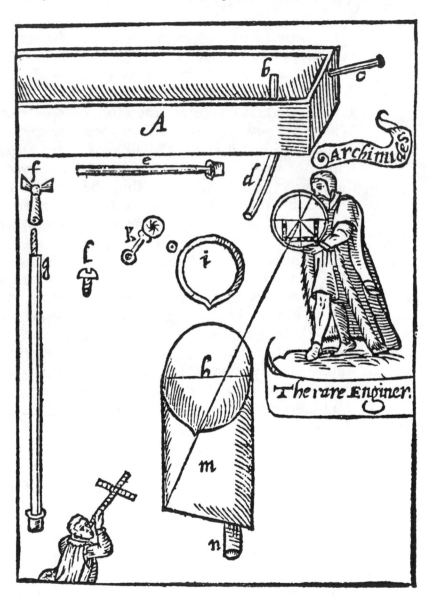

inches long; place this very close to your seat, like the pot of a close-stool; let the oval incline to the right hand.

This vessel may be brick, stone or lead; but whatsoever it is, it should have a current of three inches to the back part of it (where a sluice of brass must stand); the bottom and sides all smooth, and dressed with pitch, rosin and wax; which will keep it from tainting with the urine.

In the lowest part of the vessel which will be on the right hand, you must fasten the sluice or washer of brass, with solder or cement; the concavity, or hollow thereof, must be two inches and a half.

To the washers stopple must be a stem of iron as big as a curtain rod; strong and even, and perpendicular, with a strong screw at the top of it; to which you must have a hollow key with a worm to fit that screw.

This screw must, when the sluice is down, appear through the plank not above a straw's breadth on the right hand; and being duly placed, it will stand about three or four inches wide of the midst of the back of your seat.

Item, That children and busy folk disorder it not, or open the sluice with putting in their hands without a key, you should have a little button or scallop shell, to bind it down with a vice pin, so as without the key it will not be opened.

plot H.M.N., in the second H.K. The current is expressed in the second plot K. A special note.

In the second plot, I.L.

In the first plot G.F., in the second F. and I.

In the first plot between G.I.

This shows in the first plot K.L., in the second G.; such are in the backside of watches.

137

These things thus placed, all about *Else all is* your vessel and elsewhere, must be *in vain.* passing close plastered with good lime and hair, that no air come up from the vault, but only at your sluice, which stands closed stopped; and it must be left, after it is voided, half a foot deep in clean water.

If water be plenty, the oftener it is used, and opened, the sweeter; but if it be scant, once a day is enough, for a need, though twenty persons should use it.

If the water will not run to your cistern, you may with a force of twenty shillings, and a pipe of eighteen pence the yard, force it from the lowest part of your house to the highest.

But now on the other side behold the Anatomy.

Here are the parts set down, with a rate of the prices; that a builder may guess what he hath to pay.

		s.	d.
A,	The Cistern: stone or brick. Price	6	8
b, d, e	the pipe that comes from the cistern with a stopple to the washer	3	6
c,	a waste pipe	1	0
f, g,	the item of the great stopple with a key to it	1	6
h,	the form of the upper brim of the vessel or stool pot		
m,	the stool pot of stone	8	0
n,	the great brass sluice, to which if three inches current to send it down a gallop into the JAX	10	0

Here is the same all put together, that the workeman may see if it be well.

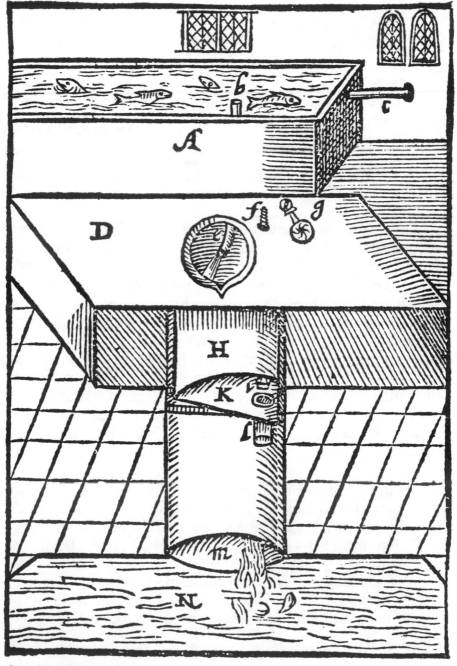

A. the Cesterne.
B. the little washer. 139

i,   the seat, with a peak devant for
        elbow room

The whole charge thirty shillings and eight
pence: yet a mason of my masters was offered
thirty pounds for the like.

... And this being well done, and orderly kept,
your worst privy may be as sweet as your best
chamber.

Sir John Harington (*1561–1612*)
A NEW DISCOURSE OF A STALE SUBJECT, CALLED
THE METAMORPHOSIS OF AJAX

This specification embodies all the main features of the modern
flushing valve-closet. One was constructed for Sir John on his
estate at Kelston, near Bath, and another was installed in
Queen Elizabeth's Richmond Palace, seemingly with some
success.

What kept the invention away from the reach of citizens
was partly the lack of interest in developing the somewhat
crude valve mechanism but mainly the fact that water in cities
had to be borne on the back of a professional water-carrier.

During the eighteenth century things began to stir again.
Experiments were made to carry water from pumping engines
along conduits to reach main streets, sometimes being piped
into great houses to fill their tanks. It was usually only turned
on for a few hours two or three days a week but it was cheaper,
and much more was available, than from the water-man.

Fixed close-stools with flushing devices began to appear.
Horace Walpole came across some in 1760, in the house of A
Lady of Fashion:

> I breakfasted the day before yesterday at Ælia
> Lælia Chudleigh's ... Every favour she has
> bestowed is registered by a bit of Dresden china.
> There is a glass-case full of enamels, eggs, ambers,
> lapis lazuli, cameos, toothpick cases, and all kinds
> of trinkets, things that she told me were her
> playthings; another cupboard, full of the finest
> japan, and candlesticks and vases of rock crystal,

ready to be thrown down, in every corner. But of all curiosities, are the conveniences in every bedchamber: great mahogany projections, with brass handles, cocks, &c. I could not help saying, it was the loosest family I ever saw. Adieu!

Horace Walpole (*1717–1797*)
Letter to George Montagu, 27 March, 1760

Fifteen years later, and a hundred and seventy-nine years after Sir John Harington's *Metamorphosis of Ajax*, the first ever patent was taken out for a 'valve closet', an invention much along the lines laid down by Sir John. It did not work very well but in 1788 it was followed by another design patented by The Blessed Bramah. Joseph Bramah's design worked well and was the most popular model for the next hundred years. The 'water-closet' had arrived.

Enormously helped by the industrial developments of the nineteenth century, and spurred by dreadful outbreaks of cholera, the problems of bringing clean water to houses and taking dirty water away again were tackled, slowly but steadily. Glazed pottery pipes were invented to make hygienic sewerage disposal practical. Iron pipes were used for water-supplies in place of wood.

A sanitary engineer, George Jennings, agreed to provide hygienic latrines for visitors to the Great Exhibition in Hyde Park in return for being allowed to charge customers a small fee, thereby inventing the penny-in-the-slot public convenience (and the expression 'spend a penny').

Pottery manufacturers devised increasingly ambitious flushing systems:

Jennings' 'Pedestal Vase' won the Gold Medal Award at the Health Exhibition of 1884, being judged 'as perfect a sanitary closet as can be made'. In a test, it completely cleared with a 2-gallon flush

10 apples averaging 1¼ ins. diameter
1 flat sponge about 4½ ins. diameter
Plumber's 'smudge' coated over the pan

4 pieces of paper adhering closely to the soiled
surface.

A simple test was that improvised by Mr. Shanks
who, when trying a new model, seized the cap
from the head of an attendant apprentice, thrust it
in, pulled the chain, saw it go and cried out
happily, 'It works!'

Lawrence Wright
CLEAN AND DECENT

By the 1900s there was a huge range of splendid 'water-closets' available, some intricately decorated, some clad in mahogany or disguised with a wickerwork seat but all with grand, dignified names.

Just as rural Americans tend to be nostalgic about the old privy in the backgarden, so urban Britishers tend to remember with emotion those fine old names like 'Belvedere' and 'Osborne'. It is one of the few aspects of last-century design that has not attracted the pen of Sir John Betjeman. However, Mr. Alan Bennett has stepped in on Sir John's behalf:

Bolding Vedas! Shanks New Nisa!
The trusty Lichfield swirls it down
To filter beds on Ruislip Marshes
From my lav in Kentish Town.

The Burlington! The Rochester!
Oh those names of childhood loos –
Nursie knocking at the door:
'Have you done your Number Twos?'

Lady typist – office party –
Golly! All that gassy beer!
Tripping home down Hendon Parkway
To her Improved Windermere.

Chelsea buns and lounge bar pasties
All washed down with Benskin's Pale
Purified and cleansed with charcoal
Fill the taps in Colindale.

Here I sit, alone and sixty,
Bald and fat and full of sin,
Cold the seat and loud the cistern
As I read the Harpic tin.

Alan Bennett (*1934– *)
PLACE-NAMES OF CHINA

The grandest of all baroque 'easences', the culmination of all advances in style and facilities since Sir John Harington's design, was built in Ulster to the wishes of a refugee from Hungary. Or so Spike Milligan tells us:

The disintegration of the Austro-Hungarian Empire hit many people, especially those who had disintegrated with it. The Count Nuker-Frit-Kraphauser was one such notable. In the hiatus that followed the assassination of the Archduke Ferdinand, and the collapse of the Empire, he had fled his native Hungary in the jade of a revolutionary night with nothing save a small suitcase with three million pounds and some silly old crown jewels, but this fortune meant nothing; his greatest loss was having to leave the great majestic family Easence. The greatest toilet in the western world and the only consecrated one in the Holy Roman Empire.

The Count Fritz Von Krappenhauser had fled to Northern Ireland, bought Callarry Castle, ten thousand acres, and a small packet of figs. For years he brooded over the loss of the ancestral abort. Finally worn out by indifferent, and severe, wood-seated Victorian commodes, he decided to build a replica of the family's lost masterpiece here in the heart of Ulster's rolling countryside. He employed the greatest baroque and Rococo architects and craftsmen of the day, and every day after; seven years of intense labour, and there it now stood, a great octagonal Easence. No ordinary palace was this; from the early stone Easence of Bodiam Castle to the low silent suite at the Dorchester is a long strain, but nothing equalled this, its gold leaf and lapis lazuli settings gleaming in the morning sun, on the eight-sided walls great ikons of straining ancestors, a warning to the unfit. Through a Moorish arch of latticed stone, one entered the 'Throne Room'; above it, in Gothic capitals the family motto, 'Abort in Luxus'. From the centre rose a delicate gilded metal and pink alabaster commode. Six steps cut in black Cararra marble engraved with royal mottoes led up to the mighty Easence; it was a riot of carefully engraved figurines in the voluptuous Alexandrian style, depicting the history of the family with myriad complex designs and sectionalized stomachs in various stages of compression. The seat was covered in heavy wine damask velvet, the family coat of arms sewn petit-point around the rim in fine gold thread. Inside the pan were low relief sculptures of the family enemies, staring white-faced in expectation. Towering at the four corners, holding a silk tasselled replica of the Bernini canopy, were four royal beasts, their snarling jaws containing ashtrays and matches. Bolted to the throne were ivory straining bars carved with monkeys and cunningly set at convenient angles; around the base ran a small bubbling perfumed brook whose water welled from an ice-cool underground stream. Gushes of warm air passed up the trouser legs of the sitter, the pressure controlled by a gilt handle. By pedalling hard with two foot-levers the whole throne could be raised ten feet to allow the sitter a long drop; and even greater delight, the whole Easence was mounted on ball-bearings. A control valve shaped like the crown of Hungary would release steam power that would revolve the commode. There had been a time when the Count had aborted revolving at sixty miles an hour and been given a medal by the Pope.

White leather straps enabled him to secure himself firmly during the body-shaking horrors of constipation. Close at hand were three burnished hunting horns of varying lengths. Each one had a deep significant meaning. The small one when blown told the waiting household all was well, and the morning mission accomplished. The middle one of silver and brass was blown to signify that there might be a delay. The third one, a great Tibetan Hill Horn, was blown in dire emergency; it meant a failure and waiting retainers would rush to the relief of the Count, with trays of steaming fresh enemas ready to be plunged into action on their mission of mercy and relief. With the coming of the jet age the noble Count had added to the abort throne an ejector mechanism. Should there ever be need he could, whilst still in throes, pull a lever and be shot three hundred feet up to float gently down on a parachute. The stained glass windows when open looked out on to 500 acres of the finest grouse shooting moor in Ulster. He had once invited Winston Churchill to come and shoot from the sitting position. In reply Churchill sent a brief note, 'Sorry, I have business elsewhere that day.' From his commode, the Count could select any one of a number of fine fowling pieces and bring down his dinner. Alas, this caused his undoing. The boxes of 12-bore cartridges, though bought at the best shops in London, had sprung a powder leak. Carelessly flicking an early morning cigar, the hot ash had perforated the wad of a cartridge.

But to the day of the calamitous fire. It had been a fine morning that day in 1873. The Count had just received his early morning enema of soap suds and spice at body heat; crying 'Nitchevo!' he leapt from his couch. Colonic irrigation and enemas had made his exile one internal holiday. Clutching a month-old copy of *Der Tag*, and contracting his abdomen, he trod majestically towards his famed Imperial outdoor abort bar. A few moments later the waiting retainers heard a shattering roar and were deluged, among other things, with rubble.

'Himmel? Hermann? What did you put in the last enema?' queried the family doctor of the retainers.

Flames and debris showered the grounds and there, floating down on the parachute, came the Count. 'People will look to me when I die,' he had once said. His wish had come true.

Spike Milligan (*1918–   *)
PUCKOON

An extraordinary aspect of this whole subject is that for something like four thousand years this place where every man and woman alive 'went' once or more every day has never, in any Western language, been given a simple, straightforward name.

A 'bath' was a 'bath' from the first, and one now visits the 'bathroom'. The hole in the ground, or the plank over the bucket, or the little shed have never been so honoured. Instead it has been referred to by a mass of coy, or poetic, or enigmatic euphemisms.

The Children of Israel went to 'The House of Honour'

The Ancient Egyptians went to 'The House of the Morning'

Monks went to the 'Garderobe' (our modern cloak-room'), or

The 'Necessarium' (later the 'Necessary House'), or

The 'Reredorter' (literally 'Room at the back of the Dormitory').

The Tudors went to the 'Privy' (A Place of Privacy), or

The Jakes (Jack's Place. Perhaps the origin of the American 'john').

The seventeenth century added 'The Bog-House' (this

146

became a word much used by builders and was the technical term preferred by most architects until the early years of this century).

When one expression became too familiar, our more genteel ancestors found themselves a new one:

> Busy in painting some boarding in my Wall Garden
> which was put up to prevent people in the Kitchen
> seeing those who had occasion to go to Jericho.

The Reverend James Woodforde (*1740–1803*)
DIARY OF A COUNTRY PARSON: 26 April, 1780

'Jericho' was originally a slang word for a place of banishment or a hiding-place. 'Jerry' used as slang for a chamber-pot is supposed to have come from a different source, i.e. 'jereboam': a large bottle.

The above, and a great many more similar euphemisms for the same thing, refer only to the place itself, the room or hut or whatever, and not to its equipment, e.g. hole in the ground, or bucket with earth in it, or marble seat over conduit. Nor do they refer to its specific purpose.

When Mr. Bramah patented his so-called 'Valve Closet' (literally 'small room with a valve') and piped water arrived, and the beautifully made device began to be installed in more and more homes to make living sweeter, one might have thought that society would have found a name for It. But no. When a nineteenth-century citizen had converted a room into one of these new-fangled bathrooms, how did he describe the Thing to his friends? 'On the left I have the bath. And on the right I have the . . .' The what?

Unhappily the growth of technology coincided with the growth of the Victorian middle classes, who became the device's main customers. And the distaste for admitting that the body needed evacuation and there was a Thing upstairs for that purpose was so strong in much of Victorian society that the Thing never did get a name. Once more, as with the Place, the Thing was referred to by a hundred evasive words and phrases.

It is a legacy from which we still suffer. If an object has just one word to describe it there is no problem. A 'bath' is a bath. We know it to be a big thing which holds a lot of water and we can get in it and wash and sing a song and muck about a bit. The word 'bath' is not heretical, although the Christian Fathers denounced baths as inducers of sloth, vanity and evil thoughts. Nor is the word 'dirty' although ladies and gentlemen once used to bath together and do naughty things therein. Nor is the word 'vulgar and horrid' because one has to sit naked in a bath and clean dirt off one's salient features. The word for a bath is 'bath' and we all happily use it, unpunished by society.

It is a totally different matter with That Which Has No Name. We have got to use one of the euphemisms, and we have to choose the right one or we *will* be punished. Perhaps the last real barrier between Britain and the Classless Society is that each social class Goes to a different place.

The Aristocracy tends to go to the 'lavatory', the Middle Classes to the 'loo', and the Workers to the 'toilet'.

The picture, however, is constantly in a state of flux. There are indications that in the last few years there has been a strong – perhaps as high as 20% – swing towards 'toilet', which has taken over from 'bog-house' as the technical term adopted by architects, builders and municipal authorities. 'Loo' is holding strong and perhaps increasing its share of the market. It seems that most of the gains made by 'toilet' have been at the expense of 'lavatory'.

All three words are a mile away from describing a porcelain bowl with a seat on it. 'Lavatory' and 'toilet' are corruptions of useful words which described entirely different things: *The Shorter Oxford Dictionary* gives the original meaning of 'lavatory' as:

1. A vessel for washing, a laver, a bath.
2. The ritual washing of the celebrant's hands.
3. A lotion.

A 'toilet' was originally:

1. A piece of stuff used as a wrapper for clothes; a towel or cloth thrown over the shoulders during hairdressing.

2. A cloth cover for a dressing-table.
3. The articles required or used in dressing.
4. The table on which these articles are placed.
5. The action or process of dressing; the reception of visitors by a lady during the concluding stages of her toilet.
8c. Preparation for execution by guillotine.

Nobody is quite sure where the word 'loo' sprang from. One school of thought holds that 'loo' is a shortened form of 'Waterloo', a jocular corruption of 'water-closet'. Another holds that it is a throwback to the old Edinburgh shout of 'guardy-loo!' when a chamber-pot was about to be emptied out of a top window. However, it seems to date back in usage only as far as the late nineteenth century, which gives credence to a private claim that the original 'loo' was Lord Lichfield's aunt:

> The story of the origin of the word 'loo' was told me by the Duke of Buccleuch's aunt, Lady Constance Cairns. Your relations feature largely in it.
>
> In 1867 (Lady Constance was not absolutely certain of the date) when the 1st Duke of Abercorn was Viceroy of Ireland there was a large houseparty at Viceregal Lodge, and amongst the guests there was the Lord Lieutenant of County Roscommon, Mr. Edward King Tennison, and his wife Lady Louisa, daughter of the Earl of Lichfield.
>
> Lady Louisa was, it seems, not very lovable; and the two youngest Abercorn sons, Lord Frederick and Lord Ernest, took her namecard from her bedroom door and placed it on the door of the only W.C. in the guest wing. So in those select ducal circles everyone talked of going to Lady Louisa. Then people became more familiar – Jimmy Abercorn told me that when he was a boy one went to 'Lady Lou' (though he had never been told who Her Ladyship was).

Now in these democratic days the courtesy title
has been dropped, and within the last thirty years
or so – only really since the war – the term has
seeped down into middle-class and even working-
class usage. But it all really originates with your
Hamilton uncles being ungallant to your Anson
aunt; who I think should have her immortality
recognised.

The Hon. Sir Steven Runciman
Letter to Lord Lichfield, 11 June, 1973

Chances are that the word 'loo' probably drifted across the Channel into our language, as so many other words did.

The Continent must have as many euphemisms as we do: *le wattair* (short for 'the water-closet'), *le double* (short for 'the W.C.'). A widespread and curious form is using the number 100. One wild explanation of this is that it is an unsavoury pun on *la chambre cent* (room one hundred) and *la chambre sent* (room smelly). Be that as it may, many old Italian hotels label it *numero cento*, as do other regions, e.g., Cyprus. The theory is that the '100' became corrupted to 'loo'.

A faintly more plausible explanation is that 'loo' is an anglicised version of the French word *lieu*, or 'place'. On seventeenth century English architectural plans the 'loo' was often marked *le lieu*, and many signs in French 'loos' still read *On est prié de laisser ce LIEU aussi propre qu'on le trouve*. In Germany they use the same word, *der Locus*.

So as far as the origin of the word 'loo' is concerned, in the words of the old saying 'you pays your penny and you takes your choice'.

The difficulty with the three main euphemisms is that they are non-interchangeable. Those who go to the 'toilet' regard the use of the word 'lavatory' as disgusting. Those who go to the 'lavatory' find the word 'toilet' deeply depressing and vulgar. Goers to the 'loo' consider the word 'toilet' to be common and the word 'lavatory' to be revolting.

The social minefield becomes ever more complex when you consider that the three social classes themselves split into a number of sub-classes and society also splits vertically into sub-divisions like male and female, extrovert and introvert, urban and rural, bright and dim, each of which clings to its own euphemism and rejects the others as being in dreadfully poor taste.

When strangers meet and a thoughtful host wishes to offer the use of his privy to an unknown guest, or the guest urgently needs to locate it, each has to thumb his way mentally through a *mille-feuille* of potentially offensive expressions before choosing the one which, on the evidence of clothes, accent, bearing, conversational style, the other is most likely to consider 'correct'.

The range of expressions is vast. It includes:

For Use in Schools:
'Please may I be excused?'
'Please may I leave the room?' (a teacher reported that one of her charges once produced the sentence:
'Please, Miss, Johnny's left the room on the floor.')

The Approach Jocular:
'Just going to see whether the horse has kicked off its blanket'
'Where's the House of Lords, old son?'
'Must go and shake hands with an old friend'
'Just going to kiss the au pair goodnight'

The Approach Hearty:
'If you're busting it's the first door on the left'
'The bog's on the landing'

For Use in France:
'*Je veux changer le poisson d'eau*'

The Approach Coy:
'Anybody seek comforts?'
'I rather want potty'

151

The Approach Oblique (from hosts who find the subject embarrassing):
    'You've had a long car journey, would you like to
    ... wash?'

The Approach Extremely Oblique (from hosts who are deeply embarrassed):
    'Would you like to go upstairs ... or something?'

The Approach Almost Non-Existent (from hosts so miserably embarrassed that they cannot bear to say anything at all):
    (Vague, nervous hand movements are made, as though testing the weight of a pair of oranges)
    'Would you care to...?'
    (The hand movements continue rhythmically until guest understands and answers. However long it takes).

Without a name it may be but the Thing now receives honour and attention because it is a household fixture on which money can be spent.

Powders in pastel colours are on sale to keep It clean and fresh.

Blocks of scented substances are available to dangle in Its vicinity so as to give the impression that It smells of flowers or citrus fruit or woodland pine.

Its seat may be soft and spongy to sit upon, or warmed by electric current.

Its lid can be made pretty with a fluffy bonnet.

And why, after all these centuries, should Its importance to our way of life *not* be recognised?

It is upon It, seated, that great books have been read, great ideas have been formulated; and will be again.

It is here, in peace and privacy, that our day begins:

    Seated after breakfast
    In this white-tiled cabin

Arabs call *the House where*
Everybody goes,
Even melancholics
Raise a cheer to Mrs.
Nature for the primal
Pleasures she bestows.

Sex is but a dream to
Seventy-and-over,
But a joy proposed until
     we start to shave:
Mouth-delight depends on
Virtue in the cook, but
This She guarantees from
Cradle unto grave.

Lifted off the potty,
Infants from their mothers
Hear their first impartial
Words of worldly praise:
Hence, to start the morning
With a satisfactory
Dump is a good omen
All our adult days.

Revelation came to
Luther in a privy
(Crosswords have been solved there):
Rodin was no fool
When he cast his Thinker,
Cogitating deeply,
Crouched in the position
Of a man at stool.

All the Arts derive from
This ur-act of making,
Private to the artist:
Makers' lives are spent

Striving in their chosen
Medium to produce a
De-narcissus-ized en-
  during excrement.

Freud did not invent the
Constipated miser:
Banks have letter boxes
Built in their façade,
Marked *For Night Deposits*,
Stocks are firm or liquid,
Currencies of nations
Either soft or hard.

Global Mother, keep our
Bowels of compassion
Open through our lifetime,
Purge our minds as well:
Grant us a kind ending,
Not a second childhood,
Petulant, weak-sphinctered,
In a cheap hotel.

Keep us in our station:
When we get pound-noteish,
When we seem about to
Take up Higher Thought,
Send us some deflating
Image like the pained ex-
  pression on a Major
Prophet taken short.

(Orthodoxy ought to
Bless our modern plumbing:
Swift and St. Augustine
Lived in centuries,
When a stench of sewage
Ever in the nostrils

Made a strong debating
Point for Manichees.)

Mind and Body run on
Different timetables:
Not until our morning
Visit here can we
Leave the dead concerns of
Yesterday behind us.
Face with all our courage
What is now to be.

W. H. Auden (*1907–1973*)
THE GEOGRAPHY OF THE HOUSE
(for Christopher Isherwood)

ACKNOWLEDGMENTS

Grateful thanks are due to the following authors, agents and publishers for permission to quote copyright material.

The Author's Literary Estate and Chatto and Windus Ltd for *The Young Visitors*, by Daisy Ashford. Faber and Faber Ltd and Randon House Inc. for 'Encomium Balnei' and 'The Geography of the House' from *Collected Poems* by W. H. Auden, edited by Mendelson. Alan Bennett for permission to print, for the first time, the complete text of his poem 'Place-Names of China'. To John Murray Ltd for 'Business Girls' by John Betjeman. Creativity Ltd, A. P. Watt Ltd and Harold Ober Associates Incorporated for *Imperial Women* by Pearl S. Buck, Copyright © 1956 by Pearl S. Buck. William Heinemann Ltd and Mrs. James L. Clifford for *Dictionary Johnson* by James L. Clifford. Dobson Books Ltd for *Nanny Says: as recalled by Sir Hugh Casson and Joyce Grenfell*. Victor Gollancz Ltd and the Estate of the late A. J. Cronin for *The Stars Look Down* by A. J. Cronin. Faber and Faber Ltd and E. P. Dutton and Co. Inc. for *Prospero's Cell* by Lawrence Durrell. Hutchinson Publishing Group for *The Collected Ewart 1933–1980*, © Gavin Ewart, 1980. The Estate of Michael Flanders, and Donald Swann, for 'In the Bath' and 'The Spider' from *The Songs of Michael Flanders and Donald Swann*. A. D. Peters and Co. Ltd for 'The Bedchamber Mystery', by C. S. Forester. Martin Higham for *A Book of Anecdotes* by T. F. Higham MA. Diana Holman-Hunt for *My Grandmothers and I* by Diana Holman-Hunt. McIntosh and Otis for a poem by Edward Newman Horn. Martin Secker and Warburg Ltd for 'Lines to a Bishop who was shocked (A.D. 1950) at seeing a pier-glass in a bathroom', from *A La Carte* by Sir Lawrence Jones; and for *Aubrey's Brief Lives* edited by Oliver Lawson-Dick. Sir Steven Runciman for permission to print his private letter to the Rt. Hon. the Earl of Lichfield. Spike Milligan for *Puckoon*, published by Michael Joseph and Co. Methuen London, the Canalian publishers McClelland and Stewart Ltd of Toronto and E. P. Dutton and Co. Inc. for 'Vespers' by A. A. Milne from *When We were Very Young*, Copyright, 1924, by E. P. Dutton and Co. Inc. Renewal, 1952, by A. A. Milne. Jonathan Cape Ltd for 'Adrian Mitchell's Famous Weak Bladder Blues' from *Out Loud* by Adrian Mitchell. April Young Ltd for The Glums episode by Frank Muir and Denis Norden. Curtis Brown Ltd on behalf of the Estate of Ogden Nash, and Little, Brown and Co., for 'Samson Agonistes' from *Verses from 1929 On* by Ogden Nash: copyright 1942 by The Curtis Publishing Company; first appeared in *The Saturday Evening Post*. Hamish Hamilton Ltd for *Historical Memoirs* by Duc de Saint-Simon: translated by Lucy Norton. The Estate of the late Sonia Brownell Orwell, Martin Secker and Warburg Ltd, and Harcourt Brace Jovanovitch Inc. for *Such, Such Were the Joys* by George Orwell. William Heinemann Ltd and the author for *Delights* by J. B. Priestley. Faber and Faber Ltd, and W. W. Norton and Company Inc., for *A Cambridge Childhood* by Gwen Raverat. The Specialist Publishing Co. in California for *The Specialist* by Charles Sale. Penguin Books Ltd for *The Cottage Garden* by Anne

156

Scott-James (Allen Lane 1981). Copyright © Anne Scott-James Penguin Books for *The Satyricon*, translated by John Sullivan. Oxford University Press for *Lark Rise to Candleford* by Flora Thompson. Hamish Hamilton Ltd and Mrs James Thurber for 'Nine Needles' by James Thurber: Copr. © 1937 James Thurber. Copr. © 1965 Helen W. Thurber and Rosemary T. Sauers. From *Let Your Mind Alone*, published by Harper and Row. Longman Group Ltd for *English Social History: The Eighteenth Century* by G. M. Trevelyan O.M. Souvenir Press Ltd for *Le Petomane* by François Caradec and Jean Nohain, translated by Warren Tute. A. D. Peters and Co. and Little, Brown and Co. for *Brideshead Revisited* by Evelyn Waugh, published by Chapman and Hall Ltd. The Author's Literary Estate and The Hogarth Press Ltd for *The Diary of Virginia Woolf*, edited by Anne Olivier Bell. Routledge and Kegan Paul Ltd for *Clean and Decent* by Lawrence Wright.

157

INDEX

IN THE BATH

by Michael Flanders
and Donald Swann

To be sung whilst taking a bath. Unaccompanied.
A percussion rhythm may be added with the aid of two
toothbrushes and an empty glass.

Warmly flowing ♩ = 104

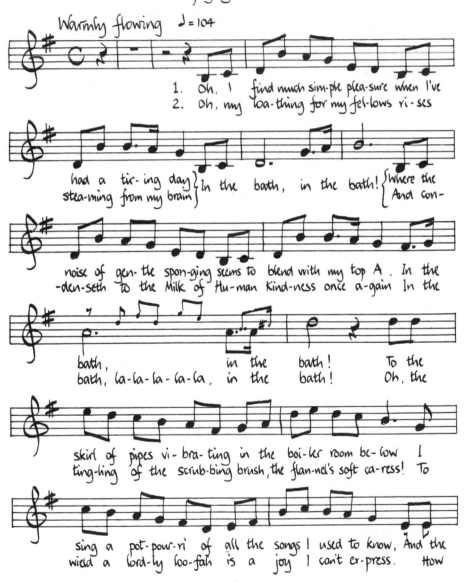

1. Oh, I find much sim-ple plea-sure when I've
2. Oh, my loa-thing for my fel-lows ri-ses

had a tir-ing day ⎱ In the bath, in the bath! ⎰ Where the
stea-ming from my brain ⎰   ⎱ And con-

noise of gen-tle spon-ging seems to blend with my top A. In the
-den-seth to the Milk of Hu-man Kind-ness once a-gain In the

bath,   in the   bath!   To the
bath, la-la-la-la-la,   in the   bath!   Oh, the

skirl of pipes vi-bra-ting in the boi-ler room be-low   I
ting-ling of the scrub-bing brush, the flan-nel's soft ca-ress! To

sing a pot-pour-ri of all the songs I used to know, And the
wield a lord-ly loo-fah is a joy I can't ex-press.   How

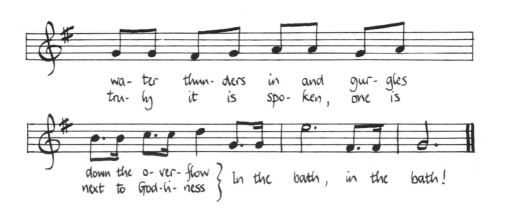

wa- ter thun- ders in and gur- gles
tru- ly it is spo- ken, one is

down the o- ver- flow } In the bath, in the bath!
next to God- li- ness

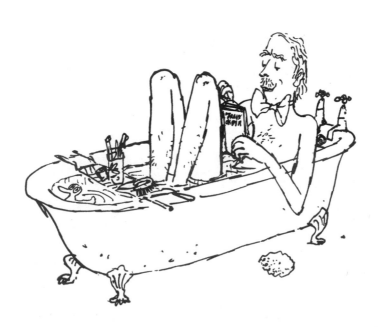

S0-AFF-126

FACING JUSTICE

For Jim:
May God bless you
this christmas. Hope
you enjoy this inside
look at how federal agents
keep us safe.

Brian Lewis

Dave Munson
DEA-Ret.

FACING JUSTICE

DIANE / DAVID
MUNSON

FaithWalk
PUBLISHING
Grand Haven, Michigan

©2005 Diane Munson and David Munson
Published by FaithWalk Publishing
Grand Haven, Michigan 49417

All rights reserved. No part of this book may be reproduced or transmitted in any form by any means, electronic or mechanical, including photocopying and recording, or by any information storage and retrieval system, except as may be expressly permitted by the 1976 Copyright Act or by the publisher. Requests for permission should be made in writing to: FaithWalk Publishing, 333 Jackson Street, Grand Haven, Michigan, 49417.

Scripture quotations, unless otherwise indicated, are taken from the HOLY BIBLE, NEW INTERNATIONAL VERSION®. NIV®. Copyright ©1973, 1978, 1984 by International Bible Society. Used by permission of Zondervan. All rights reserved.

Scripture quotations marked KJV are taken from the Holy Bible, King James Version, Cambridge, 1769.

Scripture quotations marked NRSV are taken from The Holy Bible: New Revised Standard Version/Division of Christian Education of the National Council of Churches of Christ in the United States of America. Nashville: Thomas Nelson Publishers, ©1989. Used by permission. All rights reserved.

This is a work of fiction. Names, characters, places, and incidents either are the product of the authors' imaginations or are used fictitiously. The authors and publishers intend that all persons, organizations, events and locales portrayed in the work be considered as fictitious.

Printed in the United States of America
10 09 08 07 06 05   7 6 5 4 3 2 1

Library of Congress Cataloging-in-Publication Data

Munson, Diane.
  Facing justice / by Diane and David Munson.
    p. cm.
  ISBN-13: 978-1-932902-49-5 (pbk. : alk. paper)
  ISBN-10: 1-932902-49-X
  1. Terrorism victims' families—Fiction. 2. Government investigators—Fiction.
  3. Terrorism—Prevention—Fiction. 4. International agencies—Fiction. 5. Sisters—
  Death—Fiction. I. Munson, David. II. Title.
  PS3613.U693F33 2005
  813'.6--dc22
                                    2005012060

DEDICATION

This book is dedicated to our loving and caring parents.

He has showed, O man, what is good. And what does the Lord require of you? To act justly and to love mercy and to walk humbly with your God.

Micah 6:8 (NIV)

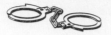

PROLOGUE

Everything about the night was black. Not a star lit the sky. The moon reflected no light. Even the revolving light atop Tour Eiffel several blocks away could not penetrate the inner sanctum of the Armed Revolutionary Cause, known for the arc of the sword they used against their enemies. It may as well have been called a Council of Death, for that was the subject at hand. In an apartment on Rue de Bologne, its minimal furnishings a stark contrast to the upscale address, sat six well dressed men on Persian rugs, between pillows and platters of figs. They spoke fervently, all but ignoring the flickering images from a laptop computer and color television on a low wooden table nearby. Tall candles reached from the floor and threw flickering light as the men talked of nightmarish things. If ricin was added to the water supply, would it kill people? How much was enough?

Clink, clink. Rail-thin as the snake he was named for, Tsouban, the Cobra, tapped a knife against a crystal glass. The men stopped talking, looked at their second in command, and waited for something to happen. When nothing did, they traded glances, the changing pictures on the television casting shadows on their faces. A twenty-four-hour news station showed protests around the world, but broadcast no sound.

In an adjoining room, a pair of eyes watched the men from the cover of darkness. They had all responded to the same coded message: *Fly to Paris. Urgent business.* All but one! El Samoud swallowed indignation at the missing explosives expert and secretly inspected his operatives. The Asian man in a tailored suit and black eye patch masqueraded as an exporter. In truth, he was ARC's cell leader in Hong Kong. To his right sat Zayed, Yemeni by birth, now embedded in New York City and sworn to do ARC's bidding. Whenever. Wherever. To

Zayed's right sat the leader from London. Others had flown from Sydney, Nairobi, and Sao Paolo.

Where was the man from Moscow? Had the meeting been compromised? Over the previous three years, El Samoud had handpicked these men. He could not afford any mistakes. Not now. In the coming days they would grow his power, make his plans succeed. The possibilities were as vast as his net worth, five hundred million dollars and climbing. But were they ready to take part in the most spectacular attack in modern history? His plan would be a greater surprise than Pearl Harbor, and twenty times as deadly.

El Samoud saw Tsouban glance toward him, then clink the glass. Even though the seventh cell leader had not yet arrived, it was the signal for El Samoud to appear. The men grew still at the sight of their leader, the hush more fitting for a funeral than a strategy meeting. Something even more deadly was about to be launched.

El Samoud lowered his wizened body, cloaked in a linen robe, until he sat crossed legged on a large pillow. No one could see his tongue flick over thin lips; a two-inch slit in the *isharb* hid all but his onyx eyes. With his left hand, El Samoud reached under the veil and slid a finger into the indentation that had been with him since he was a boy. He traced the jagged edge, excited over his plan to demolish his enemies, but reluctant to reveal too much. He closed his eyes, blocking out anxiety alive like swarming bees.

Great anger boiled beneath his skin, scarred by the British, whom he blamed for the smallpox that ravaged him at the age of three. The pock marks were not all that fueled his hate. His life had been shattered when he was eight years old, in Palestine, before Israel became a nation. El Samoud had been taking his baby brother to market in a donkey cart when a British soldier ordered them to stop. But the donkey, with a strong will of its own, careened into the soldiers.

Sounds from that day were seared in his mind and would be so long as he breathed. The donkey's pitiful wail. The soldier's pistol shot to the beast's head. El Samoud had thrown himself on his only sibling, who lay crumpled next to the cart. That British soldier kicked El Samoud in the stomach and slashed his face with a knife, shouting, "You mongrel, I'll teach you to disobey!"

Blood poured down his cheek, into his hands. When he brought home his brother's lifeless body, his mother cried for days. Her blame of him for getting his brother killed had carved his soul to shreds. Once the external wound healed, El Samoud took to wearing the *isharb.* Not long after, his daring escapades against the British became legendary. He graduated from stealing guns and ammunition, to sabotage of military movements, to murder.

El Samoud captured the attention of Yasser Arafat and became a leading militant in the Palestine Liberation Organization. His terrorist skills were honed in Lebanon during its Civil War. After El Samoud's mother and first wife were killed by an Israeli strike on Lebanon, and Yasser Arafat refused to issue an *intifada* against Israel, El Samoud birthed his own terrorist organization. Born of violence, mayhem was ARC's sustenance.

A steady diet of killing, and of moving from place to place to avoid detection, had forced El Samoud's second wife to move to Paris with his now 17-year-old son, which was why El Samoud often came to the capital of France. They lived a block away, on Rue Chevert, where this afternoon his son said he wanted to live in the largest Arab community in America. Dearborn, Michigan, to be exact. His son, the scholar, wanted to go to the University of Michigan, Dearborn campus.

El Samoud pressed the long scar, secure in the knowledge that ARC was more powerful than Arafat ever was. But, how to manage his son who would soon be a man? He dropped his hand from behind the *isharb,* which hid not only scars but a mask of pure hate. Hate for a British lieutenant, now in the House of Lords, and everything British.

Never would he allow his son to live in America. He despised them, as much as he did the British and the Israelis. They were all the same. They were his enemies. Soon, he would maim or kill that British Lord. El Samoud knew it would be so. The Presence had assured him. The taste of imminent victory was sweeter than honey from the comb. When Parliament was blown to bits, his revenge would not be complete. It would just have begun.

Besides El Samoud's mother, now martyred, only Tsouban had seen El Samoud's face without its covering. It was fitting he should. Tsouban was family, his uncle's son. El Samoud trusted his chief with his life, for Tsouban tended the secret of the scars.

Candle flames danced in the moving air, throwing a diabolic glint in El Samoud's eyes. Eyes that saw Tsouban fold his cell phone and hide it under his robe. Eyes that watched Zayed cover his mouth, hiding a yawn. With ears as acute as his eyesight, El Samoud heard Zayed whisper to his London counterpart, "Why do we wait?"

How dare an underling question his Supreme Leader? Zayed must be taught patience. A ring burst the quiet. A second ring. Tsouban reached into his robe and stalked to the kitchen.

El Samoud said to Zayed for all to hear, "Your eagerness may be a double-edged sword."

Zayed blinked his eyes, the color of tanned leather, but said nothing.

Tsouban returned with unexpected news. "Our man in Russia was followed to the Hamburg airport. He thought it safer to return to Moscow via a rental car using an alias."

Murmurs spread round the room. Distrust flashed from El Samoud's stormy eyes, but his voice held calm.

"These are perilous times. If you have to use the telephone, continue using coded messages. Even cell phones are monitored by their spies in the sky."

Nods from his commanders urged El Samoud to continue in a smooth cadence, as if reading an epic poem, "Brothers in the struggle, the world will soon fear us more. One week from today, on the anniversary of September 11, our bombs will surprise them. Terror in their hearts will blind the West to our true objectives."

Behind the veil, his cackle sounded like a gun shot. "We do much more than sow bombs. Brothers in the charitable world ensure our legacy expands to new countries. Investors send millions to help us defeat the British, the Americans, and *all* who help them."

The irony that U.S. dollars would bring down America gave him what might be called joy, in a sane person. It also rallied the faithful. El Samoud allowed the room to grow quiet, to build anticipation about why he called them.

Impatience was a prime weakness of the West. Americans especially insisted results be immediate. They knew not how to bide their time or wait for the perfect moment to strike. El Samoud considered himself smarter than they, having watched the British make mistakes in Palestine and America retreat from Lebanon. He learned to keep those crucial to his operations off guard, under constant testing.

He asked, "Are you prepared to die for our cause?"

Tsouban and the ARC's six leaders raised their fists and called, "Death to our enemies!"

Despite their uniform reply, El Samoud searched for signs of wavering. He detected none. Even though he felt more time was needed to cement the next plan, he would begin initial stages today, while he had the strength and their loyalty.

A spasm shot through his right leg. It was time to stand. To steady his cramped legs, he leaned on his right elbow. The head scarf caught beneath it. Black silk slipped below his chin. His face, with all its identifying marks, was unmasked! With a single movement, he pulled the *isharb* back in place, but not before Zayed diverted his eyes. Had he seen?

El Samoud's knees creaked. The others gazed up at him, but not Zayed. He stared at the figs. El Samoud would take no more chances. With one hand, he held the scarf in place and, to the round ball of a man sitting at Zayed's right, he asked, "Do you trust your contact in the British Parliament?"

The man scrambled to his feet and sputtered, "He is committed to our cause. As am I."

Protecting the *isharb*, El Samoud turned to Zayed. He must see his eyes, for that would tell all. "And your person in Washington, D.C. Is he loyal?"

Zayed rose to his feet and looked down at his polished loafers. In a monotone voice, as if ordering a pizza, he said, "I have two recruits. One commands our cell in Virginia. The other is highly placed in the U.S. government. Both follow my orders."

To El Samoud, this reply was unconvincing. While Tsouban gave each of the other terrorists their future targets, El Samoud drew Zayed away from the others and said, "Until now, you have been as close as my son. Why aggravate me now?"

Zayed bowed his groomed head, allowing it to hang below his shoulders several minutes. Zayed's humbleness confirmed what El Samoud thought for some time. His New York leader could be trusted with greater responsibility. Tsouban took a prearranged cue and whispered to Zayed his next assignment. As Zayed's pupils widened, El Samoud clasped his hands together, adrenaline spiking through his crippled body. The circle of violence was complete.

He had told enough. It was too dangerous to let them know more about the simultaneous attacks he planned to coincide with a Jewish holiday.

His final orders were simple. "Do not reveal each other's targets. We next meet in the Indian Ocean, the date is secret until I send for you. Begin preparations and pray. Pray our attacks will cut off our enemies' heads in one swift blow."

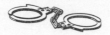

ONE

T he recruiter's warning from thirteen years ago roared through Eva Montanna's mind like a flash flood: "Few jobs have mundane moments punctuated by times of terror." This was one of those jobs. This one of those times. Alert to every sound, Eva did not move and barely breathed. In the decrepit hallway, she turned her thin body to diminish her silhouette, and pressed the white "POLICE" letters on her jacket's back against the wall.

A faint sound creaked in the distance. She strained to hear. Not footsteps. More like a loose board flopping in the wind. Outside, a storm gathered strength. Eva breathed, but not too deeply. Criminals were hiding in the building. Somewhere. Not knowing where was maddening.

"Come out!" she yelled.

The words ravaged her throat already sore from yelling. Sore from swallowing fear that frayed every nerve, especially after what happened to Jillie. *Jillie!* Sudden thoughts of her sister's death rained down on her. Eva gripped her 9-millimeter Glock, feeling something stronger than fear. Bile rose past the curve in her long throat, a mixture of a bad lunch and raw anger. Hers was not a vicious anger. It continued to hurt, like a soft bone that would not heal.

No answer to her call. Experience told her no one would. Eva's search of the storeroom had turned up only piles of empty crates. She was about to enter another room when the whistling wind blew her blond hair into her eyes, distracting her. Eva could not see! She swiped the hair from her eyes, shoved it behind her ears and into the top of her jacket.

A week ago, Eva chafed under her boss's lecture—telling her that she and the rest of the Financial Investigations Group, or FIG, must bring to justice the terrorists who acted as if the whole world was their private Wild West. It was their job, Lou Phillips said. Fresh from a cushy job as liaison to Congress, what did Lou know about what drove her? Or about terrorists? Wasn't FIG her idea in the first place after she stumbled on the financial records of the Grilled Onion restaurants?

Steady as a stalking cat, her weight shifting from one foot to the other, Eva moved toward the door. Large ammo clips drove down black jeans that hung on her hips. With each step, she closed in on her sworn enemy, the ones who cheered the plane that crashed into the Pentagon, killing Jillie. Al Qaeda, the mastermind behind September 11, had metastasized into other terrorist organizations. The Armed Revolutionary Cause was now the primary cancer, sprouting its dangerous cells around the world.

Jillie's intense blue eyes danced before her. Eva shut her own for an instant. She still struggled with the pain of knowing that terrorists had murdered her identical twin. They might as well have chopped off Eva's legs or cut out her heart. Inseparable since children, the two sisters shared more than the same features. What one did, the other tried to do. A part of Eva was empty now. There was no solace, no forgiveness. She rarely prayed. Only when Scott got restless over her apathy did she go to church with him and the kids.

Eva paused at the door. If she practiced shooting more, she'd be better prepared today. Instead, the Glock felt foreign, like when she shoved her feet into Scott's slippers. Until her transfer to FIG nine months ago, Eva lived behind a desk combing through financial records. Trying to catch white collar criminals, she shot her gun at practice four times a year. Now, she and nine agents and police officers were hot on the money trail of terrorists operating in the United States and around the globe.

In the dark hallway, shards of light fought with cobwebs to pierce through the window. It was a strange place to recall what Grandpa Marty had said when she was little and afraid. He held up her pinkie and told her of the Dutch boy who saved the Netherlands from ruin with no more than that. If a small child plugged a leak in the dike, she could bring ARC to justice. It was more than a duty. It was her destiny. Eva vowed to avenge Jillie's death.

Eva gripped the gun so tightly it felt like part of her right hand and, taking a deep breath, stepped inside. She was ready to shoot, and would shoot, to save a life. Still, a powerful vise squeezed her chest.

A scruffy guy with a sawed-off shotgun whirled to face her!

Eva fired two quick blasts. He fell backward. There was no time to think about what she had done. Others might be skulking in the shadows. She spun left. Blood pounded in her ears. Her eyes swept the room. There was no threat.

Her Glock pointed in front of her, three rounds left, Eva crouched on legs strong from running with Scott and crept to one of two rooms she still had to check. Eva burst through the doorway. Her eyes checked the room. It was empty. She sucked in a short breath, then pounced to the other side of the hallway. The door to the final room was closed. She kicked the wood, near the handle. It flew open. Eva stood face to face with an armed man.

This is it! Her brain told her to squeeze the trigger. But, before she fired the fatal blast, she saw it, on his belt. A gold badge! Eva's heart thudded. She had nearly shot a federal agent!

A sharp whistle pierced the air. The range master's voice crackled over a loudspeaker, "Cease firing. Secure your weapon."

Eva complied with his order, and answered the range master's question, "Is the line safe?" by yelling loudly, "My weapon is safe."

He must have heard because he announced to the other agents over a speaker, "You may move about."

Alone in the practice room, Eva stared at the cardboard federal agent she nearly shot. Its unchanged expression mocked her, and a chill flooded her body. Her specialty was not marksmanship it was nabbing criminals who hid money. Her shooting was improved, but she had never shot a live criminal. Could she? Was her courage a few minutes ago simply a bravado on the shooting range that would freeze under live fire?

The painted face seemed to grow grim. Like an outtake from a movie, a horrible picture blinked through Eva's mind. The sea pounded next to a beach house and a man lay crushed against weathered wood. His face looked up at her. He screamed for help. Before she could reach out her hand, he passed out. Eva squeezed shut her eyes to obliterate the image that had startled her awake that morning. Sweat once again dotted her hairline. The only difference was that this morning the man in the dream was faceless. Now, she saw he was her boss, Lou. Several premonitions had visited her in the past, but she refused to acknowledge them now. Just because they had been real then didn't mean this was real now, that her boss was in danger.

Eva assured herself that Lou was hard at work in the office and retraced her steps to inspect the other bad guy. The cardboard terrorist, knocked from the mechanical frame, boasted holes in its forehead and neck, right at the carotid artery. Her trim fingers touched the leather holster cradling her Glock. The last to shoot, Eva had grown nervous, though you wouldn't know it by her precise shooting. Eva managed a tight smile. She passed qualification.

More than that, if the target had been real, she'd be alive for Scott and their two kids, and that terrorist would no longer be a threat, which meant her aim was good enough to save another agent's life. A lilt in her step, Eva left "Scruffy" behind and threw open the door. The wind banged it behind her.

Eva went to find out if she had scored higher than her partner and could rib him about it over coffee. That was doubtful. A seasoned FBI agent, Griffin Topping was an expert shot and better at everything, an irritation that Eva mentioned to no one. Though satisfied with her first performance at the famous Hogan's Alley, she needed to get more comfortable with this range and her Glock.

A few steps inside the gun cleaning room, she learned how mundane were her concerns.

Griff grabbed her elbow. "Wanda called on my cell. Why is yours always turned off?"

Eva reached for her phone, but it was not in her pocket. Had she put it in the locker?

She asked, "How high was your score?"

He shook his head. "It's bad news."

A smile erupted on her face. She had beaten him after all.

"What, not perfect as usual?"

"Forget my score. I'm talking about Wanda's call."

"Has something happened to Andy? Kaley?"

Griff handed her his cell phone. "Your kids are fine." He wiped his thick brown moustache with the palm of his left hand, and added, "As far as I know."

Their FIG mate, Jefferson County Deputy Sheriff Trenton Nash, stood next to Griff, who was five inches taller and, at thirty-seven, ten years older than Nash. Trenton said, "It's Lou."

A shudder coursed through Eva. Minutes before, she had envisioned Lou lying on his back, screaming. Had something really happened to him?

With fear in her eyes, she searched Griff's face. "Did he—is he all right?" she managed to stammer.

Griff touched her arm. "Lou fell from a ladder, cleaning windows at the beach cottage. He's about to have back surgery."

No! Eva leaned against the table. She couldn't admit what she had seen, not yet. After Jillie died, in a moment of vulnerability Eva had hinted of her last vision to Scott. He reacted so negatively, she never told him the rest. To have it happen again! Why did she see things before they happened? She pressed the sides of her head. It was crazy, and she had no one to talk to about it.

She strode to the door calling back to her partner, "We should be there. He has no family."

Griff stopped her. "He's at Johns Hopkins. We've got another problem. When Judge Pendergast's clerk did not reach you, Wanda gave her my number."

Eva rolled her eyes. "The one day I'm out of the office, the Judge's clerk calls."

Probably the insurance case she was working on with Dan Simmons, Assistant U.S. Attorney. Because the insurance agent continued to defraud the elderly, Dan filed a motion with Eva's affidavit to revoke his bond. Did the judge want to grill her personally? Unlikely. But Pendergast was an unusual U.S. District Court Judge. He did everything by the book. Nothing got past him. Ever. Or so it seemed to Eva.

Griff and Trenton stared at her. Her eyes met Griff's. "What?"

"The shooting must have fried your brain." Griff thumped his temple with his finger. "I *said*, it's Operation Money Changer, our big raid, you know, the day after tomorrow? Judge Pendergast won't sign the warrants because Earl's affidavit fails to provide probable cause. His clerk hinted the judge might sign if you or I were the affiant. Since he's known our work for more than ten years."

Eva sighed. Right problem, wrong case. She checked her watch. Wednesday, 3:30 p.m. The judge would leave soon. They must have the warrants. The task force worked for a month to get the leads to the ARC terror cell operating in northern Virginia. She was not about to let Pendergast interfere with the operation because Earl was new to him. If Eva drove to the Court in Alexandria, she would never make dinner at church, and she had promised Scott she'd go. She made an instant decision.

Before she could reveal it, Trenton thrust forward his strong chin. "I'll prepare a new affidavit. Earl let me read the old one."

Griff snickered. "Why would Pendergast sign a search warrant based on your affidavit? He's never met you. You've been with FIG for, what, three weeks?"

Eva held up her hand. "Thanks for the offer, Trenton, but Griff's right. Griff, can you call Wanda and dictate a new paragraph with more probable cause?"

Eva's partner raised a bushy eyebrow. "There's that info the CIA gave Earl from the detainee at Guantanamo."

Eva shook her head. "Not over the cell."

"Okay. I'll be creative." Griff took back his phone, called their secretary and gave Wanda precise instructions. He nodded his head twice, then said, "I'll tell Eva."

He punched the key to end the call. "If that doesn't convince the judge to sign, I'll pen in the CIA stuff."

"Tell me what?"

"Scott wants you to get his suit at the dry cleaners. He needs it for Friday. Find your cell phone. I'm not your answering service." Griff reached the door, turned and shot back, "Lou's boss named you acting supervisor of FIG until Lou returns. Which means, Friday is your baby."

With his usual engaging smile, Trenton said, "Lou told me to cover the back entrance. But, you're the boss. Whatever I can do. I've been on raids before."

Eva flinched at the title. She hadn't wanted a promotion this way. Still, she liked the sound of being an ICE Supervisory Special Agent. It had a cold, hard ring to it. Since September 11, Immigration Customs Enforcement, or ICE, was no longer United States Customs, but an integral component of the Department of Homeland Security. The Financial Investigations Group (FIG) was a special task force created within ICE after Eva discovered links to Middle Eastern terrorists in the Grilled Onion Restaurant chain's financial records. Her mission: to find and arrest two kinds of Americans, those who gave money to terrorists and those who used legitimate businesses to aid them.

Because of Eva's sterling record of catching financial criminals, her mentor, Alexia Kyros, the U.S. Attorney for the Eastern District of Virginia, had lobbied for Eva to lead FIG. Alexia had told Eva that, soon after being sworn in as the U.S. Attorney, she realized many federal law enforcement agencies were reluctant to cooperate with one another or the local police. For national security reasons and to

prevent leaks, the feds were against permitting others to work within their offices. Eva marveled at how Alexia had convinced the FBI,
DEA, and ICE, Eva's own agency, to donate experienced investigators
to the task force concept, where each agency supervised its own task
force, under the oversight of Alexia. While located away from their
authorizing agencies, the task forces operated under the same regulations and security as the agency. Each was assigned officers from state
and local police agencies and paid supplemental overtime with funds
Alexia obtained from the Department of Justice. FIG was the ICE task
force, and Eva was now in charge.

Unfortunately, even though Alexia conceived the idea of a stand
alone task force to better marshal resources, her pull wasn't as strong
as that of U.S. Senator Russell H. Bell, the powerful Chairman of the
Homeland Security and Governmental Affairs Committee. And Lou's
uncle.

Not one to get wrapped up in the politics of career climbing, Eva
had no problem working under Lou. Besides, when FIG was born
she became Griff's partner, which was what she had wanted for years.
Not only did Griff have a hard-nosed work ethic that matched hers,
he was smart. No, more than smart. He was clever, and he had a knack
for telling a funny story when they needed it most.

As acting supervisor of FIG, Eva steeled herself for the barrage
of decisions she'd need to make. Besides Griff, who was on assignment from the FBI, and Trenton, who was on loan from the Jefferson
County Sherriff, she was now in charge of four other federal agents,
one ICE, two IRS, and one Bureau of Alcohol, Tobacco, and Firearms,
plus a Fairfax County Sheriff Deputy and a Virginia State Trooper. A
blend of personalities, each was fiercely independent. She was the
only woman. Lou kept things close, sticking to the motto, "Need
to know." He never fully briefed her on Operation Money Changer.
Lou chose Earl as lead investigator, and now the judge had tossed him
aside, so to speak.

Beyond knowing the target was Farouk Hamdi, whom Earl believed ran ARC's cell from his Columbia City townhouse, plus being
aware of the CIA's take on him, Eva was on the outer circle of the
raid plan. But two things were firm in her mind. By Friday morning,
she had to learn everything there was to know, and dinner at church
was out. While missionaries droned on about their work in the jungles,
harping that they needed money, she'd be frantic to work on Money

Changer. It all came down to the green stuff, which she tracked fifty, sometimes sixty, hours a week.

Griff and Trenton were arguing over the affidavit. Eva glanced at Griff. Beneath his moustache, his lips were pressed together, as if ready to demolish Trenton with a word as soon as he took a breath. Trenton's deep-set hazel eyes warned that he would not be ignored, and mischief played at the corners of his mouth. Eva suspected he was adept at getting what he wanted. With Lou in critical condition, it was up to her to make the transition. Right here, right now.

She interrupted their dispute. "First thing tomorrow, I'll see Lou. He may not say much, but it's worth a try. I'll tell him not to worry. He assembled the best team. Together, we'll bring down this Virginia cell. Griff, be in the office early to discuss raid plans. Now, get going."

Griff protested, "Lou gave me tomorrow off. I reserved a Cessna Skyhawk."

Eva shot him a look that said, "Don't you dare leave me hanging."

His hand on the doorknob, Griff surrendered. "I'll cancel it."

Trenton edged closer to Eva. "There is nothing more important to *me* than getting these guys. I can be in by seven."

Eva smothered a laugh. Cool and experienced, Griff could execute the raid on the fly. Trenton wanted to make his mark. She needed her team to think like one. A sudden thought came to her, and she made the second decision since her promotion minutes ago.

"Griff, you're right. Trenton is new to us. As a deputy sheriff, he's more familiar with things local. You have thirteen years experience as an FBI agent and can teach him a lot. Shake the hand of your new partner."

Eva was surprised when Griff shoved both hands in his pockets and asked Trenton, "This your first time qualifying at Quantico?"

Trenton took the dig in stride. He pushed open the door for Griff. "Am I that obvious? My dad loves this range."

Before Eva could ask Trenton about his dad, the rangemaster stepped into the room, removed a navy blue cap with "FBI" emblazoned in gold letters, and announced, "Marine One has landed. The President will address the agents and police officers training here today. Everyone is requested to join us in the auditorium. Immediately."

Eva froze next to the gun cleaning table. Her Glock was still in its leather holster, and she had not cleaned it.

As if reading her mind, Griff pointed to a row of metal lockers. "Store it until after his speech. Sounds like an order to me."

At the locker, she exchanged her gun for her cell phone, then pushed Griff out the door. "Not for you. Call me when those warrants are signed. Trenton, you and I have to stay."

Trenton laughed. "A few minutes anyway. We can sit in back, then sneak out."

Eva frowned. Such a move would be not only rude, it could be career ending. "Don't even think about it. Start for the auditorium. I've got a phone call to make."

She called Scott, left him a message that her promise to go to church was being thwarted by the President of the United States, and hung up, feeling no regret.

Eva sprinted across campus, her phone clipped to her waist band. The storm predicted by the local meteorologist was about to let loose. A streak of lightening split the sky. She counted, one thousand one, one thousand two, one thousand—thunder crashed against swelling dark clouds. That was close. The air was thick, but no rain fell. If she was lucky, she'd get inside before the heavens opened up.

Eva caught up with Trenton and Robbie, the Virginia State Trooper. Tall and beanpole thin, Robbie looked even younger than Trenton, but he was closer in age to Eva, who was thirty-eight. A thought mocked her: Even with Griff's additions, what if the Judge refused to give them the warrants? *She* should have gone to see Pendergast. The race was on. Eva had to stop the money before it financed more terror. An answer came as fast as the question. Why hadn't she thought of it before?

Eva pulled the phone from her waistband and punched in the office number. Wanda answered after five rings.

"Get me Earl."

"He went home. Sulking you might say," Wanda said, then laughed.

Eva checked her watch, which read 3:45 p.m. With mandatory overtime, they were all supposed to work until 6:00 p.m. There was nothing funny about Earl's cutting out early. So the judge questioned his affidavit. He should not take it personally.

"I'll call his cell."

Wanda laughed again, a gushing chuckle Eva found exasperating. "Won't do any good. He left it sitting on his desk."

Eva rolled her eyes. A large drop of rain fell on the edge of her upturned nose. Robbie must have gone on ahead. Trenton stood listening to her conversation.

"Wanda," Eva said, hoping the secretary that Lou had brought with him from the Hill would do what *she* asked for a change. "Call his home and leave a message for him to call me. I'll be with the President in a few minutes, or I'd call."

Eva started walking and nodded at Trenton to come along.

Wanda's ugly chuckle again. "Yeah, and the First Lady is holding dinner for me. I've got to run and get my hair done."

Keeping her frustration in check, Eva replied, "The President is about to speak here at Quantico."

"How can Earl call you then?"

"My cell will vibrate."

Eva ended the call, then rubbed her face with her free hand.

Trenton said, "My dad knows the President."

A picture formed in Eva's mind of Mr. Nash, standing in a greeting line at some political event he paid a thousand dollars to attend, shaking the President's hand. She nearly dismissed the idea but recalled Trenton's earlier remark about his dad being familiar with the Quantico range. Mr. Nash probably guarded the President at the White House.

Eva asked, "Your dad's a Marine?"

Trenton lifted his chin. "He was an FBI firearms instructor here."

That did not explain how he knew the President. She was about to ask him to elaborate, when her cell phone whirled against her waist. Eva grabbed it and without looking at the screen, laid into Earl. "You shouldn't have left. I don't care what the judge said! We need to talk. About Friday."

"It's me. You said you'd come home early this afternoon. Does this mean you can't?"

It was Scott. So much for ragging on Earl.

Eva got to the point. "Did you get my message?"

"No. I just left a meeting with the SecDef about Friday's Congressional hearing. I'm getting the kids. Will you pick up my suit?"

The dry cleaners. She had forgotten Scott's earlier message.

Eva whispered to Trenton, "Go on ahead." She returned to Scott and said, "No. The President's making a surprise speech. I have to be there. I may miss the dinner."

"It's supposed to be family time."

Scott's heavy sigh made her feel guilty. She said, "The sooner I get in there, the sooner I leave."

Eva hung up. Trenton waited for her on the auditorium steps. She fastened her blowing hair, the color of dried wheat, into a trim ponytail behind her head and caught Trenton's eye. "The rangemaster said to hurry."

Trenton removed the phone from his belt. "My grandfather was an FBI agent, too. Worked for the big man himself, J. Edgar Hoover. Mrs. Montanna, can I make a quick call?"

"Call me Eva. Not now, Trenton. We'd better get a seat."

Unfazed, Trenton punched in a number and said, "Dad! I qualified at Hogan's Alley. The President's speaking in a few minutes."

Not wanting to insult the President by being late, Eva twirled a finger for him to hang up.

Trenton continued, "You should have seen me shoot, Dad. It was awesome."

Eva held open the door and snapped, "*Now*, Trenton."

He shot her a sheepish grin, then ended the call and muted his phone. Eva walked into the dimly lit auditorium, her newest team member so close behind she felt his breath on her neck. She spotted empty seats down front, in the middle, which forced them to step over several pairs of feet. Trenton eased in beside her.

Five Secret Service agents strode to the front of the stage. Security was tighter than usual, even for Quantico. Eva figured it had to be this way, now. Her life, along with the lives of all Americans, had changed since terrorists attacked the land of the free and the brave. Her family would never be the same.

Without the usual color guard or orchestral rendition of "Ruffles and Flourishes" and "Hail to the Chief," the President strode to the podium. A sea of blue swelled like a giant wave as the audience rose to applaud. He quickly motioned for them to sit.

"You are gracious to stay late. I will get right to why I am here."

The President said something about not forgetting those who died on September 11. How could she? Her last outing with Jillie had been during the weekend prior to that awful day.

Jillie had turned from driving and smiled, "Scott's great to watch the kids. You and I need time alone with our folks."

Eva studied her twin, an Army Judge Advocate lawyer. "Scott's showing Kaley and Andy his new office, just down from yours. Mom and Dad will be thrilled to see us, even if you did cut your hair. "

Jillie's laugh was full-throated. "Wasn't it brilliant of me to introduce you two?"

"I tried to return the favor. Have you and Griff gone out since I introduced you?"

"Griff offered to take me flying some evening when Brad is out of town next week."

Eva complained, "Why date Brad, Jillie? He's no good for you."

Jillie's fingers tapped against the steering wheel. "Why don't you like him?"

Eva's memory veered to early morning, September 11, 2001, and her awful dream—Jillie was trapped in a building about to collapse. When Eva awoke, she immediately phoned her sister and, on her voice mail, left a message she'd call her at work. Eva never got the chance. The terrorists saw to that. Could she ever forgive herself for not warning Jillie?

Eva blinked back a tear and tried to shut out the "what ifs." The President strode to the edge of the stage and said, "Americans trust you to protect their freedoms. What you do with that trust matters. Because you uphold our ideals of justice, America is safer."

Then, the President made a stunning announcement. "The reward for information leading to the capture of El Samoud, leader of the Armed Revolutionary Cause, has been raised from twenty-five million to fifty million dollars."

Eva nearly shot out of her seat. The room erupted into applause. A quick smile brightened the worn face of the President. It was a staggering sum. But would any amount of money make a difference to radicals who worshiped death? El Samoud had innocent blood on his hands. Whoever turned him in deserved every penny. Last month, ARC blew up a British plane, killing one hundred high school students flying to a musical competition in Vienna. What the President said next convinced Eva he understood what she was up against.

"El Samoud hides behind a veil of secrecy. So do his operatives. They live in our communities and want their neighbors to believe they are Americans. They celebrate the Fourth of July and eat hot dogs. But, these evil ones do more. They act on their hate for us and our allies, Britain and Israel."

Eva exhaled. ARC's sleeper cells were elusive. In the black-and-white photo Eva saw of Farouk Hamdi, franchise director for the Grilled Onion, he was cleanshaven and every bit the successful entrepreneur. A diamond studded his earlobe. If it was hard for federal agents to discern the terrorists, how did the average American know of whom to be wary? In these perilous times, was there such a thing as an average American?

The Commander-in-Chief returned to the podium, his hands gripped the sides. "We must prevent El Samoud and his minions from killing those who do not follow their beliefs. In the hot light of history, they will be revealed as cowards. Cowards who stop at nothing to change the world as we know it to one filled with death and horror."

Eva felt death and horror at Jillie's funeral. Fresh grief thundered through her. Years of training suppressed an urge in her to scream, *You'll pay!*

The President put on reading glasses. "This week, I received a letter from a 10-year-old boy. His father was killed by the first plane that crashed into the World Trade Center. He writes, 'My Dad died protecting our country. My brother and I no longer have him with us to play baseball or go camping. Mom bakes bread, and I started a paper route to help. I want to be a policeman, like my Dad.'"

The President's voice cracked. His hands thumped the podium. "With your help, the terrorists who take the lives of our innocent children will soon be facing justice!"

Eva was on her feet with the others. The President should read that boy's letter on TV. The whole nation needed to hear it and believe in the mission. Some Americans had grown complacent, believing ARC and their ilk were no longer a threat. In her heart, Eva knew the awful truth. They were out there, working, planning, waiting to strike. Again.

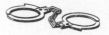

TWO

Due home forty minutes ago, Eva drove the G-car up the driveway past her light blue VW and into the garage's second stall. Scott was leaning into the passenger side of their van. She missed his back by inches. It was a good thing she hadn't stopped for fuel. So what if the tank registered below an eighth? When she left Quantico, she called to say she'd skip the dinner and stay home with Andy. Scott said "OK," but his voice sounded hurt.

Always the gentleman, Scott turned and opened her door. Eva stood on tiptoe. They traded a quick kiss.

Eva forced a laugh. "Sorry I'm late. The rain made Route 7 slick."

Scott turned his back on her.

She added, "A fender bender narrowed traffic to one lane."

"We were just leaving." Scott bent to unbuckle Andy.

"Mommy, aren't you coming?" Kaley cried from the backseat.

Okay, Scott was letting her break the bad news. Eva walked to the other side of the van, knelt on the drivers' seat, and looked back at her daughter. "I worked late. You and Daddy will have a special time together."

Scott walked Andy over, and tapped her on the shoulder. "My turn to drive."

He was not smiling. They traded places. Eva blew a kiss to Kaley, then closed the door. Scott backed the van down the driveway. Andy's fingers entwined in her left hand, Eva waved with her right. As 9-year-old Kaley's outstretched palm disappeared from view, Eva forced herself to swallow the lump in her throat. Her daughter's face was pinched, revealing that Eva had really let her down. Her daughter hadn't looked that sad since she had come home with a lost kitty and Scott found the rightful owner.

Eva whispered, "I'll make it up to you, Kaley."

A nasty voice in her head nagged, *When?* With new demands on her, Eva felt more like the rag doll her Grandmother made than like a mother or wife. Yet Eva never considered turning down Lou's job. She pressed the button to close the garage door. Griff still had not called. Either he was at the office typing a new affidavit or in Old Town, wolfing down a platter of ribs. Griff's stomach never suffered, no matter how much work he faced.

Eva and Andy went inside, and he disappeared as she rifled through the mail and papers on the entryway table. Eva stopped by Andy's room, where he sat contentedly on the floor, playing with plastic dinosaurs. At least he was not disappointed in her. She changed into jeans and an old sweater. Back in the kitchen, Eva munched a handful of trail mix and found a graham cracker to hold Andy until dinner. He skipped in for his snack. When she slid open the door to the backyard, he shot past her.

"Andrew, wait for me."

"Mommy, I'll get my shovel. Help you dig."

He reached the storage shed first. With sturdy arms, he yanked on the door. Eva placed her hand on the door to help him. Her son moved aside his tricycle and rummaged in his bucket. She chuckled. At four years old, Andy was as focused on his activities as Eva could be when she was preparing a case for indictment. Eva had stayed home tonight so she could be with him.

"Here it is!" Andy cried.

He waved a red plastic shovel above his head like a trophy, then scampered down the hill. At the bottom, he turned and splashed a grin. The beauty of her child almost made her weep. His innocence revived memories of her childhood and her Palomino horse. She fed him lumps of sugar, and Dad let her sleep in the barn when Mother was out of town.

Twenty-five years later, Eva still recalled the tears she shed at age thirteen when her folks sold the ranch and moved to Richmond. Jillie thrived in the city and could not wait to move to Washington, D.C. That was one dream that came true for her sister. A tiny briar pricked at Eva. Hadn't Mother told her it was Jillie's idea to move?

Eva's dream of starting an equestrian center for disadvantaged children disappeared with the animals. Maybe that was why she insisted on buying this rambling home at the edge of Columbia City. Their yard was expansive. Maple and pine dotted the perimeter, which gave it an aura of being miles away from the city. Scott's waterfall, which gurgled into a small pond graced with water lilies, heightened the illusion. She was a country girl at heart.

"Don't jump off the rocks!" Eva called.

She thrust the tool caddy in the belly of the wheelbarrow. Metal tools jangled as she ran past the crown of their yard to the silver maple tree that spread its luscious shade over them during family picnics. Eva looked up at the elegant branches. Drops glittered on the leaves' edges in the sinking sun. Something was wrong! The sixty-year-old tree's top was half-brown, half-green. Whatever the cause of such damage, their prized tree needed help.

Eva grew dizzy looking up. She lowered her head, and strode to the garden, which looked more like an abandoned field than a place of refuge. Where yellow mums and orange marigolds once thrived, withered heads drooped, poor sentinels in piles of decayed leaves.

Andy threw down his shovel. Arms outstretched, he twirled around the flowers, the rock, her legs. Eva longed to be as carefree. When she plunged her hands into the soil to plant crocus bulbs, she felt no sense of calm. As dirt stuck to her fingers, thoughts of her identical twin clung to her mind.

How she missed her! Eva received no counseling after Jillie died, just therapy from work. In her garden, she saw that the bond between her and Jillie never could be replaced. Was the half-dead, half-alive tree a sign of her own heart, the dead part keeping her from fully loving Scott and the kids?

When she and Jillie still lived at home together, Eva worked hard to please her parents, but mostly she strived for Jillie's praise. Life came easier for her sister, ever since she progressed to "dolphin" while Eva remained a "shark" at the community swimming pool. Jillie convinced Eva to become a federal agent, while Eva tried to steer Jillie into the perfect romantic relationship, never with any success. A pale light of truth flashed, then disappeared behind a cloud of doubt. If only—

"Ow! Mommy, it stings!" Andy cried. He swatted his face with his arms and jumped up and down.

Her motherly instincts kicked into high gear. Eva plucked him from bees that darted around his head and ran to the safety of the house. Red welts covered Andy's face, and one loomed dangerously close to his right eye. Andy cried at a full throttle. His little fists dug his eyes.

Eva hugged him. "Honey, the bees are mad because you got close to their house. When Kaley knocked over your log city, you were upset, too."

Andy whimpered, "It hurts."

Eva pressed his head on her shoulder. In the kitchen, she washed the stings with cool water and applied a baking soda paste. Andy continued to cry. Unable to comfort him, she pulled from the freezer a blue popsicle, in hopes the cold might soothe him. On her lap, she fed him the icy confection and murmured into his hair, "You're okay. Mommy's here."

A few bites later, his tears diminished, Andy shoved the rest in his mouth. Eva placed him on a giant pillow on the floor in the den to watch his favorite video of singing vegetables. Back in the kitchen, she brewed a cup of tea and grilled two cheese sandwiches. After she fed Andy and put him to bed, she'd tweak the raid plan.

Eva called, "Andy, time to eat. Turn off the video like Kaley showed you."

Her cell phone rang.

"Eva here."

"Hey, boss. Five minutes ago, Judge Pendergast signed our warrants. First, I had to relive old war stories of trials gone by. He even brought up the time when the electricity went off and I testified using my pocket flashlight."

Eva rested on a stool. Whatever Griff endured to get the warrants signed, she was in no mood to hear it. "Are we set for Friday?"

"Yup. I need to talk with you about the townhouse. I want to—"

The connection lost in the elevator, static fizzled in her ear. Eva set down the phone and went to find Andy. He lay in front of the TV, struggling to breathe. Eva lifted up his shirt. Hives marched up and down his heaving chest. The scared look on Andy's face shook her. She could handle criminals, but not anything happening to Andy.

Eva called the pediatrician. A service answered, and the woman offered to page him. Eva had no choice. In her arms, Andy gasped for breath. The next few minutes felt like hours. She held him, placed a wet cloth on his forehead. The phone's sharp rings made her jump. Eva described Andy's symptoms to Doctor Udall.

He replied, "Last month when he was stung, his reaction was slight. This is worse. Toxins are building in his system and he's making excessive antibodies. Take him to the hospital."

"We're on our way."

Eva called Scott and left a message to meet them at the emergency room. She fastened Andy into his car seat, hoping he'd bear no scars from going to the hospital as she had when her appendix burst at age ten. The doctor misjudged what was wrong and Eva nearly died of the infection.

Out on the main road, she sped above the limit until traffic congealed like the middle of rush hour. Only it was eight o'clock at night. Stuck behind a slow truck loaded with appliances, Eva's heart raced. Unable to see around it, she looked in the side view mirror. Could she pass? No. The left lane was choked with traffic.

Eva's eyes glanced to the rearview mirror. Andy's eyes were closed, his breathing heavy. Ahead, she saw boxes of refrigerators. The truck sailed through the intersection. Eva glanced at the light. It was red! She slammed on her brakes. The rounded front of her Beetle stopped in the crosswalk.

Was God punishing her for lack of faith? Maybe he had forgotten her altogether. Then Eva remembered Grandpa's hug last Christmas. Warm lips kissing her cheek, he had said, "Eva Marie, our Lord loves you and is reaching out for you. Take his hand."

The light turned green. She sped away and turned left at the street to the hospital. A block away, an ambulance roared up behind her, its strobe lights flashing. She pulled to the curb, her heart in her throat. Eva uttered the closest thing to a prayer she had said in ages, "God, protect Andy. Please!"

Later that evening, Eva worried that Scott blamed her. In their bedroom sitting area, he sat in a chair next to her, drinking tea. She had not touched hers. At the hospital, Andy was given epinephrine and oxygen. Once his breathing normalized, the emergency room doctor allowed Eva to bring him home. He was now asleep in his bed. Scott was talking.

"Sorry I never checked my voicemail. Kaley and I were having fun."

Eva blinked. She turned toward her husband and looked full in his gray eyes. "The doctor prescribed an injection to give him next time."

As if he had not heard, Scott replied, "With the anniversary of September 11 tomorrow, you'd think Kaley's teacher would have them draw pictures. Instead she resorted to politics."

Eva said, "We stick it in his thigh," and shuddered at the thought of pricking Andy.

At the edge of his chair, a thatch of brown hair over his right eye, Scott grabbed her hand. "Do you think this wouldn't have happened if you and Andy went to church with us?"

She did.

His hand rested on hers. "Don't. Last week, Andy fell off a slide while I stood by helpless. He's a curious boy who gets hurt. Tomorrow, he'll be racing his scooter."

Eva shook her head. No matter what Scott said, she tucked this new guilt in a spot she reserved for such things, where she could take it out, inspect it when needed. Eva had double-decker guilt, and it was getting hard to find room in there.

Scott changed the subject. "Kaley loved the African children's choir. She wants to visit a girl she met from Kenya. Emile Jubayl, the CEO for Helpers International, showed a video of a village where people have no running water. I grabbed an envelope to send a check. Have we met him before?"

As the name, Emile Jubayl, echoed in Eva's head, she glanced at Scott. A tall filled-out man, he was a television reporter type. When they first met, his toothy grin let loose something wild within her. She had not been the same since.

Scott set down his mug. "He goes to our church."

"Oh. That's where I heard it. You decide about the check."

Eva yawned and Scott pulled her up. His lips brushed against her hair. "We'll talk about it after your case is done."

Secure in his arms, Eva slumped against his chest. She was going to sleep standing up! His hands on her shoulders, Scott guided her into the master bath, then he handed her a tooth brush with green paste.

"I don't deserve you," she whispered, before sticking the brush in her mouth.

Scott rinsed his mouth with water. "Remember how nice I am when SecDef testifies Friday and I have to work late."

Eva dropped her toothbrush. "I've thought about Jillie all day."

Scott cupped his hands around her face. "Remember what you told me after her funeral?"

Eva shut her eyes, as if that would squeeze out the pain. "Remind me."

Scott pulled her to him. "Knowing she had accepted Jesus as her savior, you were comforted by picturing her in heaven with him."

She had to accept the unspeakable. Jillie, who laughed with her, cried with her, was dead. Heaven was a long way off, if Eva ever got there.

"Quit worrying because I work at the Pentagon. It's safer now than ever. Besides, being a federal agent is riskier than being press secretary for Secretary Cabrini."

Her face on Scott's chest, Eva enjoyed the smell of his freshly laundered sleep shirt. Caught in her throat were words to explain Lou's accident, her sudden promotion and that their family time, the little there was, was shrinking.

Scott whispered, "What did Dr. Cole tell you today? Can he help us?"

Eva pushed back. A sick feeling crashed over her like a rogue wave. "You won't like it."

A steady, beautiful look in his eyes, he replied, "Whatever he said, we'll handle it together. We always do."

Eva rubbed her face as if to hide. "I didn't go. I forgot."

His reaction was swift. "You waited a month to see him. We agreed, when the obstetrician said you could not get pregnant unless you worked less, seeing a specialist was the right course. Don't you want another baby?"

Eva turned and left him alone with his anger. She collapsed on the bed, fighting tears that blurred her eyes. With all she had on her mind, to bring this up tonight was cruel. She was still young enough to have another baby. Next year.

Scott banged shut the closet door. His heavy footsteps carried him away, down the stairs. Eva's face fell into the pillow. Her fist hit the bed. It felt so good, she throttled it again. Her cry was like a sudden squall. When it was over, Eva wanted to talk with Scott or hold him. She waited for him to come back upstairs. Some minutes passed, and she figured he was holding a grudge. Eva's mind prodded her to go downstairs and explain everything. Well, everything but the vision she had had of Lou.

Yet words of peace remained locked inside, and Eva had misplaced the key. The timing was wrong. Scott would think she was making an excuse, which would fuel him to press the issue of the baby. With extra work tomorrow, she had no energy to stand her ground tonight.

Eva went to check on Andy. She opened the door to his room and saw him curled inside his race-car-shaped bed. He was a miniature Scott, all except for his periwinkle blue eyes. They were closed now, but when they were open, it was like looking into her own eyes. Eva straightened the blanket and pulled it up to his chin.

She kissed his wavy brown hair. "Stay well, Peanut. Mommy will protect you, always."

Eva found Kaley asleep. A night light was on next to the twin bed, and a small book rested on her tummy. Eva smiled. When she was Kaley's age, Eva also read late into the night. She picked up *Misty of Chincoteague*, closed it, and turned off the light. What had Scott said about Kaley and school? There was one way to find out.

Eva returned to their bedroom, threw a robe over her shoulders. She felt silly for arguing with Scott. Not an argument, a disagreement. Eva's habit of finding the precise word for each situation made Scott kid that she should have been a lawyer.

A light shone in their shared office. Eva sauntered in. Scott was not at his desk working on testimony for the hearing as she had supposed. A file was open, a pen was on it, but no Scott. Her heart skipped a beat. She felt a sudden chill. Putting her arms into the robe, Eva checked the first-floor bathroom. It was dark and empty. The hallway took her to the formal living room. She did not expect to find him in there. It was used mostly for entertaining distant relatives and friends from church. Scott wasn't in the kitchen either. Eva found his car keys on the shelf in the back hall. This search was getting ridiculous.

Like Grandpa Marty VanderGoes, Scott was a stable man. Her relationship with her parents was strained at times, but from Grandpa, she felt love and tenderness. In many ways, he and Scott were alike. Maybe that was what attracted her to Scott. Strong yet gentle, he was a lion who could care for a lamb.

Her husband must have had a good reason for whatever he was doing. He would not purposely hide to cause her pain. Eva opened the door to the walkout level, flipped on the light, and listened. She clung to the idea that Scott was watching the news, but no television sounds drifted up from the family room.

Eva rounded the bottom of the stairs. A small lamp was on. Scott was sprawled on the leather couch, all six-foot three-inches of him. His right arm dangled toward the floor. Scott's breathing was deep and rhythmic, which meant he wasn't faking to avoid talking to her.

When Eva knelt beside him, her knees bumped something hard. It was Scott's Bible, opened to Jeremiah 29. He had underlined one verse: "For I know the plans I have for you," declares the Lord, "plans to prosper you and not to harm you, plans to give you hope and a future."

She'd never seen that one before. Did the Lord truly have a plan for her life? Scott prayed and relied on God each day, but after Jillie died, Eva stopped trusting God. Eva watched Scott breathe. He lived on dry land, while she had drifted far from what she once believed. She was out in the storm, not in a lifeboat, but in the water, clinging to a piece of soggy wood. Her eyes filled with tears. Not for hurt feelings. For her soul, which was running on empty.

Eva placed a finger on Scott's open lips, tracing their fullness. Her lips found his. He moved but did not awaken.

She whispered in his ear, "It's me. I miss you."

His right eye peeked open. Large arms gathered her to him. There was nowhere else she wanted to be. And with what would happen tomorrow, Eva would look back on this innocent moment with Scott and wonder what more she could have done.

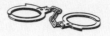

THREE

The next morning, Eva eased into the right-hand lane, one more person in the mass of humanity driving back to the office on the Baltimore-Washington Parkway. Traffic was at a near stand-still. She had been to see Lou by seven, but the visit was brief. He was partially awake, lying on his side after back surgery, and pleased she was running things in his absence, or so he nodded. It was his blessing. That was enough.

When she mentioned that Earl's affidavit was rejected by Pender-gast, Lou tried to roll over and sit up. She assured him Griff saved the day and the raid was on. Eva read Lou's file on Farouk Hamdi and was surprised at how thin it was. She had just asked Lou to connect the dots between Farouk and several calls to Paris when a nurse kicked her out of the room. Doctors' orders. Lou was not to talk about work for a few more days.

By then, she would have arrested and interrogated Farouk. Eva stifled a yawn, and blinked her eyes to moisten them. With less than five hours of sleep, it felt like sandpaper was scraping her eyes. The cell phone in the hands-free cradle beeped. It was 8:05 a.m. Probably Griff, wondering why she was late for the conference she had insisted upon to complete tomorrow's raid plans. In this traffic, she wouldn't get to her Virginia office for another hour. Eva could not have been more wrong about who was calling and why.

"Do you have your radio on?"

The anxious tone in Scott's voice sent fear coursing through her body. Eva gripped the wheel to stay in her lane, and kept her voice steady as she said, "No, I'm on my way back from Johns Hopkins. I'm stuck in traffic and I don't know anything."

His voice grew fainter as she heard him say, "Yes, Kaley, it's Mom-my." He returned to her and whispered, "Bombs have gone off all over the world. Hundreds are wounded. Not sure how many deaths. So far, none here."

"No! What happened?"

"Hebrew University is smashed. A nightclub collapsed in Australia. Suicide bombers hit both the British and American Embassies in Moscow."

Anger burned out any remnants of her fear. There would be no end to El Samoud's madness until they stopped his financial support.

"I heard you talk to Kaley."

"We're almost to her school. After I dropped off Andy, I turned on the car radio and learned what happened."

With the anniversary of September 11 just beginning in the U.S., terrorists still had time to attack here. What if they stormed a school as they had in Russia? Should Scott go home with the kids?

"Eva, " Scott said quietly, "What should we do?"

"Have you talked to Secretary Cabrini?"

"I called you first."

"Try to reach him and call me."

A car slammed on its brakes in front of her. She applied hers, missing a collision by inches.

Scott must have heard her yell out because he added, "Are you all right?"

Eva had to think. So much was at stake. By now, other drivers must have heard the news and were forgetting how to drive. There was an exit. Thankfully she was in the right lane. A minute later, her heart racing, she pulled the G-car into a hotel parking lot.

"Talk to your boss, Scott. I'll try to do the same. Call back to me in two minutes." Eva punched in the number for Headquarters. No answer. *Great!* She pressed in the number for Alexia Kyros. Eva could always count on Alexia. She answered after the first ring.

Alexia said, "The Attorney General will speak to all U.S. Attorneys by conference call at 9:00 a.m. Where will you be? I'll call you back after that."

Eva had no idea where she would be. She gave Alexia her cell number and hung up. Her phone beeped. It was Scott.

"I'm at Kaley's school. I will talk to the teacher and see if school is canceled. I reached Cabrini. He wants me in the office an hour ago."

Eva said, "I'm not to the District yet. I'll think of something. And Scott, please be careful at the Pentagon." She did not have to tell him why she was scared. They both knew what could happen today.

When Eva finally reached the office, she surveyed her building as she drove into the parking ramp at the rear. This morning she was thankful that the single story building was nondescript. Built twenty years ago to accommodate small offices in Falls Church, a busy suburb of northern Virginia, Alexia had leased it for the task forces and had gotten a bargain. The building's brick front looked like any other office building, and no signs identified the occupants, several federal task forces, including FIG.

The front entrance was locked, and visitors who were recognized on a security monitor were buzzed in. The sole rear entrance accessed a corridor that ran along the rear of the building and held separate entrances for FIG, the DEA task force, with whom Eva never dealt, the FBI terrorism task force run by Ari Rosen, whom Eva met once, and the FBI Technical Operation Group, where Griff used to work. Eva had talked with the Tech Ops supervisor, Gus Grant, in the corridor a couple of times, but she had yet to work with him. Eva now had a better idea of their activities, since Griff told of his exploits with things electronic. It also explained the cable television utility van she sometimes found parked next to her G-car. She had seen its driver, wearing a tool belt, walk in to the building and disappear into the Tech Ops office down the corridor from hers.

Before Eva got out of her car, she called her mother. With the terror alert raised, she and Scott needed help with the kids. Her folks were going to the dentist. Eva had another idea.

Ready to make her next call, she felt a cautious confidence there would be no major terror acts on the homeland. It was such a secret, she dared not mention it to Scott on their cell phones. She wanted to tell him that months before, workers who had been pouring footings for the new World Trade Center Memorial had made a gruesome discovery.

The dirt beneath their forms had been disturbed during the previous night. The foreman was suspicious and searched until he found strategically placed explosives with timers set for today's anniversary dedication. The explosives were removed. When agents learned the timing devices had been shipped as replacement parts to a Grilled Onion restaurant, the FBI scoured Eva's money laundering files for connections to ARC.

For security reasons, the incident had to be kept quiet. If ARC knew their bomb was found, they'd plant another one someplace else. A shudder pricked Eva's skin under her jacket. She wondered how many of ARC's bombers would be *eliminated* after today's bombs failed to detonate.

A knock at her car window startled her. Eva turned sharply. Griff motioned for her to lower the window.

"Nice to see you made it while the world is falling apart around us." His smile conveyed he meant it.

"Are you coming or going?" she asked.

His smile vanished. "Going, to see my friend at the FBI's Washington field office. I'll stay as long as you need me."

Eva turned off the engine, plucked her cell from its holder, and slung her long legs out the door. "Maybe we should execute our warrants today. Farouk might be planning something big, in an hour, in five minutes. Tomorrow may be too late."

"You're right." Griff replied. He ran his key card through the reader, opened the back door, and held it ajar for his former partner.

Eva walked ahead of him up the few stairs and into the FIG office. She opened the inner door in time to hear Wanda say into the telephone, "Your new boss is not going to like it."

Her hair more aflame than yesterday, Wanda set the phone down with a thump.

Eva stopped at her desk. "Lou's on his way to recovery. He said to tell you hello."

Stress lines eased from Wanda's face, giving her a younger look. "Did he get my flowers? I sent a basket of orange mums."

No doubt a perfect match to her hair color. Eva kept this thought to herself and said, "Call everyone on the intercom, Wanda, to meet at Lou's conference table in five minutes."

Wanda's face scrunched up like she was eating sour candy. "Earl just called. His car won't start. It was towed to the dealership."

Eva looked up at Griff and her shoulders slumped. If they were going to pull off executing the warrants today, everyone needed to be in place.

A step ahead of her, Griff said, "Trenton is looking for something to do."

Eva replied, "Tell your new partner to get Earl and be back by ten. No detours for donuts."

She stalked to her office, flopped in the hard chair, and called Grandpa Marty. There was no answer. Finally, at five minutes to ten, she reached him. He had been developing black and white photos for a book he was writing on the Dutch resistance in World War II.

Eva said into the phone, "I was calling to see if you could pick up Andy and Kaley from school today. Make us a batch of your famous vegetable soup. With the terror attacks, Scott and I are swamped. Mom and Dad are at the dentist."

"Eva Marie." He always used her full name. "What attacks?"

She told him of ARC's mayhem around the world. Marty assured her that he'd pick up the children from school. After telling him she would notify the school, Eva hung up the phone, comforted after talking with her grandfather. Having lived through the reign of Nazi terror, Grandpa never shrank from duty, then or now. She hoped she had a fraction of his courage.

It was Friday, 5:20 a.m. They had not executed the raid a day early. Too many loose ends. Under the guise of taking a poll about breakfast food, Griff called Farouk, who confirmed he was the homeowner. Griff put surveillance on him, and was sure Farouk remained in his townhouse all day Thursday. Not a single act of terrorism occurred on American soil. But Eva knew better than to feel at ease. ARC could attack anytime, anywhere. She needed to be ready.

The night before, Grandpa had concocted a soup with white beans, squash, and corn, which tasted wonderful. He played board games with the kids while Eva and Scott finished paperwork in the office. Scott finished telling Eva what he had started to say the day before about Kaley's school assignments. Kaley's teacher had the class write an essay about why the terrorists hated Americans enough to attack them on September 11, 2001. Kaley wrote that her mother and father worked for the government and she had no idea why people should hate America. The teacher berated her in front of the class and told her to try again!

At bedtime, Kaley had complained her throat hurt. She didn't want to go to school. That was okay, Grandpa said. He'd stay as long as they needed him. Eva was furious. When the raid was over, she'd call the teacher and the principal and blast them. Couldn't the teacher understand that some children felt so close to the terror that they couldn't detach themselves to write an essay about it?

Eva was functioning on less sleep than the night before, not ideal for the dangerous mission that lay before her. Forcing Kaley's teacher from her mind, she clutched the raid operations plan like a paper fan. Eva flattened it on her desk and made her assignments.

Outside her door, Trenton was talking to Griff. "My dad retired from the FBI after thirty-two years."

Eva pushed her chair back from her desk and walked to the door to shush them when Griff said, "Don't think you can ride on your dad's coattails here. You need to make your own bones. I've been in the Bureau more than thirteen years. Who is your dad anyway?"

Trenton's chin lifted. "Everyone calls him Duke. He was firearms instructor at Quantico."

"Your dad is the Duke Nash of flight 476 fame?" Griff drew his massive eyebrows together in a fierce frown. He glanced at Eva. "Unbelievable!"

Considered handsome by more than one young woman, Trenton flashed a smile that lit his pleasant features.

Her interest piqued, Eva swallowed a reproof. "Who is Duke?"

Griff raised his left eyebrow and shot Eva a bemused look. "An FBI legend. In 1991, a terrorist hijacked a domestic flight and ordered the pilot to fly to Egypt. The pilot convinced him to land and get fuel for the international flight."

Eva said, "There was a flight highjacked from Dulles when I was a new customs agent."

Griff's eyebrows relaxed. "Same one. In exchange for fuel and food, FBI hostage negotiators cajoled the hijacker to release a sick man and pregnant woman. That's when Duke made his famous move. He dressed like a catering truck driver and elevated the food compartment."

Eva checked her watch. "Griff, are the packets ready?"

He pointed to a group of agents talking by the coffeepot. "All team leaders have them. Trenton, didn't the hijacker have a knife to the pilot's throat?"

Before Trenton answered, Eva saw agents and officers filling the conference room and said, "We need to start the preraid briefing."

"Eva," Griff used his hands for dramatic effect, "don't you want to know what happened?" His errant eyebrow shot up his forehead. "After all, Duke is an inspiration for your new team."

Eva narrowed her eyes at Griff. Was he mocking her? She knew him well enough to know malice lived nowhere in his body. He was trying to take her mind off what lay only minutes ahead.

"All right. Make it short."

Griff slapped Trenton's back. "The terrorist let the old man and woman get on the lift. Duke rolled the food carts into the galley. With one shot to the head, he killed the guy. The pilot wasn't scratched."

Eva thrust the operations plan into Trenton's hands. "Sounds like you have a legacy to uphold. Start by making ten copies of this for me."

He shrugged and started to walk away.

Respect for Duke obvious in his tone, Griff called after him, "Your dad gave me shooting pointers some years back. At Quantico."

Eva headed back to her desk. Griff followed her and asked, "Got a minute?"

With the background of murmurs and metal chairs scraping against the floor in the next room, she said, "One."

"I watched Farouk's place last night. To get an idea of escape routes and—"

"Your point is?" Blood pounded against her temples like a bongo drum.

Griff shook his finger at her and laughed. "You're boss for two days and already you're ordering your old partner around. Be careful or I might transfer to the FBI Terrorism Task Force."

Eva did not see humor in the pretend threat. "And if you don't spill what's eating you, I'll assign you to do all post-op reports."

Griff grimaced. "Ouch. Anything but that." He grew serious. "Around eleven, a gray Dulles airport cab drove up and idled in the street. I nearly had a heart attack, thinking Farouk heard about the raid and was about to flee the country."

"You let him get away?"

"Listen! A petite, dark-haired woman climbed in the cab, not Farouk. From where I was parked, I couldn't see her face. She carried a purse over her shoulder. I memorized the cab number, but haven't been able to reach anyone at the cab company. Who is she?"

When Eva shook her head, wisps of hair broke free from her pony tail. "I have no idea. Sister. Mother. Girlfriend. Maybe we'll find out today. Time to roll."

She scrawled a note to call her grandfather when the raid was over and check on Kaley. Beside her calendar, a paperweight rested atop urgent reports she'd had no time to read. Eva touched the clear cube with a miniature building inside that she found in a box from Jillie's apartment. It now had a home on her desk.

Her throat tightened as she remembered her sister's words that last weekend at dinner with their parents, "Eva, I always wanted to be a federal agent, but I took that turn after college to the prosecutor's office. You're a better agent than I could ever be."

Eva had laughed off the compliment. "You were born a lawyer, always reasoning with me when I wanted my own way. You love defending the soldier everyone thinks is guilty and finding evidence to prove your client's innocence!"

The alarm on Eva's watch chirped. It was five thirty. She had to leave behind past hurts and take command. Yesterday, Headquarters had sent a memo advising that she was temporarily in charge of FIG. Her fingertip lingered on the cube and she whispered, "This one's for you Jillie."

Eva addressed the entire FIG task force and ten additional FBI and ICE agents that would execute Operation Money Change. "Team leaders, take out arrest photos and search warrants."

When the rustle of opening envelopes quieted down, she continued, "I have divided you into four teams. Per your assignments, you will enter four different residences in northern Virginia at 7 a.m. At the same time, ICE agents in Detroit and Miami will conduct their own raids. German authorities struck a related cell in Hamburg this morning."

Eva raised her voice above the escalating whispers. "Today we arrest Farouk Hamdi. He masquerades as franchise director for the Grilled Onion, but he really launders money for the Armed Revolutionary Cause. In league with Al Qaeda, ARC's goal is to destabilize the West. El Samoud seeks to disrupt the world's financial markets and diminish Western influence in key Middle Eastern countries. We must shut down his funding."

Eva walked closer to her group. "The Attorney General sent a memo to all supervisors. Be alert for evidence of sleeper cells. Seize cash and weapons. Look for notes, documents, and names and addresses. Yesterday, terrorists were arrested in Britain because their names were found in a terrorist camp in Yemen. Take bank records, computer discs, and backup drives."

Eva paused and surveyed. She wanted them to feel her passion to catch these guys, but a few words of caution were needed.

"Do everything by the book. Our lawyers worked hard to ensure we accomplish our mission without violating civil rights."

Sounds of groaning prompted her to hold up her hand. "The days when federal agents used to wait at a donut shop for a junior agent to arrive with a search warrant, wet with the judge's signature, are gone. There are too many civil suits for crashing in the wrong door or shooting a suspect's babysitter. We now file operational plans for approval and," Eva paused, "The Attorney General is following this case with extreme interest."

Griff let out a low whistle, which set the entire group talking.

Eva clapped her hands for quiet. "Wear your body armor. Some subjects may be armed. Any questions?"

No hands went up. Good. Eva wanted to deliver for the Attorney General and live up to Jillie's words of praise.

Trenton raised his hand. "Do we bust everyone? Even if they're not on the list?"

"And charge them with what?" Griff asked.

Trenton smiled. "My dad used to charge 'em with mopery with intent to gawk."

Familiar with that old joke, the group burst out laughing.

Eva's blue eyes became slits. "Get your laughs out now. In two minutes, it's serious business."

The chuckles subsided.

Eva said, "If you find persons for whom we have no warrants, check with me to see if there is any basis to hold them. No information will be released until indictments and search warrants are unsealed, so don't talk to the media. Be safe out there, and remember we're the good guys."

Leaving the conference room, Eva pulled her ICE raid jacket over her bulletproof vest. All of FIG's agents and police officers wore the same dark blue jacket with POLICE in white on the back.

Eva said, "My cell is on."

Trenton picked up a short-barreled shotgun from his desk and headed for the exit.

"Wait!" Griff barked. "Where you going with that?"

"You said I'm entering from the rear."

"No, you're *covering* the rear. No way we're entering from opposite ends. We'd end up shooting each other."

Trenton looked sheepish. He returned the shot gun to his desk.

Griff nudged him toward the rear office exit, and Trenton shrugged. "You're the senior partner. Can I at least drive to the raid?"

Wanda called after him, "Tough to be a rookie again, isn't it Trenton?"

Eva saw a cloud sweep across Trenton's boyish face, then disappear. His angst was understandable; Wanda exercised her mouth on the fly. Last week, when Eva banged her ankle against her metal desk and cried out, Wanda shouted for the whole office to hear, "Have you always been such a klutz?"

In the parking lot Eva checked her Glock and adjusted her bulletproof vest. She climbed in and started her car. In charge of her first raid, details pulsed through her mind at the speed of light. Who was the woman in the cab? Was Eva prepared for the unknown?

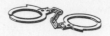

FOUR

Trenton leapt out of Griff's G-car saying, "Let's go!" and slammed the door with a thud.

Already out of her car parked on the street beside Farouk Hamdi's end unit townhouse, Eva hissed, "Quiet. The last thing we need is for these guys to get a head start or a TV news team with a copter circling overhead."

Griff opened his trunk and removed a 4-foot-long steel battering ram with handles on both sides. Trenton was by his side offering to help. Griff shook his head, then stalked up the sidewalk without his new partner.

Eva pointed to the rear and whispered Trenton, "After you hear the all-clear, come around to the front door."

Griff's surveillance had revealed a rear exit and two windows for Trenton to cover. She watched him disappear behind a clump of ornamental bushes. Robbie parked his car behind Griff's, and he and Earl joined Eva on the sidewalk. Confident she had done all to ensure success, Eva motioned for them to follow her. She jogged past Griff and was the first to reach the front door. She pounded her fist on the solid wood and yelled, "Federal Agents! Search Warrant! Open Up!"

Court rulings made them wait a reasonable period before forcing entry. One man's "reasonable" is another man's eternity. After what seemed to Eva like almost a minute, but would be argued by a defense attorney was seconds, there was no response. She grabbed one side of the ram, Griff the other, and with great force thrust it into the door jam.

Metal crashed, wood splintered, and glass shattered. They were in! Eva released the ram, drew her Glock from her shoulder holster, and led Griff, Robbie, and Earl into the dark townhouse. The strange atmosphere was unlike any home she'd spent time in. Stale air hung in the rooms. Dusty blinds shut out early fingers of dawn. Was Farouk inside, waiting with a weapon to blast them? With her free hand, Eva flipped on a light switch in the hall, which brought the sound of footsteps.

Griff shouted, "Federal Agents! Search Warrant!"

Before going down a narrow hallway, Eva angled her gun toward the ceiling, to avoid accidentally shooting one of her own. She stepped over crumpled newspapers and empty boxes toward the sound of footsteps. Her heart raced. Not knowing what lay ahead, her breath came in short bursts. This was no practice range. Danger was real. Uncertainty demanded she be careful. Shots could zing from anywhere, at any moment.

Then she saw him. An unshaven man clad in briefs ran toward the bathroom.

"Freeze!" Eva yelled.

He stopped.

"Down on the floor!"

The bald man crumpled like a paper airplane thrown with too much force. Eva pointed her gun at her prone prisoner and motioned for Earl, who was coming from the hall bedroom, to cuff him. Griff ran by, and she followed him down the hall to the back bedroom. He kicked open the door. An olive-skinned man with tangled, bushy brown hair, wearing boxers and a Washington Redskins jersey, sat on the edge of a bed rubbing his eyes, as though just awakened.

"FBI! Hands above your head," ordered Griff.

Eva was relieved to see the man raise his hands above his head. To make sure he stayed that way, she pointed her Glock at him. Griff wasted no time grabbing his arms, shoving them behind his back, and tightly securing his wrists in handcuffs.

Eva said, "Take him to the living room. I'll check the other bedroom."

She walked out of the rear bedroom behind Griff and their second prisoner. So far, they had found no weapons, but others might be armed and lurking about. Robbie, the Virginia State trooper, shouted, "Bathroom clear."

In the second bedroom a light was on. Earl must have checked it already. A computer sat on the floor, but it wasn't turned on. A double mattress, with no sheets or blankets, was pushed against the wall. She swung open the closet door, turned on the light, and peered inside. It was crammed with junk, and clothes hung from a pole on each side.

In a loud voice, Eva called, on her way out, "Second bedroom is clear!"

In the living room, the bushy-haired guy in the Redskins jersey dangled on the edge of the sofa as if any moment he'd fall off.

Griff read his Miranda rights, then asked, "Understand your rights?"

"No English." The man pushed his chin down into his neck.

Griff read the card again. "You watch too many movies. Everything I see in this place is in English."

"No English!" he repeated, shaking his curly head.

Eva stepped closer and was about to take the handcuffed prisoner outside, when Trenton rushed into the living room.

Eva motioned him over and whispered, "Have Earl check the computer in the hall bedroom."

Instead, Trenton looked at the cuffed prisoner, who glared at Griff, then leaned down and got right in his face, "Farouk, you understand English."

At the sound of his name, the man turned angry eyes to Eva, but remained silent. She saw there was something odd about his eyes. They didn't match. One was the color of a foaming ocean, deep blue with white flecks. The other was light brown, the color of ground cumin.

Trenton raised himself up to his full five-foot eight-inches and said, "Remember me? Last week, you sat next to me on a British Air flight from London. You spoke English then. I doubt you forgot how. If I were you, I wouldn't mess with Griff. He holds your future in his hands."

"Trenton, what—"

Before Griff finished his question, Eva pulled Trenton toward the messy kitchen. Among stacks of dirty dishes, she grilled, "Do you know him? What about a flight from London?"

"Hold on a second," said Trenton.

He came right back with a brown leather valise. "I wanted him to know I was on to him. His ticket to London is in here." Trenton swept wrappers and paper plates from the counter and opened this case.

As if telling an adventure story, he continued, "I was out back, ready for anything. You won't believe what happened! When you crashed in the front door, the rear bedroom window opened. I waited for someone to climb out. To arrest him."

Trenton crouched, demonstrating. "I coiled, aimed my gun. A hand appeared out the window, holding this case. Next thing I know,

it's dropped by my feet. I had enough light to see a blur of bushy hair."
Trenton cocked his head toward the man in the living room. "*His* hair.
Then he shut the window!"

"Did you open this case before now?" Eva wondered if the search
warrant would cover evidence found outside the house.

Trenton nodded. "Lucky for me it didn't explode. That guy playing dumb is Farouk Hamdi. Here's his U.S. passport. You get under
that mop of hair and this photo matches the guy out there playing
laser eye tag with Griff."

Eva's fingers flew through the valise. She found a handheld computer, a wad of one hundred dollar bills, and a used British Airway
ticket from London to Washington in the name of Farouk Hamdi.
She brought the photo to her face. There was no doubt. The mis-
matched eyes were the same. "He must be a chameleon. In the picture
I saw, he looked like a businessman."

Eva put the items back in the case and closed it. They had an arrest warrant for Farouk; she could keep him in custody.

"Good work. Put the valise in Griff's trunk to maintain chain of
custody. And in the future, do *as* I say, *when* I say. Okay?"

Trenton blinked hard.

Not wanting to get off to a bad start with him, Eva added, "After
that, search Farouk's room for any evidence he *forgot* to throw out the
window."

"Great!"

Trenton got Griff's keys and left with the valise under one arm.
Eva returned to the living room, where Griff and Farouk argued.

When he saw Eva, Farouk raised his voice and spat in English,
tinged with a British accent. "You'll see. You made a huge mistake."

Griff was about to reply when Eva said, "Forget him. After a week
in county lockup, he'll change his attitude. Their vegetable loaf is a gut
burner. Did we ID the bald guy I stopped in the hall?"

"He's a fugitive from Detroit. Earl's taking him to the office to be
interrogated."

She gestured toward the hall bedroom. "Did you check the computer in there?"

Griff moved several paces away from Farouk but kept an eye on
him. "I thought *you* searched it. You gave the all clear."

Without a word, Eva went back to the hall bedroom to search it.

Back in the bedroom, Eva unplugged the computer. She pulled open drawers, dumped the contents on the floor, and sorted through crumpled socks, computer CDs, and Arabic pamphlets. These last two she shoved in an evidence bag to be analyzed by an interpreter. Certain magazines, which Eva hoped weren't sold in stores where children saw them, she threw down in disgust. She yanked open a nightstand drawer and searched through the usual sleep aids but uncovered nothing incriminating. The pile of evidence paled next to the discard heap in the middle of the floor.

Eva opened the closet door. The light was still on. Mounds of shoes and garments littered the floor. As she patted down clothes on hangers looking for weapons, her fingers bumped something hard. Eva thrust her hand into the pocket of a leather jacket. Before she found out what it was, someone grabbed her arm!

Eva pulled back, but whoever had her arm pulled her head first into a rack of clothes. A blow to her stomach forced air from her lungs. Eva stumbled backwards. She tried, but she couldn't get her balance or reach her gun. Her feet twisted in the clothes on the floor and she fell, striking her forehead on the nightstand.

Pain rocked her stomach, seared through her head. As she struggled to rise, she glimpsed a man the size of an NFL lineman bolt out the bedroom door, his features nothing but a dark veil.

Eva opened her mouth to yell a warning. None came! Her lungs were stripped of air. She staggered down the hall, to the living room. She sat on the now empty couch and gulped air. Where were Griff and Farouk? And the man who attacked her?

Eva groped for the open front door and almost bashed into Trenton walking up the steps. "Where'd he go?"

"Your face is a mess! What happened?"

Eva heaved a one-word sigh. "Ambushed."

"What?"

Her hands shook as she pushed strands of hair from her eyes, which amplified the pain in her head. She looked at her hand. Fresh blood streaked her palm. Did she let an unknown assailant escape? Eva blew out a blast of air, relieved that her lungs worked again, and said, "We need Griff."

He was in the kitchen with Farouk, who sat on a grimy plastic chair by a table, hands cuffed behind him and a defiant tilt to his jaw. The sight of him there, daring her to mess with him, drove anger deep into her chest. She thumped her hand on the gritty table. Dirty dishes rattled, but he sat unmoved. Eva bent toward him, her eyes locked onto his.

"Who was the guy in the second bedroom?"

Griff glanced at Trenton, who shrugged, and asked "What guy?"

Farouk dangled his bare foot dangerously close to hers. An ugly thought sprouted in her mind. Eva wanted so badly to kick it. By accident of course. Eva bit down that bitter seed but was determined to make Farouk talk. Somehow.

Eva pounded the table again. "I want his name!"

Farouk motioned toward Griff with his shoulder and said simply, "That big guy said I don't have to talk. My right to remain silent."

At that moment, Robbie appeared carrying a laundry hamper filled with clothes. "I'm checking the pockets," he announced.

Eva touched the gash on her head. Fresh blood stained her finger. She needed to stop the flow.

Griff said, "Trenton, Robbie, keep an eye on Farouk. We'll be back."

He guided Eva out of the kitchen and through the back door. In the open, his questions came fast and furious. "Your head's bleeding. What guy are you talking about?"

The cool morning air soothed her hot cheeks. "Ever been run over by a charging bull? He—I don't know who—caught me by surprise and tried to kill me. He came out of the closet in the bedroom. I assume he ran out the front door. Trenton was by my car, but apparently he saw nothing. The guy disappeared."

Griff lowered his voice. "Tell me everything, quickly. We'll put out an alert."

Eva shook her head. *And say what?* Because of her negligence, a suspected terrorist was on the run, and she had no idea where or who he was. It was painful, but she told Griff the truth. She had said "all clear" earlier without checking the closet thoroughly. When she went back in, one minute her hands were in a pocket of a leather jacket, and the next thing she knew she was fighting to survive.

Griff moved fast, back into the house. "Wash off that blood. I'll ask Robbie to help you identify Charging Bull and convince Farouk to rethink his silence."

In a hall closet, Eva found a box of tissues wedged among old newspapers. Without stopping to look at those, she pulled out the last tissue and pressed it hard against her forehead. When the empty box fell to the floor, she kicked it down the hall. Back in the bedroom, her foot gave witness to internal roaring anger as she savaged the clothespile until it was spread over the floor. Eva charged into the closet, hoping to find something to identify the guy. If she'd seen his face, a police artist could sketch his likeness.

She pulled the tissue away from her forehead. The blood seemed to have ebbed. A new thought struck her. Someone else might be in the closet! Eva's hand crept to her Glock. She lowered her head below the line of clothes. She saw no legs sticking out, no moving feet. At the sounds of scraping metal, she pulled her head out of the closet. Robbie was sitting cross-legged on the floor, firing up the computer.

He said, "Maybe I'll find a lead to our escapee."

Eva liked how he said "our" instead of "your." "Robbie, find the CDs. They're on the floor somewhere."

Back in the closet, Eva patted the clothes until her fingers rested on that leather jacket. From the pockets, she pulled out two U.S. passports. One was made out to "Drury Baptiste," born July 30, 1958. His thin face had a sloping jaw and brown eyes. The other was a passport for "Richard Salem," born October 1, 1956. She compared the photos. Richard had a trimmed goatee instead of being cleanshaven. They were different men.

Eva was about to slide them in an evidence envelope when she looked again and realized that the eyes in both photos were identical. The left iris was not round, but shaped like the hull of a ship, and the brown bled into the white of the eye. Something that unusual could help identify him. She passed Robbie, deep into computer lingo, and returned to the kitchen.

Griff grumbled to Trenton, "Take this scumbag to the Alexandria City Jail. They have a contract to house federal prisoners arrested in northern Virginia."

Trenton lowered his voice. "Do I give him pants or does he go as is?"

Griff pulled him aside. "As is. When you get to the jail, tell him you have his pants. He'll believe you're his best friend."

Countering Griff's order, Eva instructed Trenton, "I want to talk to Farouk. Bring him to the office first."

Eva pressed her forehead with the palm of her hand to cover her wound and turned toward Farouk. Using a gentler tack, she said calmy, "You're under arrest for aiding terrorists. Agent Topping read your rights. You do not have to talk with us. Deputy Nash will take you to our office. If you tell us what we need to know, it may go easier for you in the long run."

Farouk swept his tongue over his lips.

Eva flipped open each of the passports and showed them to Farouk. "Is either of these the guy who was hiding in your closet?"

Farouk stared at her, lips puckered on his unshaven face. Eva thought he might say something to help them launch an alert. Instead, he spit at her feet. A glistening gob ran down the reinforced toe of Eva's black boot.

Her blue eyes burned but she did not retreat one inch. "Big mistake. They say the early bird gets the worm. One of your associates will talk first, making you the worm. Say hello to more prison time."

Eva grabbed Farouk's cuffed arm, raised him to his feet, and pushed him toward Trenton. "Take him straight to jail. Book him."

Trenton hauled Farouk outside.

Robbie ran into the kitchen, a disk in his hand. He slapped it on the counter. "This has a map of the Pentagon and a document marked "Classified." It's called, 'Risk Assessment for Fort McNair." He opened some crumpled paper. "I found these in the bathroom wastebasket: a contract for a Grilled Onion franchise, a list of cities and names, a passport photo receipt for 'Drury,' one of the names on the passport, and a slip of paper. It's got the name 'Zayed' next to a New York City number that appears to be for a pay phone."

Eva wondered, *Who is Zayed?*

Griff tapped Robbie on the shoulder. "Put those in an evidence envelope to check for fingerprints, besides yours."

Robbie dropped them and went for an envelope. Eva set the search warrant on the counter and said, "Griff, list the items seized on the back of the warrant. Then we'll secure the front door and get out of here. This place gives me the creeps."

After leaving a copy of the search warrant as required by law, and recording the messages on Farouk's answering machine, Eva held a two-by-four, while Griff nailed it across the inside of the front door. With the remaining evidence secured in Eva's trunk, she, Griff, and Robbie left the townhouse through the rear door. A petite woman clad in a tan trenchcoat rounded the corner of the condo, pen and pad in hand. Next to her, a man with a TV camera walked slowly.

"I'm Mary Katherine Kowicki of Channel 14. Call me Kat. We received a tip that a terrorist raid went on here. For the record, who are you and what are you doing?"

Griff brushed past them without so much as a grunt.

Undeterred, the reporter shoved a microphone in Eva's face. "Were these terrorists going to attack America?"

Eva blocked her face before the cameraman could get her on film.

As Eva strode away from the nosy reporter and cameraman, she said, "No comment. Any warrants are sealed by the court."

Her cell phone rang. She debated if she should answer it but clicked it on. "Eva Montanna." Too late, Eva realized she had given the reporter her name.

It was Scott. "Honey, I can't talk now," she whispered. "I'm finishing the raid. There's a reporter here."

"I'm going to be stuck at the office tonight. Can you pick up the kids?"

Eva had reached her car. She checked her watch. "I'll be there. I have to go," Eva said, then clicked off her phone.

Kat had crept up behind her. "Ms. Montanna, won't you tell me what you're doing?"

For a moment, Eva forgot she was being filmed. She turned and advanced on Kat and demanded, "How did you find out we were here?"

With a microphone protecting her nose from Eva, Kat repeated, "From a confidential source."

Eva retreated, opened her car door and said, "Then I suggest you ask your source."

As she pulled away from the curb, Eva mentally reviewed the morning's activities. Raids always involved the unexpected. Today was no exception. Besides the target, Farouk Hamdi, a surprise fugitive was arrested. Plus, an unexpected and still unknown closet dweller had escaped, leaving Eva and her team with dots to be connected and bags of evidence to be reviewed before she would know the level of success of Operation Money Changer.

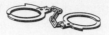

FIVE

The next morning a soft rain fell. After they had all eaten Grandpa Marty's thin Dutch pancakes for breakfast, Kaley and Andy watched the *Sound of Music* with him. Eva and Scott went to their shared office, where they read the newspaper. At least, Eva's eyes were on the print.

But her mind was on the man who got away from Farouk's townhouse. As for the mystery woman, the cab company told Griff the Pakistani cabbie dropped off a woman at Dulles Airport. He did not remember which airline. Trenton badgered Eva to meet with Farouk. Call it pride, but Eva told herself it was best to let him stew another day.

Her mind drifted to the worldwide bombings. "I can't figure it out," she broke the silence. "When those construction guys found that bomb under the World Trade Center Memorial … " Eva's voice trailed off.

She looked over at Scott. He had turned in his chair and was staring at her.

"You *knew* about that? It was a closely held secret," he said.

Eva's eyes widened. Even mentioning it could be a problem. But, with Scott's spoken revelation hanging there, would it hurt to confirm what he already knew?

She nodded her head. "How'd you find out?"

Scott edged his chair over the plastic covering on the carpet and grabbed her hand. "Our jobs intersect, and we're not allowed to know it. When I called you on your cell on Thursday with bombs exploding around the world, I wanted to reassure you that one had been dismantled in New York earlier. To admit that on a cell—"

Eva got out of her chair, sat on Scott's lap, and placed her head on his chest. He held her to him.

She said, "So did I! But we shouldn't talk about it. You never told me how your hearing went yesterday."

"Secretary Cabrini was on the hot seat for proposed budget cuts. You know how it goes. One group lobbies to purchase more F-22s, while another wants the Osprey to take precedence. It got ugly at one point. But the Secretary has no axes to grind, and I can say the rumors he's about to retire are greatly exaggerated."

Eva touched his face with the fingers. "Why is life so hard? I wish we'd plan a vacation and go!"

Scott wriggled underneath her.

"I'm too heavy." Eva rose, but he pulled her back to him.

"My knee's stiff is all. You are not too heavy and should eat more. At breakfast, you barely touched your pancakes."

Eva rolled her eyes. She leaned over and moved the shade back from the window. The driveway looked dry. The rain must have stopped. "Let's go for a walk with the kids. They love to pick up acorns and look for rabbits."

Scott stayed put. Eva slid from his lap. "Come on, big guy. It'll be fun. We'll pretend our lives are normal for a change. Forget bombs, terrorists, and not having enough money to fight the war on terror."

Scott rose slowly, holding onto his wife's hand. "I'll get some apples from the fridge."

"That's the spirit. Maybe we can take Kaley and Andy to Florida over Christmas break. See dolphins, swim in the ocean."

Eva led Scott by the hand out their office door.

"Not so fast." He grabbed her around the waist, and tickled her ribs. As she ran from his searching fingers, Eva laughed aloud. It was silly but felt good. Scott found her easily and tickled her some more.

Andy bounded up the stairs. Breathless, he jumped up and down around their legs. "Daddy, Mommy! Let me play, too!"

Scott picked up his son, whirled him above his head, then down again, like he was a human airplane. Moments later, in the midst of Andy's giggles, Kaley and Marty joined in the fun.

Marty watched Eva chase Kaley through the living room, until they collapsed on the sofa. With moist eyes, Marty whispered to Eva, "To see you and your family safe and happy gives me great joy. It's an answer to many prayers."

Her hands against his bony back, Eva hugged him hard. *He prays for us.* A feeling of wonder crept into her heart. Days ago, she reached out to her Grandfather for help, to watch the kids, make his special soup. Marty had come and stayed. More than his hands and presence, Eva saw how much they needed his unconditional love.

Church was over. Above Eva's head, rays of sun streamed through the stained-glass window, and she relished the vibrant yellow light. For the second time that weekend, she felt a snippet of happiness. The first was yesterday morning, on their walk, when she and Scott held hands. Andy found a hawk's tail feather. They planned a trip to Florida over Christmas. Kaley wanted to collect seashells on the beach with her great-grandpa. He'd come, too, of course. Not once had she agonized over the terrorist who got away.

That is, until she went to the FIG office Saturday afternoon and made herself write reports on the incident. Operation Money Changer was a success. Except for her mistake. Eva ran the names on the passports and the receipt against the national watch list on the computer. Nothing came up. They were most likely aliases.

Last night, on the way home, she had driven into the most magnificent sunset. From one end to the other, the sky was crimson red. She made a promise then and there, which she shared with Scott over dinner. This morning, she kept her word. She was in church, with her family. Grandpa went home after breakfast. Tomorrow he'd fly to the Netherlands to speak at a memorial service commemorating the invasion by Germany in 1940.

Scott walked ahead of her out of the sanctuary and toward the children's wing to find Kaley and Andy. Eva did not feel at ease in the massive stone structure. Pastor Green's sermon on forgiveness brought doubt, not comfort. Still, she lingered beneath the stained glass cross, bathed in late morning light. It held her like nothing in church had since Jillie died. A tug at her coat sleeve made her head turn slightly.

Her first reaction was to ignore it and catch up with her husband. Before she could escape, Eva met the laughing brown eyes of Kaley's Sunday School teacher, Thelma King. Because the Georgia transplant's granddaughter lived in Atlanta, Kaley had become Thelma's surrogate grandchild. She'd often drop by the house with tins of homemade peanut butter cookies or dolls' clothes she had made.

"How is your smart-as-a-whip daughter? She sure will make a topnotch Queen!" The woman's eyes danced with merriment to match her smile.

Queen? Eva had no idea what that was about, but Thelma didn't give her time to ask. Instead, Thelma put a chocolate-colored arm around a small woman with enormous dark hair and said, "Eva, meet Sari Jubayl, and her husband, Emile. He runs Helpers International."

They shook hands. As often happened when she met anyone new, Eva's investigative skills took over. She evaluated people in seconds, and Scott said he trusted her instincts more than he trusted his own. Sari's husband was as tall as Scott, older, but not nearly as handsome, with his unsmiling face and hooded, dark eyes. Eva saw Scott waiting for her by the door. The instant their eyes met, her heart contracted. She waved him over.

To Emile, she said, "My husband and daughter attended your mission banquet this week. Kaley's full of stories about Africa. She told us on the way to church that she wants to go there before she turns ten."

Emile beamed a smile. "How long will she have to wait for such a trip?"

"Well, her birthday is next July," Eva admitted.

Scott wound his way through the horde of people. When he arrived, Thelma made introductions and said, "Our pastor really preached today! Jesus forgave his enemies, and believers should, too."

Eva swallowed the quick retort that it was easier to preach than do. She saw Sari look at Emile, whose black eyes darted away. The air sizzled with tension between those two. Eva guessed they had argued before church. A thought caught her: She had no business judging other people and should stick to her own life.

Eva simply said, "It's hard to make time for the things we should do."

Emile looked at Eva, then away again as if she had struck a chord with him. Being a federal agent was tough, but at least she had job security, unlike an Executive Director of a charitable organization, who had to please a board of directors, plus fly around the country raising money. It sounded like politics, and she'd heard enough about that as a child. Eva did not want to owe anyone.

Sari said, "My son, George, is home for a few hours, then skips out when I put dinner on the table. He went out yesterday morning and still is not home." Her small smile disappeared as quickly as it had come. "Emile flies to London today, somewhere else next week. In between, he'll be home for a day or two."

Eva glanced at her watch. Scott must have read the cue; he leaned over and said, "I'll fetch the kids. We have a dinner reservation for 12:30."

Sari continued, "Thelma told me you are a police agent. You look too nice to be one."

Eva laughed at the comment, which she often heard from those she arrested.

Thelma added, "Eva gave me good advice when my nephew was arrested."

Eva replied, "Sari, I mostly gave Thelma the name of a respectable attorney."

Sari lowered her voice, "Do you mind if I ask you a question?"

Eva said, "I'll help, if I can."

Inwardly, she clenched her teeth, awaiting a tale of a speeding ticket. When people learned she was an agent, they inevitably spewed the latest story about police abuse, which had a lot to do with why she was not enamored with church.

Sari leaned toward Eva. She need not have worried that Emile would hear. He fiddled with his PDA. "The campus police are following George. Can they do that?"

Without facts, a nondescript answer was best. "If they have evidence that he violated a campus rule. What college does he go to?"

Emile walked to the door and peered out the glass. "Sari, it's about to rain."

"He studies international politics at George Mason Uni—"

Emile held open the door for her. "Now, Sari."

She thanked Eva, and followed Emile, leaving Eva by the door. The sky let loose torrents of rain.

By her side, Thelma pulled a small umbrella from an oversized bag, "That son of hers is a wild one. We may call you yet."

Thelma stepped on the slick sidewalk, eased open her umbrella. Eva closed the door before the wind ripped it from her hands. She could be wrong, but Sari reminded her of a dutiful servant being scolded by a stern taskmaster. And, as Scott said, she was rarely wrong.

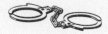

SIX

Eva stuck a red pin into the state of Colorado on the wall map and looked over her group. Whom to send? Robbie was busy with Farouk's computer and running down the names and addresses linked to the Grilled Onion. Griff took over her insurance fraud case and was tracking both the woman who got into the cab and Eva's assailant. Earl was conducting interviews, and Trenton was too inexperienced.

"Someone has to go to Denver. They busted a charity that funneled thousands to ARC. We take one down, a new one surfaces. ARC is on the State Department's list of prohibited Foreign Terrorist Organizations, but only recently have we made inroads."

Trenton twisted around on the chair. "Once I gave Farouk his pants, he got cooperative. Griff was right."

"Great, Trenton. Right now, I need a volunteer for the Rockies." Eva tapped a pin on the wall chart. She turned, and her eyes settled on Earl. It might do him good to get something new going after Judge Pendergast shot down his affidavit.

He seemed to understand. Earl stood. "I'll have Wanda book a flight."

Eva smiled. Everyone else streamed out except for Trenton.

"Can we talk about Farouk?" he asked.

Eva motioned for him to sit by the table where they had launched Operation Money Changer last week. "Have you talked with your partner? Griff's one of the best agents I've worked with, and he knows how to keep it within the lines. He can teach you a lot."

"Griff told me to run it by you."

Wanda knocked lightly on the door jamb and said, "A lady reporter is on the phone. Kat somebody or other. Says it's urgent."

Eva quickly replied, "Take her number and tell her I'll have to call her back."

Wanda disappeared without a word.

Eva snapped open her padded writing folder. "Tell me about Farouk."

"Said if I bring him a cola and cigarette, he'll provide all the details."

"That's what every defendant facing prison time wants you to believe."

Trenton flashed a smile Eva was sure swayed many a teacher to give him a decent grade when he failed to turn in his homework. "Maybe the two of us can extract something important."

She shut her eyes and rubbed her temples. Trenton's eagerness to flip Farouk did match her desire to make the strongest case. "Give me ten minutes. But I reserve judgment. He may not deliver."

Trenton headed to his office for his briefcase, and Eva pressed Griff's number. When he answered, she quizzed him, "Are you coming with us to interview Farouk?"

"Nope. Thought Farouk would open up more to the two of you. He and I didn't exactly see eye-to-eye."

"You're hoping he'll spit on my shoe again."

Griff laughed. "I forgot that. Seriously, Trenton needs face time with the new boss."

"This one time, Griff, but I want you to take him under your wing. Besides, he wants to be an FBI agent like his Dad."

Griff cleared his throat. "I've got a hunch and I'm waiting to hear from my contact at Justice."

Eva knew Griff would tell her when he knew more. She hung up. Minutes later, her phone rang. It was her mother. "Grandpa called before he left for the airport. I got the distinct impression that you and Scott need help with the kids. Dad's in meetings, but I am free for the next two days. I can be at your place in time to start dinner. How does that sound?"

"The kids will love it."

"How about you, Eva? Is it what you want?"

No. Grandpa was right, but she'd rather have his quiet ways instead of her mother's tendency to take over and make her opinions known.

Eva replied, "Mother, it would be great, if you have time."

"I'll make fried chicken. The meat is packed in the cooler, set to go."

Eva smothered a sigh. Her mother had planned it all out and called when she was ready to leave, knowing Eva could not say no.

"I'm bringing a new friend for Kaley."

"What?"

"A gray and white kitty, from the animal shelter. When I talked to Kaley on the phone last night, I told her about him. She's even picked out a name for him. Zak."

Eva was speechless. Before she could protest her mother's getting a pet for Kaley without first consulting her and Scott, her mother added, "Kaley hinted she wants to spend time with you. I hope you are not always so busy. She's playing Queen Esther at the mother-daughter banquet at church, you know."

So that was the "Queen" that Thelma was talking about! No, Eva hated to admit, she didn't know.

Her mother had a point, sharp as it was. Her job took her from special moments that soon would be gone. "Don't wait dinner for me. I have a late meeting."

"How late?" Her mother asked.

Opening her side drawer, Eva picked up an old fortune cookie and a Dutch peppermint left over from some Grandpa had sent for her birthday. So much for her stash.

"Save me a chicken leg?"

From behind a small table attached to the wall at one end, Eva faced Farouk Hamdi. His bravado from the day of the raid was dampened by an orange jumpsuit and gray flip-flops, the official uniform for all inmates. Trenton stood behind her left shoulder.

Eva wasted no time in finding out if Farouk had something to trade for leniency. "You carried more than ten thousand dollars on trips to Pakistan, Yemen, and Algeria."

In a British accent, Farouk asked, "Who told you this?"

Eva ignored the question. "You also flew to London, Germany, and Singapore and took cash to known ARC locations. It's illegal to take that much money out of the U.S. without declaring it."

Farouk stared at Eva with unblinking eyes.

Her elbows resting on the table, she said, "Your driver's license has a different name."

Farouk just blinked. Eva reminded him that the guy arrested in the hallway of his townshouse was a fugitive, and harboring a fugitive was a crime. She crossed her arms, glanced over at Trenton, then asked, "Did you tell him he faces thirty years in prison?"

Trenton leaned against the wall. "He knows it now."

Farouk sipped from the can of soda Trenton had brought him, but said nothing. Eva surveyed his thin face, scraggly beard, and mop of filthy hair. Born in Egypt and raised in London, Farouk was now a naturalized American citizen. Perhaps it was time to let him know she doubted he'd survive long in prison.

"If you cooperate, it will go easier for you. Or, you can spend the good years of your life wasting behind bars, each day the same as the last."

Farouk's left eye twitched. Eva smiled inwardly. Today, he would not spit at her.

Trenton gave his own advice. "You're smart. You help us, we help you."

"What if I know people you are interested in?" Farouk wiped his mouth on the sleeve.

"I might ask the federal prosecutor to seek a lighter sentence," Eva said.

"How light?" he asked.

Eva learned the art of interrogation from watching Griff; it was like dancing with a partner who refused to follow your lead. She'd promise nothing, yet. "Some who have helped stayed out of prison entirely. But they provided more than a name or two."

Farouk rolled the can between his palms. "A guy I know spews anti-American sentiments, protests against the IMF."

"That won't even get your sentence reduced to twenty-nine years."

"You tell me what it means when George's father, with access to millions, travels almost weekly to the Middle East."

"George who?" Trenton asked.

Farouk shrugged his shoulders.

Eva bolted from her chair and headed for the door. "Not good enough."

Farouk laughed. "When he was protesting against killing animals, I bought a double burger. We talked about how American companies rob people of their cultures."

Determined to end Farouk's cat-and-mouse game, Eva pressed the call button. "So you devised a plan to hurt America by funding terrorists? Does George aid your cause?"

From a central control room, a guard buzzed open the door.

Eva said, "We'll come back in a few minutes. Feed us this fish stew again and we're gone until we see you in court. Thirty years in the federal penitentiary is a long time for someone used to freedom and travel."

The door clicked shut behind them. Eva told the guard they'd be back.

Trenton punched the elevator button. "He's holding out on us."

"He's like most defendants, tells the least amount of information, while trying to carve the best deal for himself."

The ruse of leaving Farouk to think alone about his future gave Eva a chance to feed her caffeine habit. At the lobby concession, she poured a cup of coffee, without cream or sugar, then sipped the scalding liquid. The heat felt wonderful to her empty stomach.

"Want one?" Eva asked.

Trenton informed her he never drank the stuff. She dropped quarters on the counter, and told the blind proprietor it was great coffee.

"Thank you, ma'am. Come again."

In the elevator, Eva told Trenton only the Assistant U.S. Attorney, Dan Simmons, could reduce the charges or ask Judge Pendergast to lighten Farouk's sentence. "It won't be easy," she said, "Judge Pendergast puts the government through its paces."

They arrived at the third floor. She stepped from the elevator and drained her coffee.

"If Dan agrees, we could get Farouk released to work as your informant."

Trenton's mouth hung slightly open. "Do you mean it?"

Eva could just feel his brain whirling over the possibilities. Hers certainly was. She had thought of it on the way; it seemed like the only way to make immediate inroads into ARC, even if it was risky. Of course, Farouk had to give her *something* to bargain with.

Eva crushed the styrofoam cup, tossed it into a can outside the interview room. "We keep his passport to lessen the risk he'll flee the country. Being a naturalized citizen, with no criminal record, should make things easier. If he opens his mouth."

The guard buzzed opened the door. Trenton pulled it toward him, and Farouk nearly fell into his arms, then scrambled to lean against the cement block wall.

Eva was unimpressed by his casual demeanor. "You have five minutes to tell us about U.S. groups aiding terrorists and moving monies to ARC, or we leave. For good."

Farouk sat down and slurped soda from the bottom of his can. Eva's hand rested on the door handle. Let him think she was about to leave. Farouk plopped the can on the table and looked at it for about two minutes. No one said a word. Farouk's sandaled foot jiggled under the table.

Eva figured that Farouk wanted a specific deal before admitting anything. Eva couldn't do it. She'd find another way; she just didn't know yet what it would be. Maybe Earl would get an inroad at the ICE conference in Denver. Farouk fidgeted his other foot. Eva moved her hand to the call button. Then, Farouk sighed. Words tumbled out of his mouth. Words she could use.

"Okay. The guy in the closet was Richard Salem. He's a friend of a friend. We had a poker game going, he had too much beer and stayed the night. I don't know the name of the street, but I can show you where he lives."

Eva nodded. "Why did he have two passports?"

Farouk gave her a blank look.

She made a mental note to have Trenton learn all he could about Richard Salem once she nailed down Farouk's ARC connections. "Okay. I'm interested in who else you know."

"I move money for a Lebanese guy who supplies weapons to ARC's deputy chief, Tsouban. He is a ruthless character. He must *never* know I speak his name to you."

"And the rest of his name?" Eva asked.

Farouk wiped the back of his hand over his moustache. "Tsouban means 'the snake' in Arabic. He likes to be called Cobra and disposes of anyone he suspects of disloyalty."

She wasn't sure Dan Simmons would agree with what she was about to say, but she'd chance it. "If you enter the Witness Protection Program, you get a new identity, a new life."

Eva's periwinkle eyes did not waver from Farouk's watery ones. The thin skin under Farouk's eye vibrated as he said, "When my Lebanese contact learned I live in Columbia City, Virginia, he asked if I

knew Emile Jubayl. He's a Lebanese immigrant who runs a humanitarian organization in the same city. It reaches around the globe."

Eva tried not to show how stunned she was. Was he the same
Emile Jubayl from Helpers International, the man from her church?

"You know that guy?" Farouk guessed, his eyes narrowed to slits.

Trenton mustered the glare he practiced at home and replied,
"You talk. We ask the questions. Keep it coming."

Farouk slouched in his chair. "Emile is a smooth customer. He
runs Servant Helper or something. I saw him interviewed on TV. His
son, George, scorns America."

Eva had heard enough. "This sounds like something you saw on
the news. Time's up."

Farouk reached across the table, grabbed her wrist. "Wait."

Eva pulled her hand away as if burned by a hot stove. "Why?"

"George's old man pumps money into the Middle East like oil
from Arabia. My money guy in London says Emile gives support to
ARC."

"How?" asked Eva.

"Get me out and I'll go to London to find out more."

"Wouldn't I like to go to London, too? Get real," Trenton exclaimed.

"Listen! I can introduce one of you guys inside ARC."

Eva was wary of Farouk's sudden proposal for a get-out-of-jail-
free card. "With your arrest, your people will assume, correctly, that
you are cooperating."

Farouk replied, "My contact in London might not know. He does
not care much for America." He shrugged, as if that made his friend
less offensive.

"To lobby my boss, I need more than that. I can make it happen,"
Eva smiled, "or not."

Eva did not pressure him as she would have liked. She wanted
Farouk to see her as his ticket to freedom. Farouk's feet moved faster.
He might be trying to warm them, or he might be close to telling her
what she wanted to know. Trenton opened his mouth to speak. Eva
waved him off. Well timed silence was more powerful than words. Like
every defendant, Farouk was evaluating her, weighing his options.

At length, he looked first to Trenton, then Eva. "If I talk, do you
promise to protect me?"

Eva tapped her fingers on his arm, once. "We'll do our best." She
nodded to Trenton and said, "Write down everything."

Thirty minutes later, Farouk had admitted how he helped ARC's New York cell and brought illegal money into foreign hands, and signed a form waiving his right to counsel and a handwritten confession, both witnessed by Trenton and Eva.

Eva put the papers in a folder, then stood. "If Emile is doing what you allege, Trenton will return. We'll try to reduce your bond and get you out, which is your best shot at helping us. Speak to no one, especially cellmates. You'll have to testify. Maybe wear a wire."

It was after six o'clock. Shadows had crept over the parking lot behind the Alexandria City Jail. Eva recalled the earlier phone call from Channel 14's Mary Katherine Kowicki. Tomorrow would be soon enough to call her back. Eva hoped she would lose interest in the raid.

"Could we get a wiretap on Emile's phone?" Trenton asked.

Eva's stomach rumbled. She was in no mood for Trenton's questions. "Federal wiretap laws are stringent. We cannot waltz in," she snapped her fingers, "and get the right to listen to citizens' conversations. Corroborate Farouk's assertions first."

As Eva pressed her remote door key, she was approached by a tall man, wearing scuffed cowboy boots. He removed a wide brim hat.

"Excuse me. Y'all got any money? I came north to visit my sister. She's in the hospital for a bone marrow transplant. I used all my money to get here. Now, I got no gas to get home. I ain't a slacker."

Trenton edged toward Eva's side of the car and growled, "I've seen your kind before. You better leave."

Undaunted, Eva extracted a twenty-dollar bill from her briefcase. "Will this help?"

The man flashed her a brilliant smile. "God'll reward you, miss."

He plucked the bill from her fingers, replaced the battered hat, and swaggered away. His plaid shirt billowed like a full sail caught in the breeze. The stranger hopped in a rusty truck and spewed oily smoke as he drove down the street.

"You are a soft touch. He'll blow it on beer."

Eva laughed. "You believe Farouk is holding out. I think the cowboy was out of gas."

She opened the car door and said, "Come on. We've prison cells to fill."

Trenton got in and said, "Farouk said they were playing poker. I didn't find playing cards. Did you?"

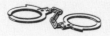

SEVEN

Emile Jubayl clicked a computer mouse to enlarge a photo of a child walking in a ditch carrying a bucket of water. He centered on the girl's liquid eyes when a knock on his office door interrupted him. His new intern, Hannah Strobel, was dressed in khaki slacks and a navy blue shirt with the Helpers' logo. She entered his office, which was filled with memorabilia from his international travel. Hannah set down a stack of papers on a small table.

He was more than satisfied with the work of the daughter of Penny Strobel, Helpers International's volunteer coordinator. A journalism major in her third year at George Mason University, Hannah was more than efficient; she was also an expert at desktop publishing. He planned to offer her a promotion to his executive assistant when her internship was done.

He pointed to the edge of his desk. "Make twenty copies of that outline. Pick up the pamphlets you designed from the printers. Take the cart with wheels, Hannah, it will be heavy."

Emile's extension chirped. He motioned for Hannah to wait before putting the receiver to his ear and listening.

"From London? Put it through."

He turned his back to Hannah, and said into the phone, "I'll get the first flight from Dulles. Wait." He put a hand over the receiver, pivoted his head toward her. "I want to see your pamphlets."

Hannah took the outline from his desk. The phone cord pulled tight, Emile followed her to the door, which he closed with a definite click. Back to his London caller, he said, "Things have reached a crisis. I wish I had never left Lebanon." He listened, then replied, "Yes, delay is unwise."

Emile hung up the phone and nudged his computer from dormant mode. The photo of the tiny girl told a story of scarcity and pain.

She carried a bucket bigger than she was. Her feet were bare. Would his donors be as moved by her needs as he was? Tears pooled in his eyes, and he knew he was right to use this photo at the fundraiser. Her wide black eyes, begging for help, would evoke sufficient empathy to open wallets. Emile needed one hundred thousand dollars. And he needed it tonight, the last day of his fiscal year.

The wait staff of the Remington Hotel cleared dessert plates from the tables, where hundreds of business leaders and politicians sipped hot coffee. Lights dimmed as two giant screens on each side of the podium descended from the ceiling. A hush rippled through the elegant room. Worry over not getting enough donations had dulled Emile's appetite. He ate little of the grilled salmon. Seated next to him, Sari finished off a slice of chocolate cheesecake in three bites.

An image of a young boy lying in a hospital bed, a yellowed sheet wrapped around his body, filled the screens. The camera panned out. He was one among dozens of injured children in a hospital ward. Volunteers in Helpers International shirts handed each child a plastic bag with a teddy bear, bar of soap, toothbrush, and toothpaste. When a volunteer gave the boy a bear, the boy tried to sit up, cradling the brown animal with his bandaged arm.

A woman's soft voice urged, "You, too, can help these sick children. Show them love by opening your hearts. They need blankets, medicine, and clothing. For twenty dollars, each child can receive these bags of hope. Please help, today."

The screens went blank. In a beige silk suit and carefully knotted gold tie, Emile walked up the riser to a podium where he turned on the new PowerPoint presentation, recently approved by his board of directors. His deep voice matched his tall stature, and Emile soon had everyone mesmerized by his narration of the pictures of children clothed in rags, standing in heaps of rubble, flies buzzing around their heads.

Eager to get to the bottom line, he clicked to the final picture. The girl who struggled with the water bucket was a perfect counterpoint to his much rehearsed story. "My parents and I fled Lebanon in the 1970s when Christians and Muslims, who had lived together for centuries, began killing each other. My older brother stayed behind with my uncle and cousin. When he wrote of hardships, I painted fences and mowed lawns to earn the money that would ease my brother's pain. There was a limit to what I could do, but not so for Wilbur Andrews, a retired physician, here in Arlington. Dr. Andrews, please join me."

The audience applauded as the 93-three-year-old founder walked to the stage without the aid of a cane or walker, his bald head held proudly. Emile thrust his arm around Wilbur's bony shoulders. He praised his efforts twenty years earlier to collect medical supplies and food in his garage to ship to the Middle East.

"Because Dr. Andrews is well known in Washington, D.C., senators and other influential people give generously to our cause. Many charter donors are here tonight."

Abrupt applause lifted Emile's spirits. So did his hopes rise that the one hundred thousand dollars were within reach. "We have grown to 217 employees at home and abroad with a new office and warehouse complex in Columbia City, Virginia. This year, we sent thirteen million dollars in food and medicine to fight poverty and tyranny in the Middle East, which many know has a special place in my heart."

Emile's arm hung around Wilbur, whose eyes were wet. Emile raised his free arm to point at the poor child whose image was frozen on the screen. His voice broke. "We, who have much, must be faithful to those with little. You can help by writing a check, not for Wilbur or me, but for the children. This child thanks you. I thank you."

Emile dropped his arm. He told the audience about gift envelopes on each table, said good night, and strode off the stage, not eager to speak to anyone. His staff would collect all the envelopes and take them back to Headquarters.

As he scooted toward the exit door, Sari caught up with him. "That was a wonderful program. It moved me to tears."

His hurried step did not slow until he reached the parking lot. It had rained during the program, and the pavement was slippery. Sari dodged puddles, tried to keep her heels dry. Emile keyed his remote and opened the doors to their champagne-colored SUV. She slid onto the leather seat. Emile said nothing to acknowledge her presence.

On the ride home, Sari had something to tell Emile. After a big event, he had his own way of winding down—silence. She glanced over at him. At the turn for their street, they passed under a bright street light. Her heart contracted. Her husband of twenty-one years wore a grotesque grimace, his eyes shrouded in darkness.

What was God telling her? Fear bubbled within her, but logic triumphed over instinct. She told herself he was simply tired. If only he would stay home and go to church with her instead of always flying overseas. She did not want to add another burden.

They were almost home. Once Emile left the car, Sari would lose his attention. She plunged ahead. "George has been gone for days. His friends are wild, with long hair and pierced noses." Sari's emotions streamed out like the waterfall the gardener installed last month in the backyard. "Do you think he is doing drugs?"

Emile pressed the accelerator, then the brakes. They turned the last corner. "Your son is nineteen. Give him a chance to be independent. George is a vegetarian. Why would he harm his body with illegal substances?"

Sari sighed. "He is *our* son. You have no idea what is going on in your own home. A week ago, I caught him sitting on the living room floor chanting like he was in a trance."

"George is like other college kids, exploring spiritual avenues. He'll come home while I am gone. Have you called George Mason University?"

"We pay his tuition, but they told me nothing. If you called, they might listen. "

Emile replied, "I'll be in London a few days."

Sari was used to his constant travel. She made a life for herself. When Emile left without warning, her days went on as before. She volunteered at the Senior Center and took silk flowers to people in the hospital. Determined to eliminate a painful burr, Sari no longer asked about his trips. Her strategy was working because Emile seemed more relaxed at home. It had taken her years to accept that, while she loved America and never wanted to leave it, he was unable or unwilling to purge their homeland from his system.

Emile pushed the garage door opener. As the door crept up, Sari decided it was not too late to call Thelma, her prayer partner. Maybe they could meet tomorrow to pray for George's safety and a successful trip for Emile, whatever he was going to do.

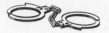

EIGHT

It was the first day of October and Eva drove along I-66, a sharp eye on her speedometer. Her lecture at ICE Headquarters started at four o'clock, thirty minutes from now, and a reserved parking place did not come with her pay grade. She was running behind because Lou had called from the rehab facility. The daily therapy was painful, and he had no idea when he could resume his duties at FIG. She gladly told him Farouk Hamdi was in custody, but not about her plans to use him as an informant. He had enough to worry about.

Almost ready to exit the Theodore Roosevelt bridge, she flipped on a radio talk show. Huge raindrops spattered her windshield. She glanced at the passenger seat. Her umbrella wasn't there. The drops became a downpour as Eva remembered that the umbrella was in her briefcase in the backseat.

Eva arrived at her street and heard breaking news. "Four thousand children marched on the American Embassy in Beirut. In Jerusalem, a suicide bomber detonated a bomb in an American restaurant today, injuring scores of people. The bomber was killed. Stay tuned for details."

Her mind overcome with pictures of smoke and screams, Eva shut off the radio. If a parking spot did not appear like magic, she'd be late. Just ahead, on the crowded street, a mail delivery truck pulled away from a meter. She pulled up, jabbed the brakes, backed the car to the curb, and put it in park. In seconds, she turned it off, and turned to grab her briefcase. Eva dug for her umbrella. It was small, but it would keep her head from getting wetter. She slammed four quarters into the meter and hurried to Headquarters on Pennsylvania Avenue, trying to keep mud off her legs.

At five minutes to four, she collapsed her umbrella and entered the lobby. To her dismay, the backs of her legs looked like they had leopard spots. She had no time to stop and clean them off. Eva flashed her badge and walked through the magnetometer. The security officer turned off the buzz from her weapon and ammo clip. She pushed the elevator button.

A man said, "The metro stopped twice. Suspicious activity on the tracks."

Eva recognized Griff's voice before she saw him. She replied, "A bomb just went off in Israel."

Griff lowered his voice as they entered the elevator that would take them to the top floor, and said, "Maybe we should take the stairs."

The doors closed them in.

"Too late," Eva decided not to say any more about Griff's secret—he suffered from claustrophobia. Instead, she wiped her legs and smoothed her plum-colored suit. When the doors opened to their floor, she steered him down the hall to the Director's conference room.

Inside, Alexia Kyros, the U.S. Attorney, was welcoming financial investigators who came from Britain, Europe, and Australia to share ideas on disrupting the money flow to terrorists. Her appearance complemented her position as the highest ranking prosecutor in northern Virginia, with her tan suit, pearls, and henna-colored hair, precisely cut.

She began the meeting with a startling announcement, "Moments ago, telephone and e-mail intercepts reveal that ARC attacked Israel and may strike here in the next twenty-four hours. Bridges and monuments might be bombed, which makes the District a target."

Eva caught her breath. Alexia should cancel the conference. It would be hard for them to focus on illicit money trails with a possible bombing on their minds. But Alexia had a different idea.

"Acting Supervisory Special Agent Eva Montanna will give an *abbreviated* briefing on Operation Money Changer. ARC's Hamburg cell was broken up the day our arrests occurred."

Alexia left Eva to face a nervous audience shifting on their chairs. She decided to get their attention. "In four hours, we netted thirty-three terrorists in D.C., Miami, and Detroit, a cache of illegal weapons, and seized two million dollars in various bank accounts. Are ARC cells operating in your cities? That's what we need to know."

Griff handed each investigator a list of terrorists operating ARC cells in European cities. Eva began highlighting the strategies her team used to uncover financial crimes, when Alexia raised her hand at the back of the room.

Eva concluded, "ARC gets profits from illegal activities, like cigarette smuggling. Their hands are deep into cocaine trafficking in Columbia. A chain of vegetarian restaurants owned by a Lebanese con-
glomerate is a front for ARC to skim the proceeds to buy weapons
for terrorists. Grilled Onion Restaurants are cropping up in Europe,
America, and Hong Kong."

A deep scowl etched on her brow, Alexia ended the meeting.
"Another bomb threat was phoned in for the Capitol. These happen
with some regularity, but I would not want you to be complacent. Be
alert as we have to be."

Ready to leave, Eva was stopped by a wiry gentleman with salt-
and-pepper hair. With a Union Jack pin on his lapel and tortoise shell
glasses, all he needed was a tweed jacket to look as if he stepped from
a British movie.

In a clipped British accent, he said, "Brewster Miles, British Counter-intelligence. Pleased to meet you."

"Are you with Scotland Yard?" Eva asked.

Brewster handed her a card, which identified him as working for
MI-5, Britain's counterpart to the FBI. "I specialize in international
terrorism cases. Cut my teeth on our own Irish Republican Army."

Griff shook Brewster's hand and said, "Your accent sounds like my
Dad's. If it had not been for my Mom's persuasive powers, I might be
MI-5 instead of FBI." He pulled out his wallet and edged Brewster's
card between a fold.

"But you sound American." Brewster's smile showed he meant no
offense.

"Like Winston Churchill, my Dad married an American. He grew
up in Cornwall. Fell in love with my Mom when he visited America.
She refused to leave."

Eva turned to Griff. "You never told me your Dad wasn't a native
New York, like you."

Griff just shrugged.

Brewster took off his glasses and put them in his suitcoat pocket.
"Griffen Topping sounds English. Our Admiral Topping, who served
with honors in World War II under Winston Churchill, hailed from
Penzanz, a port city in Cornwall. He's a national hero. I say, are you
related?"

Griff bobbed his head, stuffed both hands into his pockets. "The
admiral was my grandfather. He's no longer living, but my grandmother still lives in Penzanz. I try to visit every year."

An idea overrode Eva's desire to get home. "Brewster, we have learned of an ARC contact in London. How long are you in town? Maybe we could discuss it over coffee before you leave."

Brewster glanced at his watch. "I fly out tonight at eight thirty." His ice-blue eyes twinkled. "I have time for a pot of tea, if both of you do."

"I know just the place." Eva smiled at Griff, who detested tea almost as he did much as elevators.

Some blocks away, the colonnade in front of the State Department was jammed with protestors who carried signs denouncing capitalists. George Jubayl fit in with the crowd. His brown hair was stringy, and the tee shirt he wore had a target bullseye superimposed over a caricature of the President. George pulled a "Sink the IMF" banner from a backpack by his feet. A few celebrities and rock stars posed for pictures. George waved to his new friend, Barnard, the mountain climber who had traveled to every peak higher than 10,000 feet and climbed them all.

This day was a pinnacle for George. He had found a reason for living, to make the world a better place for the helpless. Next week, he'd quit George Mason University. He was sick of being stifled by his mother and ignored by his father. They had no idea how kids taunted him in high school for being an Arab. Even the coach kept him off the soccer field. So what if his ankle was weakened after he broke it? He could have played anyway!

If his father knew he was here, he'd have a coronary. George felt a stab of pain. Emile cared more about having money to fly around the world than about him. A plan welled in his tortured brain. If he moved out tonight, Dad wouldn't notice he was gone. Not for days, maybe weeks. Mom loved him and would be sore at his going. But she did not have a clue. George echoed Barnard's Buddhist chants, imagining he rose above the George Washington Monument. *His namesake. What a joke!*

If he left, he could quit sitting around with the kids his mother invited from church. They believed a bunch of nonsense he'd never hold as true. But where would he go? Lebanon? His mother, the total American, wanted nothing to do with her homeland, while his father could not stay away. *I'll fly to London and see Aunt Reni. There's a lot of important protests—*

A policeman's sharp whistles halted his mind's travels. "You have one minute to clear out! You're blocking the government of the people and will be arrested for trespassing. Move!"

A protestor shouted in George's ear, "Down with America! Death to Israel!"

The woman, her hair fuzzed like a dandelion gone to seed, knocked a sign against George's head and ripped his cheek. The peace George felt moments ago turned to rage.

He shoved his face in hers. "Watch what you're doing, hag. That's my head!"

George thrust her away so the sign no longer threatened his eyes.

A younger man with a shaved head pushed George. "Leave my Granny alone!"

George fell. His shoulder slammed on the concrete. Pain shot through him. He rose and shook his fist. "You'll pay for that!"

Eva was awed by the Willard Hotel's posh surroundings. President Ulysses S. Grant had often smoked cigars in the hotel lobby. Anyone wanting to petition the government found him there and pitched their plans. Thus, the term "lobbyist" was born. Today, the President could go nowhere without a full Secret Service detail. As Eva sipped Oolong tea with lemon, she watched Griff doctor his tea with two lumps of sugar and a dollop of cream.

Brewster was well into his second pot. He stirred in cream. "Thanks for the best cup this side of the Atlantic."

"My parents honeymooned here," Eva said.

"You grew up in Washington, D.C.?" Brewster asked.

"Virginia. Then I went to a small Christian school in the Midwest, Wheaton College."

Eva buttered her raisin-studded scone, feeling uneasy. If the Capitol was hit, Scott could be in it. She checked her watch. By now, he was home, eating dinner with the kids. That thought calmed her down.

Griff was talking. "Mom was born in Puerto Rico, grew up in New York. With my dark hair and Bronx accent, I've had my share of undercover work." As usual, Griff shifted the topic from himself and back to work. "Brewster, what do you know about the Lebanese community in London?"

"Can you be more specific?" He poured a dash more cream in his cup.

Eva kept her voice low. "Our arrestee, Farouk Hamdi, claims Emile Jubayl finances terrorists via a Lebanese connection in London."

About to ask if Brewster knew Jubayl, Eva turned her head to the window in response to sirens outside. The piercing sounds grew louder. Eva thrust down her scone, just in case. Jillie had not gotten out in time! But the sirens diminished. She sat back into her chair, still on the alert.

Brewster put on his glasses and looked at a man and a woman sitting nearby, reading a menu. "I have to be careful. MI-5 knows of Emile through his family. His cousin, Duma Jubayl, is a wealthy banker in Beirut. Emile's sister, Reni Jubayl, is the president of the bank's London branch."

"Are they connected to ARC?" Eva insisted.

Brewster gave a little shrug. "We have long suspected the Beirut bank is not only tied to ARC, but Hezbollah as well. We have yet to find enough evidence to charge anyone. Without clearance from superiors, that's all I can say."

Brewster's dilemma did not lessen Eva's need to know more. "Emile raises funds in churches, including mine, for his organization, Helpers International. My husband went to an event with our daughter and wants to contribute. Emile sent a letter asking to meet with us. Do they support ARC?"

Griff interjected, "Eva, you didn't tell me this. I don't trust what Farouk says."

"Neither do I. That's why I hope Brewster can tell me something."

Brewster did not hesitate. "I strongly suggest you not write a check."

Eva replied, "That says a lot. If we develop the source in London, will you help?"

"I'll see what we've got on Farouk," Brewster said.

Sirens again split the air.

His tea cold, Griff handed Brewster his card. "Most likely a traffic accident. When I'm in your neighborhood, we'll skip tea and go to your favorite fish and chips place."

Their waitress interrupted, her eyes wide with fright. "The police said a bomb exploded at the State Department!" The young girl wrung her hands. "I hope no one was killed."

Zayed walked down the gangplank of the rickety freighter. His feet ached in his leather shoes. When he leaned over to loosen the laces, the backpack fell from his shoulder and hit his head. He set it on the dusty ground, surveying the quiet street for a taxi to take him to the village of Hadibu. Zayed saw none. He trudged on, certain he would be late meeting the man who would drive him to El Samoud's villa.

Instead of being on this hot, pitiful island, Zayed longed to be in New York, personally putting in motion ARC's next attack. El Samoud had summoned him to Socotra, an island off the coast of Yemen, but demanded Zayed transfer from one freighter to another.

Hadibu was deserted. Who dared call this forsaken place the Island of Happiness? Yet, he had to admit, El Samoud was a genius. ARC soldiers could meet on the island, which was visited only by the occasional scientist studying the rare Frankincense trees, and go virtually unnoticed by western authorities. The CIA and MI-6 had probably never heard of it! Reminded of his constant efforts to outwit the two spy agencies, Zayed spat on the ground.

The convertible jeep was parked on a side street. He recognized El Samoud's driver. The tank-sized man probably kept an AK-47 under the front seat and permanently dealt with anyone who got out of line. Zayed climbed in the back of the vehicle without a word. They ascended the road, dodging rocks and crater-sized holes. Dust rose in small whirlwinds, coating Zayed's face and hair with a thin sheet of grit. They stopped outside an iron gate set in a high wall of stone, protecting ARC's new headquarters, a mud block villa perfectly situated on a hill overlooking the port.

The driver asked in broken English, "Travel long?"

"No," Zayed lied. "I come from Yemen."

The jeep parked haphazardly near the edge of a cliff. Zayed saw the small freighter on which he arrived moored in front of the Crescent, a trawler El Samoud had bought to allow him to travel anonymously.

The driver handed Zayed a small stone.

"What is this for?"

"Throw over cliff. If reaches bottom, you live long life."

Zayed smoothed the stone with his fingers. "And if not?"

The driver shrugged. He got out to watch.

Zayed stepped out, then tossed the stone. It disappeared in the brush halfway down the cliff.

"Too bad. Now I will tell you what I could not." His English improved. "The others came yesterday. You are late. El Samoud said the last to arrive had to throw the stone. If it did not go to the bottom … ."

"What do you mean?"

El Samoud's driver remained as silent as the stone Zayed had thrown. Zayed walked to the iron gate. A guard with a turbaned head and rifle slung low over his shoulder motioned him in with the tip of his gun. Inside the villa, a strong smell of incense burned Zayed's nose. He followed the guard and tried not to sneeze. They entered a large, beautiful room where the six other leaders sat on a blue rug. Zayed filled the empty place in the circle.

ARC's Supreme Leader appeared from behind a Persian rug hanging over a door, concealed in his customary black robe and *isharb*. His second in command, the Cobra, clapped his hands together. "At last, Zayed appears. The others gave their reports. Now it is his turn."

El Samoud stared at Zayed. He arranged his bony body on a plush pillow, then said, "I began to despair you found another loyal cause."

Zayed felt irritation flow toward his leader. It was not his fault that it took him weeks to get here; El Samoud had directed every step. To humiliate Zayed before his comrades was not honorable. Despite an empty stomach—he had eaten nothing since yesterday—Zayed rose and bowed low. He licked dry lips.

"Everything is ready. I met with my man before I left." Zayed did not speak Farouk's name. "He has a highly placed source in the Homeland Security Department. I await your instructions."

El Samoud pointed to a bottle of *ma* and allowed Zayed a sip of the water. "You helped test our new method of travel. We must elude authorities as much as possible. All future travel will be by vessels. Seaports are less scrutinized."

The others nodded at Zayed as if he had accomplished some great feat.

El Samoud looked at his soldiers, one by one, until his eyes rested on Zayed. "Our attacks on the anniversary of September 11 were successful, except for New York."

Zayed choked on the water and nearly spit it out. Surely, this was a trick. He had personally seen the bomb placed under the World Trade Center Memorial as it was being built. It should have exploded on September 11, the day it was to be dedicated, killing thousands. What mystery had surrounded him since he stepped on Socotra? Zayed reached for more water, but his hands froze in midair.

El Samoud said, "September 11 was a rehearsal. Our next attacks will be massive. Each one of you knows a portion, because together we planned your individual parts. What you do not know is that each attack will occur at the same time on March 14, the day the Jews will celebrate Purim. All targets will be destroyed at the same time!"

The others chanted, "Brotherhood of the Blood." Zayed's lips moved, his heart raced. He had always hoped for such a grand plan. Why wait for Purim? March was a long way off.

Sitting cross-legged, El Samoud explained the rationale for his plot. "The Jews' ancient infidel Queen saved them from the great martyr Haman." His hands lifted empty air, "I bring Haman back to life."

El Samoud stood and began to pace around the circle of cell leaders. His veiled head shook as his voice rose. "Where Haman failed, I will not. We must destroy the Jews. We will succeed against them and their infidel allies."

Zayed listened to every word El Samoud spoke, until he noticed his leader repeated himself. Zayed had heard him rant in other meetings about the crimes British soldiers committed against his people and how he hated Jews, Americans, and the British. El Samoud stopped walking and stood across from Zayed, where he could see his eyes, which looked so fierce there was no way Zayed wanted to cross him. Would El Samoud be satisfied with his efforts to support ARC in New York? What was the meaning of that stone? Zayed wondered if he should be on guard against ARC's leader, when El Samoud sat once again on his pillow and gestured wildly with his hands.

"Twenty-four hours before you launch your attacks, my words will be broadcast over television and the airwaves. When you hear me, say, 'Destroy the Satans of the world,' you will know to act."

When the shouts stopped, El Samoud continued. The Tower of London and Parliament, gone. This time, New York City will be nothing but dust. Christian sites in Israel will be obliterated."

El Samoud laughed and took a *sikkin* from a golden sheath hanging under his black robe. When he ran a finger over its deadly point, Zayed shuddered. He knew nothing of the new plan. Was El Samoud now going to kill him?

El Samoud's eyes glittered like black diamonds, as he said, "Enough about other targets. I will tell you each separately your mission."

He stood more slowly this time, and pulled Zayed aside. "You are elevated to Lebanon. You have a special assignment with the British Ambassador in Beirut."

Relief washed over Zayed. He would not be killed. Still, the truth hurt. He was no longer the leader of the New York cell.

"Succeed there and you erase your blunder."

Which blunder? The long journey? The bomb not going off in New York? Glimpsing the leader's face that time in Paris? Scared to ask any questions, Zayed exhibited only loyalty. "When do I leave?"

El Samoud's finger rested on the point of his *sikkin*. "Now. Your ship is ready."

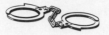

NINE

Trenton watched his still agile father climb out of the cuddy cabin of the boat, aptly named the *Enforcer*, and hoped he would be as fit at sixty-two.

"Give me a hand covering her," Duke Nash said to his 27-year-old son.

On separate sides of the U-shaped dock, father and son pulled the canvas toward the boat's stern.

Trenton started to speak but stopped when his Dad pointed to the snaps. "Fasten those. I want to keep her snug from the chill and salt breeze."

Trenton liked to please his Dad, so complying with his order came easy. He was in no hurry to leave his father's company or the air, which was balmy for the first week of October. As he secured one snap at a time, he mentioned to his dad that he had only two more quarters left at George Mason before graduating.

"I like the sound of that," said Duke.

"The FBI recruiter did, too. He gave me an application. It asks for every address I've lived at. Does that mean an agent will interview all our neighbors?"

Duke glanced at his son. "Are you worried that Mr. Wilson will reveal that you flattened his tires after he refused to let you take Missy to the prom?"

A deadpan expression on his face, Trenton strummed his fingers on the fiberglass gunnel. "I drove through the old neighborhood. Mr. Wilson moved."

Duke grinned. "Then you have nothing to worry about. My contacts will help. The FBI's number-two guy used to be my junior partner."

Trenton failed to hear. His dad's set jaw convinced him not to ask the question bottled up inside.

Duke pushed the last snap in place. "It's tough to get accepted into the FBI. Build a good record on the task force, and you'll have to finish your degree first."

Trenton wished he could accelerate things and become his family's third generation of FBI Agents. "I have more regular hours at FIG than I had at the Sheriff's Department. So," Trenton flashed a smile, "I signed up for an extra class at George Mason."

Duke pulled on the canvas to make sure it was tight. "Your grandfather and I would be proud if you join the Bureau."

A gull landed on the dock and shoved its black beak high in the air for a piece of fish. Trenton almost asked the question, but his Dad spoke first. "Remember Marshal Owen, my best friend in charge of security for the stock brokerage. He got every one of his employees out of the second tower of the World Trade Center. But he went back in." Duke shook his head.

Trenton rolled his eyes. Not again. Dad had to accept Owen's death.

Duke's face muscles twitched. "Your grandfather never thought he would live to see another act of terror after Pearl Harbor. His heart gave out after watching those twin towers collapse to the ground."

Trenton felt terrible about his grandfather's death. Their family was getting smaller all the time. First his sister, then grandmother, now grandfather. All gone. His mom hadn't yet asked if he was dating anyone new. But she was bound to when he went inside. She always did.

He changed to his favorite topic. "An FBI agent on my team said the Patriot Act allows retired agents to be rehired without taking a hit on their pensions."

"So?"

Trenton chuckled. "Since you retired, the feds are tracking down terrorists by following their money. I'm on a big case. An ARC money guy is going to work as my informant." He did not say Farouk might not be released from jail. "Maybe I can help settle the score for Mr. Owen and Grandfather."

Duke tugged the mooring line, and the screaming gull flew off. Calm descended on the dock, but not inside of Trenton. He posed his question to Duke's back.

"What if the Bureau won't hire me?"

Duke remained bent over.

"Dad—"

Duke faced his son. "I heard you. That will not happen. Your mother and I believe in you and pray for your future."

Before Trenton objected, Duke held up a large tanned hand. "I know you are not with us on that, but we pray anyway. We did what we could to show you the truth while you were growing up. Someday, you may see the wisdom in it."

Duke reached into a rope locker on the dock and drew out a green object. He tossed it to Trenton.

"My GMU cap! I've looked all over for it."

"You left it in the boat the last time you were here."

Trenton placed his favorite ballcap on his head. Duke threw an arm around his shoulder. "What you said about rejoining the Bureau to fight the war on terror, I'm game, if you get in."

Sari clutched two plastic bags with one hand and opened the back door with her key. As she pressed the button to close the garage door, the kitchen phone rang. Sari set down her groceries and hurried to answer it. Emile was back in London and could be calling.

"Hello," she answered, slightly out of breath.

Silence, then a screeching noise.

"Is anyone there?" Sari asked.

She heard a grunt, then "Mom?"

"George? Where are you?"

"Mom, I was at the State Department protest with Barnard. I learned how bad the IMF is from some kids at school."

Sari's heart contracted. "You sound funny. What happened?"

"They arrested me. I'm at the D.C. lockup."

Numbed by the thought of her son in jail, Sari collapsed in a chair by the kitchen table. *Lord, help me and my son. He is lost!* She tried to keep her voice calm so that George would not guess how scared she was.

She said quietly, "Tell me everything."

"It was peaceful. You would like Barnard. He's like Gandhi."

"George, forget Barnard! Why were you arrested?"

"A lady smacked me with her sign. When I moved her away, her grandson slugged me. I fell. My shoulder hurts, like when I broke my foot."

George's mother heard him say, "Give me a minute."

"Mom, this place is a pit! Can you bail me out?"

George stifled a cry. He sounded pathetic and alone. She'd wait to ask about the bomb at the State Department until he came home.

Instead she said, "Your father is not here."

George stopped crying. "Where is he now? He's never around when we need him."

"He flew to London. Your grandmother is ill."

"Oh."

George sounded unconcerned, and Sari wondered when he'd changed. He used to love getting packages from Emile's mother and often wrote her letters. Now, he never asked about her.

With no knowledge of jails or criminals, Sari could only think to say, "I will pray for you."

"I know that, but can't you get me out of here?" George wailed.

Sari held in her sobs until she hung up the phone. Her only child was in trouble, and she felt powerless to help. She had an overwhelming urge to call Emile. But he was at the bedside of his mother at a hospital in London. To give him the bad news about George would be a mistake. Sari decided not to call his cell number. From within her came an answer.

She wiped her wet eyes and put the yogurt and cheese in the refrigerator, leaving the canned goods on the counter. Thelma's nephew had been in jail. She would know what to do. Sari picked up her keys, went back out in the garage and got back in her car, all the while asking God to give her strength.

On Monday of the following week, Eva pointed to one of many diplomas on the wall. "Look, Trenton, Dan graduated from George Mason before he went to law school at the University of Virginia. Maybe you'll follow in his footsteps."

The federal prosecutor, Dan Simmons, leaned over his desk. He was stocky and losing his hair, but his dark eyes shone with wisdom in his cherubic face.

He turned to Trenton, "Thinking of law school?"

Smiling, Trenton said, "I've got to graduate from college first."

Dan waved two pages of yellow legal paper in front of him. "You convinced Farouk Hamdi to waive his right to an attorney before giving his statement."

Trenton shrugged. "I guess he wants out of jail."

Eva slid the papers from Dan's hands and directed his eyes to the bottom of the first page. "Farouk admits here that he took money from terrorism supporters and made deposits of just less than ten grand each."

Dan nodded. "A clever scheme. The banks are mandated to report to the Treasury Department deposits of more than ten thousand dollars." He skimmed over the rest of Farouk's confession, "Good work, Nash."

Eva agreed. "Trenton complements our team."

Trenton looked pleased. "We want to get Farouk out on bond as my informant."

Dan's reply was swift, "Will he wear a wire in meetings with ARC members? Can we trust what he says?"

Prepared for this battle, Trenton replied, "Farouk links Emile Jubayl and his son, George, to the funding of terrorist sympathizers in Lebanon and elsewhere." His eyes flashed. "Helpers International should be shut down and their assets seized. Farouk will help us put Jubayl behind bars."

Dan raised both eyebrows. "The aid organization, Helpers International? My mother volunteers there."

Her face grim, Eva nodded.

He asked her, "Are you as eager as Trenton is to launch a full-scale investigation on a religious organization?"

Eva tented her hands. "I first reacted as you, but our country is no longer the same. Everything and everyone are suspect."

Her words sounded a note of sadness in the musty office. It clung in the air like heavy dew.

"I believe my own mother is exempt from scrutiny," Dan declared.

Trenton said firmly, "Several heads of charitable organizations have pleaded guilty to funding groups on the State Department's list of prohibited organizations. Is Emile any different?"

"That remains to be seen," Dan said.

Eva was due at an agency head meeting in less than an hour and wanted Dan's answer before she left. "Farouk's contact in London knows Emile. If Farouk gets out, he can attend a prearranged meeting in London with that financier. Also, Farouk says George bragged that his father knows militants in Lebanon, including Hezbollah. It is illegal for Americans to deal with that organization."

Dan swiveled in his chair. A loud squeak permeated the room. "Mere association is not enough to prove one is a terrorist."

Eva winced at the sound. Last night over steaks that Scott grilled, she prepared for Dan's objections. It had been another quiet dinner. "It may prove to be more than that. Farouk's London connections could reveal other American links to ARC. The meeting is scheduled in three weeks."

Dan tapped his pen on a legal pad, as if deep in thought.

Eva added, "It is risky, but worth doing. "

Dan pulled on his bottom lip. "I'd need evidence beyond your informant's claims of Jubayl's involvement."

Trenton pitched another tactic. "When that bomb exploded at State, George Jubayl was there. Fifteen people were hurt. He's being held on a twenty-thousand-dollar bond for assaulting an old lady. A detective said George denies knowing about the bomb, but I think he does. The guy hates America."

Eva told Dan what Brewster had told them about MI-5's suspicions of Emile's extended family. While her next words might cause Dan to reassign the case, she had to tell him. "Recently, I met Emile. He and his wife go to my church."

Trenton immediately changed direction. "Let's make Farouk a double."

Dan looked askance. "A what?"

Because Eva and Trenton had discussed this, she explained, "He pretends to work for their side, and collects the proof we need to convict Emile and his terrorist friends."

Dan silently massaged his lip. Eva nodded at Trenton to give him time to think.

At length, he said, "Eva, prepare a subpoena for Emile's home and office phone records. We have three weeks, so move quickly. If there are calls to forbidden groups, we'll apply for a pen register warrant."

"What is that?" Trenton asked.

"A machine that records all numbers of Emile's incoming and outgoing calls." Dan slid Farouk's statement in an accordion folder, then reached for the phone. "I have to be in court in ten minutes to pick a jury on our insurance agent case. Griff's a great fill-in for you, Eva."

Trenton was not finished. "I have another idea."

Dan held the receiver, but did not punch in the number. "Go."

"We contribute ten thousand dollars to Helpers International as a way for me to meet Emile." Trenton glanced at Eva.

She looked up from her note pad, her pen jabbed the air. "That might work."

Trenton's face radiated a smile that was short-lived.

"I don't have funds for that," Dan said.

Trenton countered, "Last year, the Drug Enforcement Administration used my informant to buy five ounces of cocaine for ten grand, which gave him credibility to topple higher targets. Why can't we spend that same amount of money to get inside a terror group?"

Eva headed off Dan's certain protest. "You just said Griff is great. With his experience working undercover, he could pose as a sympathizer and make a contribution using an undercover name and Detroit address. If Emile accepts funds designated for prohibited terrorist groups, we'll have him. I'll find the money in my budget, somehow."

Dan thought a moment, then replied, "Eva, We've worked together for ten years. I trust your judgment. Create an undercover bank account and send a check. Keep me informed."

Four days later, Eva had just returned another call to Kat, Channel 14's reporter. They were playing phone tag and Kat was "it." As Eva replaced the receiver, she looked up to see Trenton in her doorway. He asked if she had a few minutes. She motioned to him to sit in a chair across from her desk. It was past six o'clock and she was ready to go home.

Eva leveled piercing eyes at Trenton. "How's the case against Emile? The clock is ticking if we want Farouk to get to London."

He held up a stack of papers a few inches thick. "Good news, for a change."

"That looks more like work."

"They're phone bills for Emile's home phone and Helpers International." He spread out several computer sheets. "These show every number called from his phones."

"Do they match numbers in our intelligence data base?"

Trenton smiled. "Someone at Helpers called Beirut."

Eva's day had exploded midmorning. Kaley fell off the balance beam in gym class. The result was a gash to her head. Fortunately, Scott was able to take her to the emergency room for stitches.

Her eyes on the numbers, she said, "So? Much of their humanitarian aid goes to the Middle East."

"This call went to ARC's top money man."

Emile might be knowingly supporting terrorists, or there could be an innocent explanation. She had seen Emile in a crisp white shirt walking with his wife last Sunday in the church parking lot, looking like the other believers.

"Was there just one call?"

Trenton admitted there was.

"I would feel better if there were a series. Any incriminating calls on the home phone?"

"I'm still checking. There is one from the jail, which could be from George. Is this enough for Dan to get us a pen register?"

"Stay on it." Eva picked up her purse and keys.

Their meeting at an end, Trenton walked out with his stack of evidence.

Eva called after him. "Tomorrow, wear a shirt and tie. We're going to the grand jury."

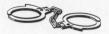

TEN

While Trenton accelerated up the entry ramp onto the Capital Beltway, Eva checked her seatbelt. She had asked Trenton to drive her G-car to the federal Courthouse in Alexandria.

"Stay in this lane. You'll get off before the Wilson Bridge."

Much to Eva's discomfort, he quickly changed lanes and increased his speed. With one hand on the wheel, he asked. "What's it like testifying before a grand jury?"

"Did you ever testify before a county grand jury?"

Trenton's eyes were glued to the rear bumper of the car ahead. "No. I did testify at preliminary hearings before a judge. That's how we charged defendants."

Eva put her hand on the dash as if that gave her more space from the car in front of them. "We agents like the federal grand jury. Some defense attorneys complain it gives us too much power to decide if someone should stand trial."

Trenton jerked to the left, stepped on the gas to pass an offending car, then roared in front of it. He asked easily, "Do we wait while Dan selects the jury?"

"No!" Eva strained forward against her seatbelt. Trenton was over the speed limit. She unclenched her teeth and said, "Once citizens from the Eastern District of Virginia are sworn in, they serve a couple of days each month for eighteen months."

He checked his mirror and changed lanes. A car cut in front of them.

Eva yelled, "Watch it!" She promised herself she wouldn't ride with Trenton again. Ever.

Unperturbed, he asked, "Do you think we'll get the pen register today?"

Eva removed one hand from the dash and rubbed her face. She

doubted they'd make it in one piece. "We present our evidence. Dan asks the grand jury to vote on our subpoenas for bank records. Afterward, Dan approves our pen register warrant and asks the judge to sign it."

"The grand jurors don't approve that?"

Eva turned to Trenton. He was catching on. "Right. Later, Dan may ask the jurors to vote whether Emile should be indicted. If he is, an indictment is returned and arrest warrants are issued. He would be tried by a separate jury."

Traffic thinned, Trenton eased off the speed. "Defense attorneys won't question you today?"

Eva's other hand relaxed from the dash. "There is no way for the targets to know or cross examine what we say. Our testimony and conduct in there must be above reproach."

"A defense attorney told me that being assigned to the Feds was like working for the gestapo."

"Some defense lawyers get kicks out of telling stories and making citizens believe that the federal system is unfair. Your friend should spend a few days watching the nonexistent legal system in Cuba."

"He's not my friend. How about Harlan Scribbs, former U.S. Attorney, now a defense lawyer? I testified in a case where he defended a former police officer who took money from the drug fund."

Eva pointed ahead. "Thankfully, this is our exit. Go to Old Town. If we have time, I'll take you to a great spot for Reuben sandwiches." She added, "Before I drive back."

Trenton missed her attempt at humor. He stopped at a red light. "Where next?"

"Park in the ramp on the right."

Eva rolled her eyes. "Dan expects me to testify, but after seeing you drive, you can handle it."

"Great!" Trenton's smile grew wider.

"For all the grand jury's power, they knit in their seats, lean back in chairs against the wall. Business owners, stay-at-home moms, and retired folks get well acquainted. If there's a birthday, we might get a piece of cake. Don't be offended if they eat while you testify."

Trenton entered the parking garage and pushed the button for a ticket.

Eva warned, "Rule 6 (e) of the U.S. Criminal Code requires the grand jury's work to be absolutely secret. That goes for you and the jurors."

Trenton eased into a second-level parking spot and turned off the ignition. He handed Eva the keys and asked, "Can I tell you what goes on in there?"

They got out, and Eva locked the car with the remote. As they hurried down the ramp, she said, "There are exceptions, like advising your boss."

Trenton broached a new subject. "When I tailed Jubayl, he was talking on a cell. Can we get his cell phone records, too?"

Trenton was walking ahead. He turned. Eva stood on the sidewalk, hands on her hip.

"You tailed him?"

"When he left his office. Why would he visit a gemologist in Vienna?"

"Did Griff give you permission to put surveillance on him?"

"Do I need an okay?" He shrugged. "When you and Dan approved my investigation, I decided I should investigate."

Eva started walking again. "Funny. You need supervision."

"Sorry. I'm used to working on my own. There was a diamond symbol on the office door. A gemologist works with gems, right?"

"Maybe he was appraising his wife's wedding ring for the insurance."

"Can I tell the grand jury what I saw him do?"

Eva pulled open the federal Building door. "We have one minute to get up there. Run!"

Dan poked his balding head out of the grand jury room, saw Eva, and asked, "Ready?"

She nudged Trenton's arm and said, for his ears only, "Skip your surveillance, for now."

Dan eyed his new witness. "After you are sworn in, I ask you questions."

Trenton caught his breath. "Eva explained everything."

Inside, he was greeted by smells of coffee and cinnamon. The grand jurors were spread about the room. Some smiled, some nodded. One younger woman with bright yellow hair looked bored. Dan sat next to a clerk at a long table and pointed at the empty chair for Trenton.

A pretty young lady with a headset and control panel sat between the table and the jurors. Trenton grinned at her. Her fingers poised above the device, she returned his smile. Eva was right. This grand jury would be fun.

The clerk said, "Raise your right hand for the oath."

Trenton complied.

She asked, "Do you swear your testimony before this grand jury will be the truth, the whole truth, and nothing but the truth, so help you God?"

"I do."

Dan began his questions. "State and spell your name for the record."

"Trenton Nash, spelled N-A-S-H."

"By whom are you employed?"

"Jefferson County. A deputy sheriff, I am assigned to the ICE Financial Investigations Group."

Trenton answered Dan's questions about the Armed Revolutionary Cause and his investigation of Helpers International. Dan asked, "What was found in Mr. Jubayl's home phone records?"

"He called Beirut, Lebanon." With Eva's warning not to tell about surveillance, Trenton wondered if he should say more. He decided to let Dan ask what he wanted to know.

"Mr. Jubayl was born in Beirut, right?"

Trenton replied, "Yes. This call was to one whom we suspect is ARC's top financier."

Two Grand Jurors shifted in their seats. Then, a man in a bow tie looked directly at a woman with red hair piled atop her head. She returned the man's look.

Dan checked off a column on his legal pad. "How will you follow up?"

Trenton guessed Dan did not want him to say more about the phone calls, including the one to the jail, so he answered exactly what he was asked. "We need a subpoena for his personal bank records."

"I will seek authorization from this jury when you are finished." Dan said. "Do jurors have questions?"

A young man with a tattoo on his forearm asked, "If I'm stopped for speeding in Jefferson County, can I drop your name?"

Everyone in the room erupted into laughter, except Dan.

"How about a serious question?" Dan repeated.

The red-haired lady slowly raised her hand, and the man in the bow tie nodded. She said, "My name is Penny Strobel. I work at Helpers International. Will that affect my service on this grand jury?"

"*That* is a serious question." Dan's lips formed into a tight line on his face. "Let's discuss it in the conference room. Everyone else may take a lunch break."

Trenton got up from his chair and waited for Dan. His stomach churned, like when he ate too many hot dogs. Who was this lady, and why was she messing up his case?

Dan and Trenton walked into a conference room down the hall, where Eva was drinking her second cup of strong coffee. She looked up and was about to ask Trenton how he liked being a witness when she noticed a strange woman, red hair piled atop her head.

Dan shut the door. "Eva, this is Ms. Strobel. She works at Helpers International." He nodded at her. "Please explain what you do there and what interaction you have with Mr. Jubayl."

A look at Dan's face told Eva this was a problem. In fourteen years working with federal grand juries, she had never encountered a juror who knew a target. What would Dan do? Their whole case was in danger of imploding. And Trenton looked like he would explode.

Penny wiped her hands on her black slacks. "I coordinate hundreds of volunteers, but don't have much contact with Mr. Jubayl. My daughter Hannah works with him daily."

Eva hoped her shock did not show.

Dan said evenly, as if he often faced the issue, "Ms. Strobel, did you tell your daughter about the grand jury?"

The woman looked unsure for a moment, then said, "I told her I was called to serve. I did not talk about anything I have heard."

Dan looked relieved. "That's right. You took an oath to maintain grand jury secrecy under *all* circumstances. I am not trying to scare you, but if you reveal what you heard about your employer, you could face a contempt charge and possible jail."

Penny's delicate face was flushed. "As a Christian, I take my oath seriously. You can trust me not to tell a soul, not even my daughter. Can I stay on the jury?"

Eva wanted to comfort her. But Dan was running this show. She let him reply.

"Your eighteen months of service will be over soon. It's best we end it today."

Penny's face fell.

Dan added, "If you do not step down, you would have to leave every time this case is presented. That could disrupt the whole system." He closed off further argument by shaking her hand and saying, "Thank you, Ms. Strobel. Please get your things and see the clerk for your pay."

Dan, you're being rough. We need her cooperation. Eva need not have worried.

Penny assured them, "I understand and will honor my oath. Good day."

When she left, Dan wiped his brow. "She could have put up more of a fuss."

"You seemed cool enough," Eva said.

Trenton shot back, "What about my case? If she slips up and tells Jubayl what she knows, it will ruin everything!"

Eva said, "Dan, we could bring her before Judge Pendergast to reinforce the secrecy rules. What will you tell the others when she fails to return this afternoon?"

"I need lunch." Dan picked up his briefcase. "Join me for a burger?"

"We should get back to the office and move this case along," Eva said. She glanced at Trenton, who shrugged. His appetite must have disappeared, too.

"It's your empty stomach, not mine. They have spicy potatoes." He looked hopeful.

Their case was in danger of being compromised, and Dan thought only of food. She shook her head.

Dan snapped shut his briefcase. "I trust her. Pendergast might scare her from ever wanting to serve again. We'll leave it be. I'll explain Penny was excused because she knew a possible target and find out if anyone else is acquainted with Helpers International."

Eva had not even considered that possibility. Maybe it was naive to trust her, given that her employment was at stake.

Trenton was a step ahead of both of them. "I'll interview Ms. Strobel and develop her as an inside informant."

Dan and Eva chimed in unison. "No!"

"Bu—" Trenton protested.

Eva interrupted his plea, "No. But it is time for you to visit Farouk."

"Dan, can I tell Farouk you will recommend he get out on a bond?" Trenton asked.

Dan smiled. "We could talk over lunch about what I need to make that happen. Afterward, I'll have the bank records subpoenaed for you."

Trenton turned his electric smile to Eva. "You did promise me a Reuben."

"Mom, I practiced my lines for Queen Esther all week." Kaley set down her fork on the plate of chocolate cake and licked her lips. "But I don't feel like a queen."

Taken aback by her daughter's maturity for her nine years, Eva compared Kaley to the other daughters in the church fellowship hall at the mother-daughter banquet, some of whom were in her daughter's class at school. She should let Kaley invite the girls over for a party sometime.

Eva patted Kaley's hand. "You were wonderful. I am proud of you. But we have to go. I have an early morning meeting."

"We have to finish our cake," Kaley insisted.

"I'll find something to wrap it in. You and your brother can share it tomorrow." As tears gathered in Kaley's eyes, Eva added, "How about renting a movie on the way home, for tomorrow night? You love *Anne of Green Gables.*"

Her blond head swathed in a gold scarf, Kaley nodded in resignation. Eva slipped away before more objections came. She felt bad enough having to leave early. Nearing the kitchen, she was stopped by Thelma King.

"Kaley sure made us believe she was Queen Esther."

"Thanks," Eva held out her hand, which Thelma folded into her larger one. "Kaley will be glad to know you thought she looked like royalty."

Thelma turned to Sari Jubayl, who stood next to her. She nudged her side. "Ask her."

Eva noticed Sari's eyes were puffy and red. She'd been crying.

Sari blew her nose on a white handkerchief. "It's my son. He's in jail. Emile is out of town again. What should I do?"

Eva froze. George Jubayl was not implicated in funding terrorists. But Sari's questions could easily lead to Emile. Eva had to end this.

"Sari, I am very sorry. I really cannot talk about it now. Kaley and I have to get home. Perhaps you should call an attorney for your son. He or she can advise you."

Thelma threw an arm around Sari's shoulder. "That's what I told you she'd say. Now, do it."

Sari could not mask her confusion. "But George is innocent. If he hires an attorney, won't that make people think he's guilty?"

Eva replied, "Under our Constitution, everyone has a right to a lawyer. If he can't afford it, one will be appointed for him; perhaps one has been already."

Thelma dropped her arm. "The court appointed one for my nephew. He was good."

Sari looked up at this. "Was he cleared?"

"No! He 'fessed up like he should and only did a year in prison for passin' a bad check."

"Prison?" Fresh tears wavered on her lashes like raindrops after a storm.

Eva waved in farewell. "Listen to Thelma. She's a good friend. Kaley," she called, "We're leaving now."

She turned to get her daughter, but heard Sari say, "I need money from the bank for George's bond. Could you go with me to the jail and pay it?"

Pangs of guilt hit her. Eva glanced back. Thelma reached out a gnarled hand for Sari to take and said, "We'll go to the bank in the morning. I'll drive you to the D.C. jail. I know the way."

Eva steered Kaley out of the Fellowship Hall and to the parking lot.

"You forgot my cake!"

"I will buy you candy at the video store. Please get in the car."

Kaley slid on the seat and Eva shut her door. Walking over to the driver's side, Eva thought about Sari. If she was this upset about George, what would she do if Emile was charged with aiding terrorists and went to prison for the rest of his life? Eva rarely witnessed the personal side of her cases. The closest she had ever come was when a businessman's wife collapsed in court after he was sentenced to ten years. This was different. This was someone *she* knew. Eva did not like the lump in her throat.

"Don't you think so, Mommy?"

"What, honey?"

"Queen Esther was courageous when she said, 'If I perish, I perish,' and went to see the King, even though she might have lost her life."

"Why did she do that?" Eva hoped Kaley thought she'd been listening.

"The Bible says her uncle believed God put her there for 'such a time as this.' They prayed, and Esther's people, the Jews, were saved. Mrs. King said that's why Jewish people celebrate Purim. We are going to blow noisemakers and celebrate, too."

They reached the video store. Eva turned off the van, absorbed with the memory of Sari Jubayl's large dark eyes and the even darker rings beneath them. Kaley ran ahead in her costume and yellow flip-flops and quickly found her movie. Eva paid for the film and chocolate bars and thrust the change in her purse.

On the way home, a painful thought struck her: She had few friends. Her mother said friendships were like creating a garden. It took time to plant and water the seeds before harvest. If she was not investigating Emile, would she have stayed to talk with Sari? Probably not.

Eva felt odd leaving, but it was improper to be too friendly. Maybe, someday, she could make it up to Sari. Eva glanced over at Kaley in the passenger seat, her head slumped against her arm. She was sleeping. *I need to tell her I love her, more often.*

In a moment, her mind veered to her cases. Earl had flown to Denver to help in the new indictments against the sleeper cell. Griff would be in court for a few more days. When Eva had returned to the office from the grand jury, she'd called Lou to check on his progress and get an idea when he would return to FIG. A nurse's aide answered. Lou was sleeping. That did not sound good. It was Eva's job to manage Trenton's assertiveness—it was a fine line she had to walk between encouraging him and reigning him in.

They arrived home. The front porch light was on. She pictured Scott reading, waiting for her. She should have picked up a comedy to watch with him. They needed more fun times, just the two of them. Scott had not asked her again about a baby, but she knew he thought of it.

Eva pressed the garage door remote. George's presence at the bombing linked him to it, and maybe to his father's activities as well. If father and son were involved, Sari had to know something. Even though the family went to her church and Eva felt sorry for Sari, she had to find the truth, no matter how painful.

Later that evening, after Eva tucked Kaley and Andy into bed, she found Scott downstairs in the family room reading a biography about Winston Churchill. A book in her hand, she smiled and sat next to him on the couch. Marty had sent her this book about Corrie Ten Boom and how she was miraculously saved from the concentration camp in World War II. After reading a chapter, Eva rested her head on Scott's chest. He continued reading. She did not feel like talking. In moments, she sensed her head was slumping downward. Her body felt heavy. Eva breathed in deeply the peace in her home.

In moments she was asleep. A woman dressed in a yellow silk robe and headdress walked beside her in a beautiful garden. She looked like Kaley in the play, but she was older, with large brown eyes. With two hands, she took off the scarf wound around her head, and her red hair flowed around her shoulders. The woman beckoned Eva to sit under the shade of the tree, then touched Eva's hand. She spoke three words so softly, Eva could barely hear. *Save my people.* That was all. She walked away. Eva ran after her until she came to the water. There was no one there.

"Honey, are you all right?" Scott shook her awake.

Eva's mouth felt dry and her tongue thick. She sat up and looked at Scott.

"You were breathing funny, like you were out of breath."

She said, "I was running."

"I never remember my dreams. You seem to recall everything."

Eva replied, "I'm going to get some water. Want anything?"

Scott pulled her up. "Time for bed. Turn on the stairway light and I'll turn off this one."

Her fingers touched the switch, and she wondered at her dream. The woman was a mixture of Queen Esther, Kaley, and Penny Strobel. What did it all mean?

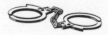

ELEVEN

E arly the next morning, Trenton swiped his magnetic card and entered the rear door of the building. He walked down the hall, past the FIG office, and knocked against a locked steel door. It was opened by an agent wearing jeans and a shoulder holster thick with a gun.

Trenton held up his government credentials. "Agent Grant?"

The agent opened the door. "Follow me."

Anxious to discover what secrets lurked in the FBI's Technical Operations Group, Trenton wound around desks cluttered with a lineman's work belt, wire clippers, and hard hats. He heard many stories from Duke about wiretaps and eavesdropping. This was his chance to experience it firsthand.

A heavy man limped over to Trenton. "I'm Ralph Grant, Group Supervisor. Call me Gus. Eva said you would stop by. It's this way."

On the way to the adjoining room, Gus stopped. Trenton banged against his arm.

Gus asked, "A deputy sheriff has no authority to enforce federal laws. You been sworn in as a FIG officer?"

"I'm official. What's wrong with your leg?"

Gus rubbed his knee. "Blew out my knee playing soccer with the young guys. I need an operation. No way I want to go under the knife if I don't have to." With a wave, Gus entered the wire room. "Pen registers are in here. Next year, we're going high tech." Gus sighed. "It's too bad. I love these old machines."

Trenton blinked his eyes in the almost total darkness and searched for the machine to help prove his case. He heard nothing and saw only small red, green, and yellow lights that peered at him like laser guns. There was no other sign of the important work being done in such secrecy.

Gus turned on the overhead lights. The spell was broken. Tables laden with electronic equipment and power strips lined the perimeter. Gus hobbled to a gray machine the size of a microwave oven standing on end.

"It's usually quiet in here. But when your Mr. Jubayl makes a call, this pen register springs to life and records all numbers to and from his phones." Gus motioned to a door with an official looking sign, *Court Authorized Persons Only,* and said, "In the monitoring room where we tap criminals' telephones, it's always noisy. The courts require us to monitor those conversations as they occur."

Trenton's eyes found what he was searching for: the court order taped above a machine, *U.S. vs. Emile Jubayl.* A jolt of glee filled him. He stared at the order, which was sealed from the public. Even the media couldn't find out about it. Trenton started to plan what he'd tell Duke.

Gus turned the machine, exposed the rear. A genius with all things technical, Gus pointed to an electrical junction. "Judge Pendergast ordered the phone company to run this wire from Jubayl's home line. The pen register prints out every number called by and received at his home." Gus laughed. "The family hasn't a clue we know who it is the instant a call is made."

Trenton let out a low chuckle.

Gus continued, "That's not all. If the Court does order you to listen into a conversation, I move the equipment to the monitoring room and connect a tape recorder and speaker at this electrical junction."

Gus carefully pushed the pen register back up against the wall, then wagged a finger. "Remember, because most of Helpers' employees are not suspects, Pendergast refused to let you monitor outgoing *business* calls. You need more evidence."

A green light glowed on the machine. The inside mechanism clattered so loudly that Trenton jumped, as if he'd been caught doing something forbidden.

"What was that?"

"It's a call coming into Jubayl's home. Someone just picked up a ringing phone."

Paper tape advanced out the front of the register. Gus tapped a digital reader above the tape and said, "The caller I.D. shows it's from the D.C. police lockup. Does someone in Emile's family work there?"

Trenton leaned forward and checked out the tape. *Cool!*

He replied, "His son is in jail for bashing a protestor at that State Department demonstration. Maybe he set off the bomb."

"The one full of nails?"

Trenton nodded.

"Stay on 'em, Nash." Gus pressed a button on the front of the pen register, and the printer spewed a stream of paper tape. "Each morning, remove the tape for the previous twenty-four hours. Initial and date it. Have the analysts check each call."

Awed by the gadgetry, Trenton was sure he would master it in a day or two. Gus flipped off the overhead light and limped out of the wire room. Trenton couldn't resist looking back. The lights glowed red, like eyes of wolves waiting for their next meal. He felt certain they'd help seal the fate of Emile Jubayl, whom he was certain was a terrorist masquerading as an honest businessman.

Trenton caught up to Gus, who said, "See my secretary for your own key."

"Registered parcel for Task Force Officer Trenton Nash," said Wanda, her hair plastered with more spray than usual. "My, aren't you special."

"Got a big date tonight?" Without saying he was glad it was not with him, Trenton seized the package and turned it over. The return address was from Detroit! Trenton laughed. Griff, the veteran FBI agent, had taken his advice and sent the 10-thousand-dollar donation to Emile using an undercover name and address.

He strode out of Wanda's eavesdropping range. He did not trust her. Maybe it was because once he saw her after work with a guy who looked just like a drug dealer he'd arrested. Maybe it was her hair, dyed the color of a tangerine. It did not seem real. Plus, his dad had drummed it into his brain: An agent should never let secure information leak to anyone without a need to know.

Well out of Wanda's eyesight, Trenton ripped open the envelope and pulled out a sealed plastic envelope. Inside was a letter with the Helpers return address and a custody receipt from the Detroit agent who retrieved it from the undercover post office box.

Trenton donned latex gloves, broke open the sealed envelope, and carefully drew out the letter addressed to Mr. Ashur Wadi, Griff's undercover name. Trenton did not read it until he had photocopied it, resealed the original in a new evidence envelope, and returned to his office and shut the door. His eyes absorbed the few sentences:

Dear Mr. Wadi:

Your generous $10,000 gift to Helpers International will help children in the Middle East. We have programs supported by Middle East refugees in Detroit, and I often travel there. May I show you what your gift is funding? I called the telephone number on your letterhead, but there was no answer. Please call the number on my enclosed card to arrange a time for us to meet.

Emile's signature was scrawled at the bottom.

"Yes!" Trenton's cry echoed off his office walls. He hurried to find Eva and tell her that Jubayl had not only swallowed the bait, he was hooked.

Emile Jubayl dimmed the overhead light and tried to ignore the incessant noise and movement in the crowded Boeing 777 cabin. He secured headphones against his ears and turned up the volume to Wagner's *Ride of the Valkyries*. He would declare nothing on the Customs form. After all, it was not like he purchased the stone. It was a gift. One he would not tell Sari about. His wife was full of questions, but she was the last person Emile would confide his secret to.

Eyes closed, Emile decided not to declare the watch, either. It was from his mother. The government had no right to know about such a personal item. A nudge on his arm. He ignored the old man sitting next to him in the middle seat. Another tap.

Emile sighed and lifted the right ear phone slightly. "What is it?"

"You dropped your Customs form," the old man said gently.

Emile snatched the paper from the aisle. "Thanks."

He prepared to snap his earphones in place when his seat partner offered him a box of peppermints from the Netherlands. Emile's hand wavered over the box. If he took one, the man might take it as an invitation to tell him his life story. Yet his mouth had a dry ache that came from not eating. The in-flight meal was hours ago.

"You are kind." Emile put the round mint in his mouth, ready to return to his music.

"A good deed lives in the heart, my Aunt Deane used to say. She is in heaven now."

The compassion in the man's voice drew Emile to him. They shook hands, and Emile was surprised that the elderly man's grip was firm and strong. "I'm Emile Jubayl, CEO of Helpers International. Our motto is a life helped is a life saved."

The old man's dark eyes shone behind silver glasses. "Marty VanderGoes is my name." He removed his glasses and looked at Emile. "I may have gotten a pamphlet in the mail about your work in the Middle East." Marty shut his eyes for a moment. When they opened, his face beamed. "Yes. I was so impressed, I showed it to my pastor."

Emile shoved the headset in his seatback pocket and, for thirty minutes, told Marty things about his dreams for Helpers that he had not shared even with his Board. As the flight attendant announced they should prepare to land, Emile mentioned his mother's heart problem.

"The giver of life knows our every need. Are you a believer?" Marty returned the trifocals to his long nose.

Unsure how to answer, Emile stared at his manicured hands. A believer in what? He did not want to offend a potential donor.

A smile burst on Marty's face, remarkably without wrinkles. "I was raised in America by a churchgoing family. At eighteen, both my parents died within weeks of each other. I was sure God had abandoned me. I moved to Holland to live with my Aunt Deane. Her deep love of Christ sustained us during the Nazi occupation. But that is a story for another time."

Emile looked sharply at Marty's black eyes and black and silver hair. "Are you Jewish?"

Marty shook his head. "My parents were born in The Netherlands, in Zeeland, where the Spanish occupied the land for generations. My Aunt and I worked for the Dutch underground in World War II. The Lord gave us opportunities to save many Jewish lives. Why do you ask?"

A male flight attendant announced, "Fasten your seatbelts and prepare for landing."

Emile took Marty's card. "Would you like to visit Helpers sometime? We have a lot of ways to volunteer."

Marty said, "I'm always interested in the Lord's work. My time is spent between the Netherlands and northern Virginia." He pressed

Emile's forearm with his hand. "I will pray for your mother's heart. If I can help, please call."

At his touch, warmth surged through Emile. He tucked the card in his wallet, with no idea he had just poured his heart out to Eva Montanna's grandfather. He put away Marty's question, was he a believer, more focused on the chance to turn him into a donor than to examine the state of his own soul.

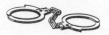

TWELVE

A stiff breeze blew fallen leaves around Hannah's feet. She zipped up her jacket, a perfect match to her long auburn hair, opened the car door with her key, then heard a voice say, "Excuse me, Ms. Strobel."

Hannah looked around the student parking lot. Over her left shoulder she saw a man, a stranger, walking toward her. She felt a tinge of panic. How did he know her name? No one else was in the parking lot. Classes had already started.

She was about to get in her car and drive away when the man, who she guessed was in his late twenties, said, "I'm Deputy Sheriff Trenton Nash." He pulled out a leather credential case and added, "Don't be afraid."

Dressed in a jacket and jeans, he did not look like a policeman. Trenton flipped open his official identification for her, and she scrutinized his picture. She read the words *United States Department of Homeland Security,* which were scrolled above an embossed eagle with wings spread.

"I'd like to ask you some questions," he said.

Puzzled, Hannah checked again around the lot. "Have I done something wrong?"

"You may have information to help me in a case I am investigating. Can we talk?"

"I don't know." Hannah peered at Trenton's I.D., which he left open. "I have to be at work in an hour."

"At Helpers International. You're not closed for the holiday?"

"How did you know I work at Helpers? Hannah pulled her keys from the lock, crunched them in her hand, but kept the door open. "Why are *you* working on Columbus Day? It's a federal holiday."

Trenton flashed her an enormous smile. "Because crime never takes a holiday. Can I buy you a soda at the Commons? I'll explain how you can help me."

Hannah glanced at his good-looking face and beautiful white teeth. He seemed legitimate. "Ten minutes is okay, but I don't drink pop."

"Pop?" Trenton flipped his credentials into his back pocket.

She laughed. "Sugary stuff with fizz. That's what we call it in the Midwest, where I grew up. I like mocha coffee."

Trenton held open the heavy glass door to the George Mason University Commons, where students gathered to eat and talk. He said, "I attend classes here, too."

Surprise brightened Hannah's eyes. If Nash was a student, maybe that was why he acted more casual than the police officer who almost gave her a ticket the day before for running a red light. "What's your major?"

Even though he didn't usually drink coffee, Trenton ordered two mochas. "Administration of Justice. And yours?"

"Journalism. This semester, we're focusing on photojournalism. My mom just gave me a five mega-pixel digital camera with a ten power optical zoom."

"Wow. I wish I had one."

She glanced at his face to see if he was teasing. She asked, "Are we in any classes together?"

"No. I would have remembered you."

Trenton led her to chairs over by the window, away from a group of loud students, and explained his role with FIG. "Please keep our conversation confidential," he said.

"You said I did nothing wrong." Hannah coughed. She had drunk the coffee too quickly and burned her throat.

"But Helpers International may have. That's what I need to find out."

Hannah set down her coffee on the small table. "Helpers International lifts up oppressed people all over the world. The people who work there are like me."

"What do you mean, like you?"

Hannah cleared her throat to try to explain things. "When I was eleven, I made a decision that changed my life. Jesus became more than a Bible story. He became real in my life. He influences the way I live each day."

Trenton shifted in the chair. "Other charitable groups have gone down for supporting terrorists. A religious label means nothing."

Hannah stiffened at his rebuke. "My mom works there, too." She took a small sip of coffee. It was still too hot to drink. Hannah held the cup between her hands and said, "My faith is more than being religious."

Before she could explain, Trenton asked, "Your mother is Penny Strobel?"

Hannah nodded. "Why?"

"She knows of my investigation, but took an oath of secrecy. Do not try to question her."

"If it is secret, why can you tell me?"

Trenton finished his coffee in two gulps. "I'm not telling what I know. I'm asking what you know."

Hannah perched on the edge of the chair. This was a real case, not something from the newspaper. She should approach it as a journalist. "Can I tell my mom I talked to you?"

"Please don't, for now. Security reasons."

Hannah's green eyes widened. She had to know more. "Okay, how can I help?"

"Tell me what you do at Helpers." Trenton took a note pad from his back pocket. "I'm going to take notes."

Hannah said, "My job is nothing glamorous. I copy papers, sort mail, run errands."

"Tell me about your boss, Emile Jubayl."

"He is all business, and nothing like his son George."

Trenton stopped writing. "You know him?"

Hannah nodded. "He was in my world history class this term and once came to the college group at church. I want to say this right," she paused. "He sympathizes with everything anti-American. Emile is not like that."

"But your boss sympathizes with the Middle East?" Trenton asked.

From what she had observed at Helpers, Emile did. "Yes," she said.

Pen in hand, Trenton asked, "How does he show his sympathy for the Middle East? Does he have visitors from there, or does he travel and make phone calls to Middle Eastern countries?"

Hannah scowled. This was getting complicated. She thought she'd stick up for Emile and that would be it. Nash was as persistent as her cat when he wanted food. "We have projects all over the Middle East, and in Africa, too."

"Where, exactly? Who are the people that visit?" Trenton prodded.

Hannah pursed her lips. "I'm really not sure. Lebanon, he's from there. Palestine, and Jordan. I think Kenya, Egypt, and other places. The directors travel to our headquarters. They don't invite an intern to their meetings, if that's what you mean."

Trenton stretched out his legs and folded his arms behind his head. "I don't want to accuse anyone at such a longstanding organization without reason." He leaned forward, looked into her eyes. "After September 11, for the good of our nation, we follow every lead."

Her heart was mixed with emotions. Hannah wanted to help, but should she tell Nash more about Mr. Jubayl? She wished her mother was here. Then, Hannah realized there was someone more important she could ask. She lifted a silent prayer to God for wisdom, then opened her eyes. Trenton was gazing at her. He was protecting the country. It was right for her to tell.

In a low voice, she said, "I was in Mr. Jubayl's office when he received a phone call. From London. It sounded like a crisis."

"What did he say?"

"He closed the door, but I heard him say, 'Delay would be unwise' and 'I should have never left Lebanon'."

"That's all you heard?"

"Another time, I passed by his open door and heard Mr. Jubayl speak in what sounded like Arabic." Hannah checked her watch. "Oh!" She stood. "I have to get to work, especially if I'm forbidden to say why I am late."

"Anything else?" Trenton rose from his seat.

Hannah shook her head.

"Thanks for talking with me. May I call in a couple days, in case you remember more?"

She wrote her cell phone number on a piece of paper and handed it to him. "On Wednesdays after five I teach a class at church to the children."

"Does Emile Jubayl use a cell phone?"

"Doesn't everybody?"

Trenton smiled. "Do you know his number?"

Hannah thumbed through her planner. "Give me back that slip." She wrote his number.

Trenton reminded her, "Keep our conversation confidential."

"You can trust me."

Trenton opened the Commons door for her. "Can I walk you to your car?"

Hannah did not look back at him and said, "All right, but hurry. I don't want to lose my job because I'm helping you."

Eva rolled her chair away from her desk. She was reading Trenton's pen register warrant applications to track Emile's private line at Helpers International and his cell phone.

"How do you know these are Emile's numbers?"

Trenton's face was lit with a grin. "His direct phone number is listed on the business card he sent in the letter to Griff's undercover P.O. Box. The other number is his cell phone."

Impressed by Trenton's ingenuity, Eva smiled. If asked, she'd admit he reminded her of a young Griff, only more confident. "Good detective work. How did you get the cell number?"

"From a new source I developed within Helpers International."

Eva leapt to her feet. "You were not to contact Mrs. Strobel."

Palms open, Trenton defended himself. "She is *not* my informant"

She needed to stay on top of this case. "Who is it, exactly?"

Trenton's chin was slightly raised and he looked at Eva. "I assured the source I will not reveal the name or gender."

Detecting a note of respectful defiance in his tone, Eva didn't want to challenge him at this point and quash his enthusiasm. ICE needed more agents as dedicated as he, not fewer.

"Okay, I'll let that stand, for now. Tell me, what can this source give you in the future?"

"My source is placed highly enough to give me updates of Emile's activities and will protect the confidentiality of our inquiry."

Eva nodded. The telephone on her desk rang. It was Griff.

He said, "I've got good news. The jury found that insurance agent guilty on all counts. Dan and I are going to celebrate over ribs at Roy's Place in Old Town. Want to come?"

"I can't."

Maybe she *should* go and invite Trenton along to spend more time with him. She noticed Griff was never around his junior partner, either. She put her hand over the receiver.

"Trenton, want to go with me for ribs? Griff and Dan are celebrating. Another bad guy bit the dust."

"Sure."

She returned to Griff, "Okay, Trenton and I will both be there. Say," she checked her watch, "in one hour."

Griff replied, "Guess who was on camera filing a news story with her station?"

Eva moaned, "Kat. I can never reach her."

"She recognized me and asked about our search of the townhouse in Columbia City. I told her to talk to you."

"Thanks a lot."

Eva hung up. At some point, if Kat kept persisting, Eva would have to agree to give her background information, at least. To Trenton she said, "On our way, we'll bring these pen register applications to Judge Pendergast to sign. Hopefully, we can get them for both lines. Farouk's meeting in London is just over a week away. We have to convince Dan to let him out on a bond."

Eva got her warrants. The results were enough for her to finagle a meeting several days later with the FBI's Assistant Director for Counterterrorism, a former colleague of Trenton's father. Eva, Griff, and Trenton sat at a round table in Nathan Barlow's office. Barlow stood by the window, his back turned on the FIG group. Trenton shot Eva a hopeless look.

Eva defended Trenton's request to go to London with Farouk. "Sir, trust us to do everything possible to keep an eye on our informant."

Barlow came away from the window, took his seat around the table. "Can you assure me Farouk will produce what he says? Would this Cobra risk meeting in a public place?"

Eva explained, "When the Cobra is not selling arms around the world, he is with El Samoud. Farouk is scheduled to meet Cobra in a few days."

Trenton began to say, "Farouk's information has—"

Eva overrode him. "Cobra is clever. To make sure he is not followed, he travels through Amsterdam on his way to London. El Samoud trusts him for a reason. The Soviets trained him in counter-intelligence."

"He'll disappear if he sniffs surveillance," Trenton added.

Eva's glance said, *You just ruined your chance.*

Maneuvering through the FBI ranks for more than thirteen years, Griff had faced many bureaucratic logjams. He said, "Mr. Barlow, your trajectory in the Bureau is legendary. This sounds like a case you would have worked."

Eva thought Nathan's chest swelled beneath his shirt.

Barlow replied, "In a case like this, I would ask the Legat in London to provide hands on support."

"What's the Legat?" Trenton asked.

Griff's bushy eyebrows rose and fell. "FBI jargon. He's the agent in charge of the FBI office at the London Embassy. Also known as the Legal Attaché."

Reflexively, Eva touched her eyebrow. "Sir, with backup, Trenton can handle Farouk. Our goal will be for Farouk to meet with Cobra and convice him to meet, sometime in the future, with an undercover FBI agent posing as a new recruit. Successes involve risks, many greater than this. If we hesitate, we are that much further away from ARC and their terror plots. I am not willing to take a chance on another September 11."

Before he could reply, Nathan's phone rang. He reached a long arm across his cluttered desk and grabbed the receiver. "Barlow here." His head nodded vigorously. "It's in writing?"

Silence. Barlow's jaw muscles tightened, then relaxed. "We'll do everything to catch the killers." He hung up. His voice turned to steel. "ARC struck again."

Eva's hand flew to her mouth. The Pentagon! Was Scott safe? She asked, "Where?"

Barlow looked unhappy. "The British Ambassador to Lebanon was kidnapped yesterday. The Attorney General issued an internal memorandum to pull out all the stops on any case hinting at ARC involvement. Nash, looks like you're a key player. Use extra vigilance."

He turned to Eva. "Have an operation plan on my desk ASAP." Barlow gave a final order, "As the FBI agent in the group, Griff is to contact the Legat. Tell him I said he is in charge and will provide close support and surveillance. That's all."

Eva motioned for Trenton and Griff to follow her from the room before Barlow changed his mind. Griff shut the door behind him and caught Eva by the arm as Trenton strode to the elevator.

"Between the two of us, I know the Legat. We will definitely need Brewster's help. I'll call MI-5, and give him the details of Trenton's arrival."

Eva replied, "Barlow would have shot us down, if it wasn't for you. Let me know what Brewster says."

Trenton pressed the down elevator button. "What are you two talking about?"

Griff slapped his partner on the back. "Come to my office. We'll call the Legat together. I want you to develop a good rapport with him. Agent Lanning takes some getting used to."

Zayed held the British Ambassador's head under water for another twenty seconds, then let it bob to the surface. Ambassador Cook coughed, spat water through his mouth.

"Do you agree?"

Cook shook his head. Zayed cursed the prisoner and plunged Cook's face under again. Whatever the ARC operative tried, nothing worked. The diplomat better crack soon.

When Cook did not submit to demands, Zayed withheld food. For the last two days, Zayed had deprived him of water. The Ambassador, lips parched and bleeding, still said no.

El Samoud's orders were clear: Make Cook agree to pressure Britain to release three ARC soldiers standing trial for murder, or kill him. Zayed grew impatient with this man. But killing him too soon might mean losing his own life. That Zayed was unwilling to do for this hardened Brit he held captive in the Bekaa Valley. He could not forget his Supreme Leader's ominous promise, "Succeed there and you erase your blunder."

Zayed now hoped water would change Cook's mind. If he had known this would be the result, he'd have gotten that stone he threw to the bottom, somehow. Then, El Samoud would not have ordered him to Lebanon, and Zayed would be in New York, at home. He grabbed a chunk of hair and pulled up the Ambassador's face from the tub of cold water.

Zayed put his hand on the Brit's head, ready to thrust him under again. "Tell your Prime Minister to release our soldiers from jail!"

The former British spy, who endured worse on the field, spat out water and the words, "Torture will fail." Cook's courage on the field was the main reason he sought and received the posting to Lebanon, a desolate and difficult place.

Zayed pulled back his hand, prepared to strike the bony face, when a new method leapt to his mind. He clapped his hands. An armed guard appeared, dressed in black pants, shirt, and face mask.

"Bring me towels, a fresh robe, and hot tea."

When Cook was dry, Zayed motioned to the rug, and they both dropped onto it and sat cross-legged.

Zayed announced in perfect English, "It is time to talk."

Cook gulped down his tea.

Perhaps, Zayed had starved the Brit long enough. "Your country is the reason Israel became a nation. Britain shares the blame for the plight of the Palestinians. Unless your Prime Minister agrees to ARC's terms, you are a dead man. Do you like the sound of that as much as you do your tea?"

"Could I have another cup?"

It was a reasonable request. Perhaps the Brit needed something to eat. No, he would wait for that. With a wave of the hand, Zayed spoke in Arabic to the guard. They waited for more tea.

When it was brought, Zayed said to Cook, "You did not answer my question."

The Ambassador finished the second cup of tea, then replied, "You believe your cause is just. But you kill innocent people, who know nothing of you or your cause. The civilized world will not bow to terrorism. In the end, you will be defeated. Good will prevail."

Zayed spit his tea behind him on the stone floor. "Bah. Who decides what is good? I say it is good for Britain to release my friends, before it is too late." He smiled, his face looking older than his thirty-two years. "For you."

Cook returned Zayed's glare, then said, "You are an educated man. You spent time in Britain, I think, but I detect an American accent. New York, if I am not mistaken. How long did you enjoy the freedoms you now want to obliterate?"

Zayed swallowed. In the apartment where he lived for two years, he stood under the warm shower for ten minutes and swam in the pool. ARC recruited Zayed because he was an architect and expert in building technologies. How did Cook discern so much about him?

Cook straightened his legs in front of him and leaned toward his captor. "An educated man is usually a smart man. He uses reason, not raw emotion, in deciding which path to take. Life is more than the toss of a stone."

"How did you find out about the stone?"

"We know more than you think. Right now, a special operations team is on the way to rescue me. They could be here in another hour. If you kill me, they will hunt you down and finish you off."

"I do not believe you." Zayed said these words boldly, but mention of the stone shook him.

A British spy must have infiltrated Socotra. Maybe that taxi driver who gave him the stone worked for British Intelligence. If Cook knew about the stone, he probably knew Zayed had seen El Samoud's face. Was this posting to Lebanon a trick by the Cobra to get rid of him because he knew too much? Zayed had to find out if his life was in danger.

He waved away the guards. "Get something to eat and leave us alone."

He was about to ask more about the stone when Cook said, "I have a proposition for you. Think carefully. Your life depends on it."

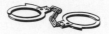

THIRTEEN

It was Halloween in America. But Trenton was in London watching double-decker buses stream down the street. From his vantage point at the old-fashioned window, he found the constant motion invigorating. Soon, Farouk would meet with the Cobra. Griff had helped him prepare questions for Farouk to ask about Emile and ARC's Virginia connections. Inwardly Trenton was seething. Farouk had played with his PDA on the entire flight over and kept the overhead light on. Why Eva had allowed him to bring it, after ordering Trenton to download it, was beyond him. Especially since she refused to let him bring his gun. Too much hassle she had said, because the Brits do not permit guns. They would have confiscated it as soon as he landed.

A tap on the hotel room door surprised him. He'd not ordered anything from room service. Farouk was asleep in the lone chair. Trenton went to the door and peered out the security lens. Two men he did not recognize, clean shaven and in navy jackets, stood in the hall.

"Nash, open up. We're here to make your trip worthwhile."

Trenton cracked the door open an inch, leaving the chain lock in place.

"We're friends of Griff." The tall man snapped open, then shut, his FBI credentials, and placed them in his pants pocket along with his hands.

It was Agent Lanning, the Legat who Griff cautioned him about. Trenton glanced at Farouk, whose mouth had fallen open, then closed the door and removed the chain.

He greeted them warily. "We were to meet you at the American Embassy."

The same height as Trenton, Lanning had a face that was all-American. He shook Trenton's hand, then motioned with his head to a shorter man with a buzz cut.

"This is my partner, Agent Quinn. We didn't want your companion," Lanning flipped his head toward Farouk, "seen entering the embassy. Quinn will stay with Sleeping Beauty. You and I will meet somewhere privately." With his hands still in his pockets, Lanning jerked his head toward Farouk. "Bring his passport."

Trenton had paid heed to Eva's warning that he was to hold Farouk's passport at all times. He patted his inside jacket pocket. "Griff introduced us on the phone last week. He said you've spent more time in London than in Washington."

"Quinn, call the Bureau office at the embassy. Advise them our package arrived."

Lanning's head jerked so quickly toward Farouk and then back to the door, Trenton cleared his throat to keep from laughing. He'd never known a person to gesture with their head instead of their hands. To him, the Agent acted like one of those bobble-head dolls in the back window of a car.

"Agent Quinn," Trenton changed gears. "We just arrived and ate little on the plane. When Farouk wakes, let him order breakfast from room service."

Quinn shrugged and wordlessly took up Trenton's post by the window.

The elevator stopped at each of the six lower floors. Since several people got on, it was a quiet ride. At the lobby, Lanning nodded his head toward a crowded coffee shop.

Lanning wound his way to a back corner table and sat, facing the room. Trenton took the opposite chair, but he felt uncomfortable. Police officers don't like to sit with their back to a room. They each ordered a black coffee from a waiter Trenton was sure looked like an ex-cop. Trenton sampled the bitter brew. British coffee was disgusting. He called the bulky waiter over and ordered a cheap English breakfast.

The chap brought him a plate full of eggs, bacon, sausage, and baked beans. His eyes on his food and away from Lanning's ever roving head, Trenton found the aroma more pleasant than the taste. He flicked the broiled tomato off his plate, swished the sausage into the tangy beans, and shoved an enormous bite into his mouth.

Lanning whispered, "What does Farouk claim he can do?"

Great sense of timing. A swig of coffee washed down his barely chewed food. Trenton brought Lanning up to speed on Farouk's intelligence and briefed him on the planned meeting.

Lanning drained his coffee cup. "That's what I needed to know. Griff was short on details. But then, he's not here. We'll have Farouk and the Java House covered. Now, let's go."

Trenton looked longingly at the half-eaten breakfast. While he had not asked for Lanning's help, he had better get along with him. His dad had told him it was prudent to have someone watch your back.

Though the elevator was empty, they still rode up in silence. Trenton considered asking several questions, then changed his mind. Lanning was like Duke Nash, blunt and in command. He was in charge, so Trenton would let him set the tone.

He punched in the security code to the room, pushed in the door, and was met by the smell of grilled meat. There sat his informant, at a white-covered cart, eating steak, eggs, and fried potatoes. Trenton decided Lanning was one of those guys who lived on adrenaline. He, on the other hand, was brought up by a doting mother who cooked his favorite meals.

He tore his eyes from Farouk's steak. Was this the same hotel room he left awhile ago? Unfolded newspapers and clothes were strewn over the double beds. A sock was thrown on the window sill, near where Quinn drank a cup of coffee. An open suitcase blocked the bathroom door. Trenton folded the *London Times* and sat on the bed. He had a peculiar urge to call Griff and tell him he was right about the FBI's London office. They couldn't even babysit a guy for twenty minutes without the room being torn to pieces.

Several hours later, per Lanning's instructions, Trenton looked out from the Grilled Onion but was forced to stand to see the Java House across the street, where at any moment Farouk would meet with the Cobra. Lanning neglected to tell him that the lower halves of the cafe's windows were covered with curtains. *Could these guys get anything right?* he wondered.

Drinking his cola, Trenton saw Farouk put his hand on the coffeehouse door. Farouk looked to his left. A turbaned man approached him. Trenton had to squint to see his face. The man was squat with a large head, but Trenton couldn't make out his features. Was he the Cobra?

The Grilled Onion windows were filthy. No wonder his view was blurred. He could see Farouk sitting on a stool. Trenton blinked. The green-turbaned man passed by Farouk but did not stop. Nor did he take a seat. Trenton strained to see if they exchanged words. His view was blocked.

Trenton moved his head. A woman walked by the cafe window. She had raven black hair that flowed around her face and down her back. Her hand held something. His eyes followed a leash to a large Rottweiler. That woman looked like his sister Tena! How could it be? The years dropped like falling acorns. He was fifteen again.

Trenton's horse pawed the ground. He turned in his saddle to watch his sister's horse pull up to the fence and stop. "Take her back to the stream, Tena. Then, run her hard. Show her you're the boss."

Trenton's mind refused to replay the horrible accident. Remorse still gripped him after these twelve years. He envisioned her pale and bruised face in the hospital room. Tena never recovered from the fall; she died of a cerebral hemorrhage. Trenton never rode a horse again.

Sweat beads clung to his forehead. He threw off his jacket and carried it outside. A cool breeze flooded him with welcome relief. He tried to focus on Farouk. Wait! That woman with the dog was taking his picture.

His first thought was to get the film. Trenton lunged for the tiny camera, small as a cough drop box. Her dog growled and bared long, white teeth. His hand fell to his side. He had no gun to shoot the beast.

Trenton stepped backward. The girl shoved the camera in her purse. Her dog strained on the leash, snarling at Trenton. She pulled the Rottweiler over to a black taxi and got in. Trenton ran to hear her destination. All he picked up was barking.

He memorized the taxi's number. Could she be an ARC lookout? Trenton swiveled his head toward the Java House. When he realized he was losing his grip, he felt disgust, which quickly turned to panic.

Farouk was not on the stool! Was the woman part of an elaborate escape plan? Trenton ran across the street, dodging another black taxi. He peered in the window. Breath blew out of him like a deflating balloon. His informant was inside, next to the man in the turban. Were they talking? He could not go in. Part of the plan. Trenton withdrew from the window, checked his watch as a tourist might. He sauntered slowly by the window. Farouk held a piece of paper and he seemed to be reading.

Trenton pretended to study a map he pulled from his jacket pocket. Moments later, Farouk walked out of the Java House. According to plan, Trenton fell in behind him. He did not see Lanning or his promised backup, but they were to follow Trenton and Farouk back to the hotel. They descended the stairs to the underground tube to take them to Liverpool Station. There, they would board another train to their hotel. Farouk turned slightly and held up his right thumb.

All must have gone well. The train whisked to a stop and the doors opened. Farouk sat inside the door. The doors closed with a *shwoosh*. Farouk fumbled with his handheld computer. Across the aisle, Trenton kept an eye on his charge, his mind disturbed by the woman who looked like Tena. Why did she take his picture? Maybe she was a tourist snapping the vibrant Muslim quarter.

Whatever her purpose, Trenton was rattled. He had to get Farouk to the hotel and debrief him right away. The train slowed to a stop. Farouk catapulted from his seat. He was out the door and onto the platform before Trenton left the train.

This was the wrong stop! Among the crowd, Trenton caught sight of Farouk's maroon plaid shirt, then it disappeared. His eyes desperately searched the crowded platform for Farouk or his colorful shirt, but he only saw people ascending the stairs from the tube, and passengers going in the opposite direction.

Another train was about to depart. Trenton stepped toward it. The doors closed, the train pulled away. Trenton scanned the moving cars for any sign of a plaid shirt. He sprinted up the stairs, skipping two at a time. In the daylight, he was surrounded by a flood of pedestrians, but no Farouk. And no Lanning.

Deputy Nash wiped his mouth with his hand. He knew Farouk could not get far with only a photocopy of his passport. But what about the Chunnel? Farouk could hop in a vehicle and get into France under the English Channel. Neither Griff nor Eva had considered that possibility.

A sick feeling washed over him. It would be impossible to explain this mess to Eva. Trenton descended the steps into the tube. His instincts said Farouk would not be so stupid as to become the subject of an international manhunt. He felt better, then recalled the obvious. Farouk Hamdi was more than his informant. He was ARC's financier, an alleged terrorist.

Trenton continuously scanned the crowds for Farouk. Finally, he hailed a cab. On the way back to the hotel, the driver pointed out several landmarks.

Fed up with the turtle's pace, Trenton leaned forward. "Mac, if you want to earn a five pounder, cut the gab and get me to Hotel Felix pronto."

Farouk better be there when he arrived. Trenton did not even want to think what he would do if he wasn't.

From a bright red phone booth, Farouk looked outside for Trenton, then punched in a series of numbers. Into the receiver, he said, "Meet me as planned. I am alone."

He found a cab for hire. "Tower of London. Hurry."

Farouk glanced out the back window to see if Trenton or the London FBI agents were behind him. No other cars turned when they did. He smiled in victory. At London's most famous tourist site, he paid the cabbie, then meandered to a fish-and-chips wagon near the attraction where several wives of King Henry VIII had lost their heads.

On a bench across from the entrance, Farouk sipped a bottle of sparkling water and ate a wrapper of hot chips. A costumed guard gave directions to a young woman. She wasn't the one he waited for. Satisfied that no FBI agent was among those waiting in line, Farouk finished his small meal and threw away the empty containers.

He checked his watch. Time to take his place in line. He had to be at the Jewel House in less than three minutes. One minute later, Farouk moved with the crowd to glimpse the spectacular Jewels of the English Crown. The graceful Queen Mother's Crown caught his eye. The largest diamond he had ever seen dominated the setting. It was the Koh-i-Noor, or Mountain of Light.

Farouk felt a slight pressure on his arm. She had come. He had not seen her since the day before his arrest. Camille had flown out the night before, and he hoped she knew nothing of Eva Montanna and her band of agents. She hugged him fiercely.

Camille was beautiful, dressed in an expensive black linen pantsuit. He saw she was wearing the pinpoint diamond earrings he gave her in Virginia. Pointing to the Queen's diamond, he said, "I will buy you such an exquisite gem. If all goes well—"

"Shh. You have spent too much time in America if you believe I care for such things." Camille whispered into his ear, "I wish we could steal that diamond and use it to help El Samoud. They say that whichever woman possesses it will rule the world."

He replied, "It is wonderful to see you."

She took hold of his hand. "We have the present. Let us open it like a precious gift."

Farouk knew then he would do anything for her. He'd make the U.S. government allow her to emigrate or refuse to help them.

Hand in hand, they strode across the Tower green where so many had lost their heads, and found a seat on a far bench along the brick wall.

"If only Great Brain would lose its head," Camille said. "The diamonds it boasts of today will soon be part of its end."

He squeezed her hand. "I fly out at seven tonight. Will you come with me?" Farouk did not want Camille to suspect his new role as informer.

Camille shook her head. Dark hair fell across her black eyes. "I return to Paris. Our leader moves final pieces into place."

"When?"

"Soon." She pushed a strand of hair behind her ear and pulled a handheld computer from a black leather bag, a perfect match to her shoes.

Farouk eased his computer out of his pocket, turned it on and made a few notes. He set it between them on the bench. He slid Camille's PDA from her long fingers. Did she miss him as he missed her? On that bench, a decision was before him. How was he going to resolve his legal predicament and convince her to help the U.S. government? He looked in her eyes and saw only determination for her cause. After the first Gulf War, Camille's father and brother recruited her into ARC. Could she ever leave it? Thoughts of remaining with Camille were only momentary. He had to return with Trenton. That was his best chance of gaining his freedom, her freedom, and the 50-million-dollar reward to finance their life together. He needed more time to work it all out his way. Her hands slipped from his.

"I return in a week, " he said, his voice dull with defeat.

Camille picked up his small computer from the bench, placed it in her purse, and left Farouk there, with only her fragrance to keep him company. Minutes later, on the way back to the hotel, Farouk rehearsed the story he'd tell Trenton.

Trenton paced up and down in his hotel room. If Farouk was not back soon, he would be forced to notify Agents Lanning and Quinn. The thought of dealing with them under such circumstances was unnerving. Trenton flipped on the television, found a cable news channel. He stared at Farouk's passport.

His informant could be in a million places, which meant Trenton's career was over. He would never be an FBI agent now. He lifted the receiver to call Eva, then stopped. Back home, it was just seven in the morning. Better to give her bad news at the office and not at home. He'd wait another hour. No need to transfer his panic to her. He hung up.

In frustration, Trenton threw the passport on the bed. It was his idea to bring Farouk to London. Maybe he should forget him for now and go to Reni Jubayl's bank. But that could tip her off. Besides, he had no authority in England to do anything about Emile's sister. Trenton went to the window. His hands balled into fists, he watched the street and willed Farouk to return.

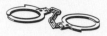

FOURTEEN

"How could you get lost? You said London was your backyard." Trenton wanted to shake his informant by the collar, but tried to stay calm.

Farouk plopped in the chair, seemingly unconcerned over Trenton's worry. "Well, now I'm back."

"Stand up," Trenton ordered, his blood pressure climbing.

"What?"

"Get your carcass out of that chair." His cheeks hot, Trenton stepped closer.

Farouk stood and shrugged. "Now what?"

"Raise your arms." Trenton patted down Farouk's body for weapons and contraband.

Farouk moved back and objected, "What are you doing?"

"Deciding whether I take you back in handcuffs, or have your bond revoked when we get to Virginia. Empty your pockets on the bed."

The wait for Farouk had taken a toll on Trenton's usually cool temperament. He was in no mood for games. Farouk emptied his pockets on the bed. Trenton combed through the contents, frisked Farouk's body, and reached inside each of his pockets. He picked up the personal computer from the bed. He shot Farouk a cynical glance.

Farouk reached for his PDA. "That's my handheld. You told me you already looked at the contents."

Trenton handed him the computer. If Farouk was up to mischief, evidence wouldn't be found in his pockets. He motioned to the stuff on the bed.

"Pick it up. We check out in thirty minutes for Gatwick Airport. Tell me about your meeting with the Cobra."

"Can I clean up first?"

Farouk did not wait for an answer. He sauntered into the bathroom and closed the door.

Trenton sighed. It would take a miracle to get back to the states with Farouk in tow. He shoved his worn socks, tee shirt and the *London Times* into his carry-on bag. He even tossed in a few postcards from the hotel. He had just set his bag by the door when he heard a light knock.

His eye to the peephole, he saw Agents Lanning and Quinn in the hall, wearing the same navy jackets. Trenton swung open the door, ready to find out where these two clowns had been the whole time Farouk was on the loose.

Lanning stepped into the room, with Quinn behind him and said, "We got called to the Embassy or would have been here sooner. The whole place was in an uproar."

Trenton narrowed his eyes. "About what?"

Quinn walked over to the window. Lanning's eyes scanned the room and he asked, "Where is Farouk?" Informed by Trenton he was in the bathroom, he continued, "Ambassador Cook, who was kidnapped in Lebanon, escaped across the border to Israel. Israeli soldiers found him bloody and beaten, but alive. He was aided in his escape by ARC's New York cell leader, a guy named Zayed."

Before he could stop himself, Trenton's head snapped toward the bathroom, and he said, "We're almost ready."

Lanning said, "Quinn and I will take you to Heathrow after we debrief him."

Trenton scowled. "We fly out of Gatwick. Our shuttle leaves in twenty minutes."

"Change of plans."

Lanning was his usual terse self, but Trenton was almost used to his oddities. With a few long strides, he listened outside the bathroom door. The water shut off and Trenton banged on the door.

"You are needed out here. We have guests."

Farouk stepped into the room holding a towel around his jaw. When he dropped it to the bed, Trenton was stunned. Farouk's beard and mustache were gone.

"What's with the clean face?" Trenton asked.

"I am getting rid of anything reminding me of jail. I do not intend to go back." Farouk sat on the edge of the bed. "You'll agree when you hear how my meeting went."

"Let's hear it, Sherlock," Lanning baited. "Did you tell him you have a new recruit?"

Trenton held his breath for Farouk's answer. Getting an FBI agent of Middle Eastern heritage introduced into ARC was the reason Barlow let him come to London with Farouk. Now, Farouk must be able to convice the Cobra that the undercover FBI agent he would bring to a future meeting was really an ARC sympathizer.

Farouk cracked each knuckle on his right hand. "I did not meet Cobra. He stayed in Paris and sent a subordinate. I return to the Java House a week from today. Then, I will be taken to meet the Cobra." He cracked another five knuckles. "He knows nothing of my arrest. I intend to keep it that way."

Trenton was speechless. He had suspected that the turbaned man was not the Cobra. The woman with the vicious dog. It all made sense. The Cobra did not trust Farouk and had him watched. Maybe that was why Farouk ditched him. He took a circuitous route back to the hotel in case he was being followed.

"Nash, are you going to keep tabs on that guy," Lanning's head bobbed toward Farouk, "for a whole week in London?"

Trenton's informant said, "They think I'm going home. I gave him my townhouse number to call."

Farouk then placed his hand on the telephone.

Trenton snapped, "Get your hand off that. You can't call anyone from here."

Farouk looked hurt. "I'm starved."

Trenton looked at Lanning, who said, "Go ahead." He picked up the receiver. "What do you want?"

"Double burger with pickles, fries, and large coffee. Make sure they send up catsup."

Trenton ordered four of the same to be sent to the room. With his whole case taken over by Lanning, Trenton figured he may as well eat.

Eva checked her watch. It was 9 a.m. She had just gotten off the phone with Lou, who was about halfway through his rehab. He sounded tired, and when she tried to brief him on their cases, he seemed disinterested. When she hung up, Eva concluded it would be hard for Lou to get up to speed once he cameback. Had Trenton tried to call while she was on the phone? Eva calculated the five-hour time difference with London. Perhaps Trenton and Farouk were on the way to Gatwick Airport.

Wanda did not answer Eva's buzz. The FIG secretary was—well scatterbrained came to mind. With Lou out, Wanda was always gone when Eva needed her. Eva knew governmental regulations made it nearly impossible to get rid of an incompetent employee. But since Wanda had confided that she found it hard to handle the pressures of law enforcement, Eva hoped Wanda would find her way back to Congress, where she felt more at home.

She turned on her computer and waited for it to come alive. On the secure system, she had an unopened e-mail from Brewster titled, "Urgent." Eva read it and was most interested in what he wrote about Farouk. That required her immediate action. Later, she would have time to follow up on his revelation that Ambassador Cook, who had been held captive in Lebanon, managed to escape with the help of an ARC operative named Zayed, who was now cooperating with MI-5. Eva recalled that Robbie had found a scrap of paper with that name on it at Farouk's townhouse. Eva typed a short reply to Brewster. She deleted both and called Griff's extension. There was no answer. Eva tried Wanda again, and this time she answered.

"Please connect me with Trenton at the Felix Hotel in London."

Eva hung up and waited, more concerned now that Trenton had failed to call her this morning as agreed. What was going on over there? She should have gone with him. But that was the cost of being a supervisor. She had to direct others, and it was not always possible to get them to do things as she would.

Her phone rang. She hit the intercom button. "Trenton?"

"He checked out thirty minutes ago," Wanda said.

"Call Griff on his cell. Tell him to get here. Then put me through to the Supervisor of Customs at Dulles Airport. It's going to be a long day." *And night.*

Farouk left the window seat and climbed over Trenton for the third time since their airbus departed from Heathrow. This time, Trenton followed him. His arms folded, he stayed in the back of the plane until Farouk came out of the restroom, wiping his hands on his pant leg.

"Are you sick or something?"

"I hate to fly." Farouk stuck out his lip. "A drink might settle my nerves."

"I'm on duty and you're not going to drink. When we land and clear Customs, we have to debrief."

Back at their seats, Farouk slumped down by the window. He edged a pillow under his head and shoved on earphones. Trenton was free to do paperwork, but dread rolled in his stomach. Soon, he'd tell Eva that Farouk did not meet with Cobra and that they would have to return to London in a week. When she learned that Trenton lost sight of Farouk for two hours, she'd never agree to let him go again. Trenton finished his notes.

A flight attendant handed them plates of lasagna and salad from the dinner cart.

"Is it vegetarian?" Farouk asked.

She smiled. "All those meals are gone."

"I can't eat meat!" Farouk was not slumping now.

What was the guy up to? At the hotel, he inhaled that hamburger.

"I am sorry, sir. Would you like more rolls and another salad?"

Farouk yelled at the flight attendant to bring him a proper meal.

Trenton stood in the aisle and said, "I'm sorry, but he's agitated. He's afraid to fly."

He glared at Farouk, mouthing for him to be quiet. Trenton felt breath on his neck. He turned and stood face-to-face with a hefty man in uniform. Trenton stepped back.

The copilot leaned toward Farouk, pointed a finger at his face and said, "You calm down, or the police will meet this flight when it lands."

Farouk started to choke. The attendant gave him club soda, which quieted him for the moment.

Trenton urged the copilot to the galley area where he opened his credentials and explained, "Confidentially, I am undercover. That passenger must not know he's being watched. If necessary, I'll have him arrested when we land. Your flight crew can relax."

"You promise to keep an eye on him?"

"Yes, sir."

The copilot glanced back at Farouk and returned to the cockpit. Trenton replaced his credentials.

Back at his seat, he grabbed Farouk's arm and hissed, "You eat that lasagna, with as much gusto as you did that burger or I will personally see that you are a guest tonight at Alexandria City Jail. Your bond will be a thing of the past."

Farouk drained the soda and put on his headphones. He did not talk during the rest of the flight. Tired of Farouk's antics and glad for a moment of peace, Trenton ate his meal until the plane hit a patch of turbulence. Trenton kept his tray from sliding to the floor, and the plane steadied. He turned off the overhead light. Headphones on, a jazz track played in his ears. Another trip to London with Farouk would truly be a sacrifice. But for his country, he'd do it.

After the dinner trays were collected, a flight attendant handed them Customs' declaration forms.

Trenton said to Farouk, "Fill it out and sign it. We should have no problems clearing Customs at Dulles."

Eva had said she would grease the wheels at Customs, but Griff warned against special treatment. If anyone who knew Farouk saw him walk through, it could get around that he was cooperating. A sax solo soothed his aching head. Wouldn't it be like Griff to give them a hard time? Just to make things look good.

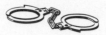

FIFTEEN

Hundreds of people crammed the Customs area at Dulles. Trenton walked ahead of Farouk, who still had not spoken a word. That was okay. With Farouk silenced, they stood a better chance of breezing through.

Trenton asked over his shoulder, "Did you fill out the Customs form?"

Ahead of them, a flight crew was searched.

Farouk said, "Yes. I have not seen that before."

"The terrorism security levels are elevated to orange."

"Oh, yeah."

"Agent Montanna took care of your name on the watch list." Trenton gazed slowly around, but he did not spot Eva or Griff.

Farouk fidgeted with his Custom's form, his eyes darting around the room. "I should have gotten some sleep."

"Settle down." Trenton knew that furtive head movements triggered an Officer's attention.

The form rolled in his hand like a baton, Farouk asked, "You have my passport, right?"

Trenton eyed his troublesome informant. When the Custom's Inspector motioned Trenton forward, he handed Farouk his passport. To the official, he gave his own passport and form.

"Anything to declare, Mr. Nash?"

"No, ma'am."

"What was the nature of your travel?"

"Business."

The inspector scanned the bar code on Trenton's passport. "Welcome home." She handed Trenton his passport and waved him through.

Trenton walked a few steps, turned, and waited for Farouk to clear.

Farouk gave the inspector his passport and declaration form. Trenton watched the inspector scan the bar code and check the computer monitor. She thumbed through the pages of Farouk's passport and looked at his declaration.

"Nothing to declare, Mr. Hamdi?"

"No," he said.

"What was the purpose of your travel, Mr. Hamdi?"

"Pleasure."

"It was a long way to fly, for such a short amount of pleasure. Set your backpack on the counter and open it."

The inspector unzipped the pockets, then pulled out clothing and toiletries.

"No camera?"

Farouk shook his head.

"Not the sentimental type? Most tourists bring back pictures." She examined his handheld computer, then ordered, "Boot it up for me, sir."

"The battery is dead. I forgot to bring my charging plug." Farouk put it into his pocket. The inspector wiggled her finger. She wanted it back.

Trenton could not hear what was being said, but he didn't like the looks of this. The inspector pushed the items back into the backpack, zipped shut the pockets, and looked over her shoulder. She spoke into a microphone attached to her white shirt. Instantly, two plain-clothed Customs agents appeared. They stood on each side of Farouk and escorted him to a secondary search room.

This was not supposed to happen. Where was Eva? Some foulup on the watch list. Trenton followed at a discreet distance. He scanned the crowd. If Farouk's associates were in the Customs area, his cover was blown. Someone grabbed Trenton's arm. It was the copilot, who slapped him on the back.

"You kept your word and had that creep arrested. Thanks for your help."

"Whatever!" Trenton shrugged off the guy's arm.

An officer in uniform guarded the door to the search room. Trenton showed his credentials and tried to move past.

The officer held up a hand. "Sorry. Can't let you in. Sit there."

His frustration in check, Trenton sat and waited, like a nonmember of the club.

Ten minutes later, Eva walked out of the search room. Griff, too. He had not seen them arrive. Eva's face was grim. She crooked her finger at Trenton to follow them to another room. Inside, she sat on the edge of a small desk, hands on her hips. Eva's blue eyes were stormy.

"I was puzzled why you did not call me from London as arranged. When I received a secure e-mail from Brewster, I knew the answer. Farouk met no one inside that coffee shop. How long was he out of your sight?" Her lips formed a thin pink line.

"I was going to call," Trenton sputtered. "I didn't want to worry you. What could you have done from Virginia? He got on the wrong train and returned within the hour. I think he thought the Cobra was trailing him. The whole thing was a test-run. The Cobra sent him a note via a courier. Farouk goes back to meet him next week."

Eva raised her brow. "The man in the green turban. Do you have the note?"

Trenton felt like he was being interrogated. "No. I saw Farouk read it in the Java House."

Griff said, "Sorry buddy. MI-5 tailed Farouk to the Tower of London. He met a female, who may be an ARC suspect. They exchanged PDAs. Is this all news to you?"

"He didn't." Trenton folded his arms across his chest. "The FBI would have told me."

Eva resumed command of the postmortem. "The FBI was fooled, as well. For some reason, Lanning was not aware of it either." She looked into Trenton's eyes. "It gets worse. Farouk's PDA was full of cut diamonds. He's still financing terrorism. ICE agents are taking his statement, now."

Trenton crammed his hands into his pockets. He felt like a failure. He wanted out of there! But first, he wanted Eva to know what happened. "Lanning was called to the Embassy, something happened to an ambassador. He didn't give me *any* backup. On the plane, I gave Farouk the Customs forms. Did he declare the diamonds?"

Griff interjected, "He's been arrested for smuggling."

Eva put her hand on the doorknob. Trenton guessed she was done grilling him, for now.

She said, "This is not my doing. Barlow wants him charged."

"What about my case?"

Eva touched his arm. "He's no use as a snitch, now. Go home, get a few hours sleep. Then report to the office about ten tomorrow. You'll have a lengthy report to write."

Trenton wriggled his arm away from her hand. He wanted no pity. "I wrote it all up on the plane. I know nothing about diamonds." His face hard as a stone, he said to Griff, "That FBI Legat is worthless. If he had done his job, this never would have happened." He turned back to Eva. "I can make a case against Emile Jubayl without Farouk. Remember, my infor—"

Eva opened the door. "We will talk tomorrow."

He mastered the anger burning at his core and asked, "Did MI-5 find out if Farouk met with a woman with a large Rottweiler? She took my picture."

"Put it in your report. We'll try to find out." Eva walked out of the room.

Griff said, "Trenton, Farouk is double dealing. He's working for ARC. We don't know what intelligence he shared with them."

Trenton walked away and promised himself that Farouk would not outwit him again.

His will hard like iron, Trenton did not go home. Farouk made him look like an idiot. Emile would not get the chance. He drove straight to the office. In the parking lot, he used his cell and called Hannah Strobel. She agreed to meet him in an hour at GMU. At least the day would not be a total loss.

Trenton used his key to get into the wire room, which was dark. He flipped on the light and laughed. Paper tapes streamed out from the three registers like favors at a child's birthday party. The one connected to Emile's private office phone boasted a two-foot-long tape. The home register's tape crept like a serpent across the table, down to the floor, and under the table. The tape from Emile's cell phone was half as long.

He rolled up each tape, secured them with paper clips, then ripped them from the machines. On each, he wrote his initials, the date and time. After snapping off the lights, Trenton looked back at the power lights on each machine and those red eyes hunting his prey, Emile Jubayl.

"I'll be back," he whispered.

The door was about to close, when he heard *click, click, click.* The door shut with a bang. Desperate to find out about the call, he thrust his hand into his pocket and pulled out the key. Trenton reopened the door, hurried inside, and rushed to the clattering machine. He heard a dialing out tone from the machine on Jubayl's home phone. A number flashed on the display. Tomorrow, he'd ask the analyst to check it.

He set the rolled tapes on the analyst's desk, and penned a note that by tomorrow afternoon, he needed the phone numbers collated by date, time, and name of each person or organization called. Each subscriber's name had to be compared against their intelligence files. Tonight, there was nothing more for him to do. Trenton locked the door, confident that, if his next meeting went well, by this time tomorrow he'd be typing a warrant for the arrest of Emile Jubayl.

Trenton reached for his wallet to pay for their mocha coffees. Hannah stopped him.

"I can buy my own."

"Then let me buy pizza and beer this Friday night," Trenton replied.

Hannah gave the cashier two dollars and pocketed her change. "I don't drink beer and don't go out with guys who do."

He noted her icy comment, picked up his coffee, and found their usual seats by the window. It was too dark to see the last of the leaves turning rusty orange. This fall, there'd been no time to fish with his Dad. His life was his job. Despite flying for more than eight hours and having little sleep or food, he had to compensate for dropping the ball with Farouk. Trenton's questions to Hannah took on a sharper tone.

Before she took a sip, he fired, "Does Helpers give money to causes not approved by its board or donors?"

Hannah's green eyes sparkled in the bright lights. "You seem to have forgotten. I'm an office intern, not a board member."

Trenton humored her with a begrudging smile. "Have you ever heard anything like that?"

She whispered, "Do you have Mr. Jubayl's office bugged?"

Trenton leaned forward. "What do you know?"

She studied him, then said softly, "I overheard a donor argue with Mr. Jubayl over a project."

He was finally onto something! Trenton removed a spiral notebook from his back pocket. "What projects? Why?"

"I was on the computer outside Mr. Jubayl's office. In a heated voice, a donor accused Mr. Jubayl of supporting a cause with which he did not agree, and implied other donors would not approve. Then, Mr. Jubayl closed his office door."

Trenton looked up. "I don't suppose you heard where the funds were going."

Hannah sported a laugh. "Helpers can't afford solid wood doors. I could hear."

Trenton's pen was poised above his pad. "Well?"

"Understand, when a major donor complains Helpers is not following the Great Commission, Mr. Jubayl listens."

This seemed noteworthy. Trenton wrote on his pad, "Great Commission. Who are members?" He remembered his Dad's stories about meetings of the mafia's Appalachian commission.

He was so absorbed in thoughts of his imminent triumph that he did not hear her say, "He said funds were going to the wrong groups."

Moments later, he looked at her with an air of expectancy, "Tell me more."

When Hannah repeated the donor's complaint, Trenton replied, "By wrong groups, did he mean terrorists?"

Hannah sighed. "I was having a little fun with you. Christians give aid so people will see the love of Christ."

Trenton gazed at Hannah. Her eyes held a heavy weight.

She said, "Jesus told his disciples to tell people of all nations the truth about him and to teach them to obey his commands." She sat back in her chair, looking a little sad. "I may have misled you, Trenton. That's what Christians call the Great Commission."

A barrier came between them. Trenton stood, shoved his notebook back in his pocket. "That's it? No connection with terrorism?"

Hannah got up and reached for his arm. "Don't go. I'm trying to figure it out myself. The complaint was that Helpers reaches physical needs but not spiritual. You keep suggesting something sinister is going on, but, Deputy Nash, you have failed to reveal any evidence of it."

The way she said "Deputy Nash" seared through him like a hot knife. He wanted her respect more than any woman he had known, except for his mom. Why? A more powerful voice inside him said he was wasting time.

He shot back. "And you have failed to *provide* evidence of it, like I asked. Your religious faith blinds you. Most Christians are hypocrites. After my sister died, our minister blamed me, saying I was going to hell.

I was fifteen. Forget that I bothered you. Live your life with a veil over your eyes. Someday, you'll see I am right. Good day, Ms. Strobel."

With rigid shoulders, Trenton walked away from her and failed to see Hannah's eyes follow him out the Commons. His only thought was that she, too, played him for a fool. He would show her, show them all. He would not stop until he captured the American terrorist.

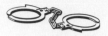

SIXTEEN

On Monday of the following week, Eva, Griff, and Trenton were in Dan Simmons' office to decide if and how to go forword against Emile.

Eva wished Dan would hang up the phone. She was anxious to hear his opinion on Emile's case. Griff toyed with a wire puzzle on a corner of Dan's desk. If the case fizzled, Griff was experienced enough to handle it. She was not so sure about Trenton. He stared out the window, arms folded, just like Nathan Barlow had done a few weeks ago. Her newest officer had worked tirelessly, but, with Farouk's deception, the balance of the scale was thrown back in Emile's favor. Besides that one phone call to Beirut, what evidence pointed to his guilt?

Dan set down the phone, an enormous smile on his face. "Better make this quick." He reached into a side drawer, pulled out a handful of cigars, and slid them across the desk. "My son was born yesterday, on November 7, my wife's birthday. They are coming home from the hospital today. His three sisters are thrilled."

Griff and Trenton took a cigar.

Dan said, "Eva, take one for Scott."

To be polite, Eva plucked a cigar and put it in her briefcase. But there was no way she was giving that cigar to Scott and rekindle the painful issue they had seemed to put aside for now. With Dan in a happy mood, Eva laid out the evidence for and against Emile. Dan took notes. At length, he set down his fountain pen.

"Midge Hopper came to see me." For Trenton's sake, he added, "She's the AUSA that prosecutes terrorism cases with the FBI's Terrorism Task Force. They want Farouk as an informant on a different case."

Trenton wheeled around. "Are you going to let them steal him out from under me?"

Griff put down the puzzle. "Forget Farouk. He stiffed all of us."

Dan raked a hand through his sparse hair. "We should question Farouk's veracity. However, with the Attorney General's directive to bring terrorists to justice, it may be too soon to close Emile's case."

Eva saw her chance. "Farouk's bond is revoked. He will be in jail while he awaits trial. I think we should see how Emile reacts to Griff."

Dan asked, "When is the undercover meeting?"

Griff replied, "We waited to see you. I will call Emile this afternoon and arrange it."

Eva thought she saw a shadow pass over Trenton's face. His eyes narrowed. Did he think Griff was taking the case out from under him?

"What's the plan?" Dan asked Griff.

"Offer him a large a donation, gain his confidence, then see what he does."

Trenton sprang to the center of the room. "The undercover donation was my idea. Right now, nearly a hundred calls from Emile's home, cell, and business phones are being analyzed by intelligence. I'll have the results by three."

Eva needed to find a way to appease Trenton. "Your idea was a good one, which is why Griff, with years of undercover experience, is meeting Emile."

Her words had the opposite effect. Trenton exploded, "You mean, I blew it in London and Griff won't. I did all I could to stay on Farouk. I searched him, too! Who knew he would trade his PDA, which we checked, for a hollow one?"

Eva's heart went out to Trenton. Every one of them in that room had been disappointed by the results of an investigation or a judge's ruling against them. "I blame myself for letting you go with him. I should have gone along or sent Griff."

His cheeks puffed out, Trenton raised his chin. "My source inside Helpers is giving me information."

Eva glanced at Dan. "Trenton, it better not be Mrs. Strobel."

"It isn't." Trenton's eyes were slits. "Trust me."

Emile checked his office door. It was tightly closed. He was glad for the new phone system, which prevented another from picking up the line and listening in when he called out. He punched in the number from memory. After being routed through a series of extensions, he finally reached his party. He identified himself, then listened to the man on the other end who gave him instructions.

"I am not sure I can handle what you describe," Emile replied. He listened another minute. "That sounds radical."

The sweat began as warmth under his arms. The more he heard, the moisture grew to streams running down his arms. Using his chin to cradle the receiver to his ear, he peeled off his suit jacket and loosened his tie.

"It appears I have no choice but to do as you say. Tomorrow, I have an important meeting in Dearborn, Michigan, which I must keep. Then, I will do as you say. But I can stay for no more than a week. My absence could have serious consequences for my agency."

Emile hung up the phone. If he was to be gone for that long, he had to tell Sari something. But what?

Early the next morning, Eva buzzed Griff. "Come to my office."

Griff reluctantly set his carry-on case on the floor and picked up the phone. "I'm about to leave for Reagan National. My flight to Detroit leaves in three hours."

Fingering the encrypted transmittal, Eva said, "I'll be as brief as the hot information I just received from Brewster will allow. Of course, if you want to walk into a meeting with a possible terrorist without—" Eva heard a click.

"Hello?"

Nothing. The line was dead. Smiling, she returned the receiver to the cradle of the intercom. Griff rushed into her office, leather case slung over his shoulder.

"You got me. What's up?"

Eva's smile faded. "You warned us about Farouk. I had hoped you were wrong. You weren't." She pointed to the computer screen. "Brewster says MI-5 and Scotland Yard searched the apartment of the woman whom Farouk met at the Tower of London. She is not the one who snapped Trenton's picture. Brewster said he could find nothing out about her and that she was probably a tourist."

"And the woman Farouk met?"

"Camille de Berg. She and Farouk swapped computers. It's likely their meeting was prearranged. They fund ARC through an elaborate diamond-smuggling scheme."

Griff slid the case from his shoulder to the floor and sat on a chair opposite her desk. He picked up the paperweight with a miniature Windsor Castle inside. "I bought one like that once," he said casually.

Eva watched him set it down. Should she mention it was Jillie's? When Eva invited Griff and Jillie to dinner, she had hoped they would hit it off.

"How does their scheme affect my undercover meeting with Emile?" Griff asked.

Eva spoke as rapidly as her Glock fired at the range. "Camille and other sympathizers steal jewelry. They remove, then send, the diamonds to Farouk in the U.S. They cannot be traced. He sells them on the New York diamond exchange. Farouk returns the illicit funds to Camille via wire transfers of less than ten thousand dollars, to avoid bank reporting requirements."

Griff's eyebrow shot up over his left eye. "You haven't mentioned Emile. Is his sister, Reni, involved at the London bank?"

Eva checked her watch. "You better get to the airport. Camille has an account at Reni Jubayl's bank, but it is one of many. In Camille's computer, MI-5 found links to ARC and El Samoud. Also, Brewster and MI-5 are continuing to debrief Zayed. At this point, he admits Farouk was his subordinate in Virginia but insists he knows nothing of Emile Jubayl. He claims he never heard of him."

Eva picked up the paperweight. With her palm, she smoothed the domed surface. "So far, no links to Emile, which makes your meeting with him all the more critical."

Griff grimaced. "If I don't get incriminating evidence against him, our case disappears."

She replaced the weight on a stack of papers. "Like a snowflake on a warm windshield."

Griff rose, picked up his case. "I could draw Emile out about London."

"It might raise a red flag."

Griff hiked the bag on his shoulder. "Eva, could you drive me to the airport? I won't make it otherwise. The FBI is supposed to staff the undercover office. When I called this morning, no one answered."

Eva shut down her computer and grabbed the car keys from her top drawer. "Griff, that was Jillie's paperweight."

Griff's other eyebrow shot up his forehead. "I bought her one at Heathrow Airport on a trip back from seeing my grandmother. She had talked of meeting her sometime …" His words fell away like a crumbling shoreline in a storm.

Eva should have kept her mouth shut. Griff lost his wife to cancer. When Jillie died, Eva never asked how he felt. She was too locked in her own grief. Eva motioned to him to follow her out the door. "I've wanted to say something, but never knew exactly what."

"Me, too," was all he said. His knuckles that gripped the shoulder strap were white.

"Jillie was more than my identical twin. She was my best friend. I'm glad you and she were friends, too." Eva wiped away threatening tears.

Griff nodded to Wanda, who was smoking outside the back door.

"Have a safe trip," she called after them.

When they reached her G-car, Eva opened both doors with the remote. She gladly changed the subject. "Unless Emile brings up London, forget it for now. Camille's in custody. Brewster cleverly dangled in front of her the fifty million reward for El Samoud's capture."

Griff asked, "Did Trenton brief you on Emile's phone records?"

"The analyst said he'd finish this morning."

"Maybe Trenton doesn't realize I'm meeting Emile today."

"I haven't seen Trenton yet. If I learn anything new, I'll call you on your cell."

Pastor Greene passed out prayer request sheets. "Break up into two groups today. This group prays for missionary requests. Thelma, your group for family requests."

Sari moved her chair next to her friend's. After each of the six persons in their circle prayed for some who lost jobs, another who fought drug addiction, and even a baby with a brain tumor, Sari started to cry. Soon, the others started weeping softly. The needs of their fellow believers were huge, and they felt the burden to pray.

Sari choked back a sob. "I have an unspoken request. I cannot say what it is."

"God," Thelma's rich voice began, "Help Sari face whatever challenges are before her. Meet her at the point of her need. Show her you love her. In Jesus's name, Amen."

Sari wiped her face with her palms and dug a crumpled tissue from her pocket. *Lord, help me through this. I cannot do it alone.*

Trenton raced out of the wire room and down the hall. He stopped by the FIG office door, shoved papers under his arm, and swiped his key card. He burst through the door and blew past Wanda, who smelled

like cigarette smoke. He went straight to Eva's office. It was empty.
Disappointed, Trenton slowed his pace and went to his own office.
Wanda might know where Eva had gone. He punched in her exten-
sion number.

"She drove Griff to Reagan National so he wouldn't miss his flight.
I heard you were supposed to give him some phone information."

Trenton rustled the papers in his hand. "I have it right here!" He
called Griff's cell number, but got his voicemail. He tried Eva's cell
and got her voicemail, too.

Wanda shrugged. "I have his flight number somewhere."

Trenton didn't wait for Wanda. He found the number to the airport, and after a series of prompts he finally reached a person who
agreed to page Griff Topping. Trenton was put on hold. Five minutes
later, no one had answered his page.

He slammed down the phone and grabbed his jacket. As he ran
out of his office, Trenton almost knocked Wanda down as she walked
in with Griff's flight number. Trenton asked her to call the airport
again while he called Griff on his cell, with no success. Was that Eva's
voice he heard? He walked into the outer office and found her and
Wanda joking about her son Andy's costume for a harvest party at
church.

"His little head fills only half of Scott's old football helmet," Eva
said.

When Wanda giggled, Trenton had enough.

"I am sure he is cute, but Eva, I've got to reach Griff."

Eva's face turned to granite. "Is it the phone calls?"

He jerked his head toward her office. Eva took the hint. He followed her. Careful not to let Wanda hear about the case, he closed the
door behind him.

"Emile made two calls to someone in Hezbollah in Lebanon. With
that earlier call to ARC's money man in Beirut, this is more than a
coincidence. I can't reach Griff on his cell."

Eva rummaged in her side drawer. Trenton shifted from one foot
to another. What was with Eva? She was usually one step ahead of
him.

He repeated, "One call from his cell and another from his office
private line. Both to someone in Hezbollah. They have to be Emile's."

Eva popped a piece of white candy in her mouth. "When Griff
lands in Detroit, maybe he'll turn on his cell. Meanwhile, I'll leave a
message on the undercover voicemail."

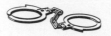

SEVENTEEN

Griff turned the doorknob to the specially leased undercover office. It was locked. He inserted a key he'd received via courier from the Detroit FBI office. Inside, it was dark. Griff flipped on overhead lights and called. To his surprise, no one replied. Where was the undercover FBI agent who was supposed to be his secretary?

Griff opened his leather case and took out his undercover nameplate engraved with the name Ashur Wadi. He walked from the reception area to an interior office complete with a desk, long table, and several chairs, then put the name plate on the cherry wood desk. The Detroit FBI agent had told him the recording equipment was in a small room next to this office.

In that room, Griff inspected the special video camera, which was attached to the backside of the wall of the undercover office. Aimed through a pinhole in the wall, it was focused on two chairs that faced the undercover desk. Griff inserted a memory card into the recorder. Would the hidden microphones pick up his conversation with Emile?

A door shut in the outer office. A man said, "Hello. Anyone here?"

At the words, a column of green volume lights scrolled across the indicator. *Yes!* The microphones worked. Griff hustled out the side room, through the office, and into the receptionist area, expecting one of the agents. Instead, there stood an elegantly dressed man who looked at home among the leather couches and chairs, expensive artwork, and crystal vases.

Griff asked, "May I help you?"

The visitor extended a manicured hand. "I am Emile Jubayl. My plane arrived early so I came on ahead. I hope you do not mind."

Griff replied, "Pleased to meet you. I am Ashur Wadi."

They shook hands. Griff was surprised that Emile's comportment was that of a gentle humanitarian, nothing like the stereotypical terrorist he imagined was their target.

Griff apologized, "I just returned late from an appointment and found my secretary left unexpectedly. We can talk at my conference table."

Emile followed him to the undercover office, where Griff motioned for him to sit in the chair facing the wall with the camera.

"Get comfortable while I find coffee."

The agent who was supposed to record the meeting was also a no-show, so Griff rechecked the equipment in the tech room. He intended to sit on the chair opposite Emile, which was more casual than sitting behind the desk, and because he did not want his head in the way of the camera. Fortunately, Griff had worked with such devices for years. Like watching a crime show on TV, Griff observed the monitor as Emile sat on the correct chair and gazed about the room. The camera's view of Emile was good, but Griff needed to pull his own chair more to the side.

Once Emile believed Griff was a philanthropist interested in helping the Middle East, Griff thought he would reveal his terrorist sympathies. In the kitchen area, Griff's hopes for coffee faded. None was made, and he'd been gone too long already. In a small refrigerator, he found two bottles of sparkling water and snatched two glasses that looked clean.

He put the water, glasses, and a tin of cookies on a tray and took them into the office. Griff placed the refreshments toward the front of the desk, then turned his chair slightly, ensuring his head would not block the camera's view of Emile. As though following the script in Griff's mind, Emile stood slightly and moved his chair toward Griff. *Perfect angle. Now sit there.*

"I am sorry, but we have no coffee. My mother sent molasses cookies from New Orleans." Griff should have tried one to see if they were stale.

Emile replied politely, "I had two cups of coffee on the plane. May I set up my PowerPoint on your desk?"

Griff moved the tray to the conference table where he poured the water and arranged cookies on a plate.

Emile powered up his computer. "Mr. Wadi, I sent a letter thanking you for your large donation. Many poor people in the Middle East appreciate it."

Griff took his assigned seat and played his part. "Call me Ashur." But he was unprepared for Emile's grilling.

"How did you find us? With no previous contact, your generosity amazes me."

Griff reached for an answer he thought would require no further explanation. "I have always been concerned about the welfare of the people in the Middle East."

"Why?"

From his briefcase, Griff pulled out a solicitation brochure supplied by Trenton. "A gentleman left this with my secretary. Knowing my interest in supporting organizations such as yours, she saved it for me. After our college intern did some research, I decided that Helpers International is a worthy cause."

"Your name is familiar," Emile suggested, "mentioned to me, possibly by Abu Mohammed, an Arab philanthropist. He also lives in Dearborn." Emile leveled his black eyes at Griff's clear gray ones. "Surely, your paths have crossed."

Concerned Emile might invent a name to test him, Griff smiled. "I meet so many people in my line of work and travel much. Abu Mohammed. Hmm." Griff arched his left eyebrow. "I may have met him somewhere, but cannot be sure."

Griff sipped his water, and without another word, Emile showed pictures of some of Helpers' well-digging, food, and hospital projects. Emile stopped at the photo of the little girl carrying the water bucket in the Lebanese village and mentioned several other large donors from the Dearborn area.

Mindful that Emile might have laid a trap, Griff refused to admit he knew them. "You must be thankful for concerned patrons. Now you have another. I am willing to contribute more money. I see that you do good work."

Emile looked at Griff and asked, "What is your proposal?"

With the camera recording Emile's every facial movement, Griff expected the next frame would show Emile's gratitude. Griff offered him, "One million now, and another within the year, all to help Lebanon."

Emile's smile was magnetic. "It is my life's work, as you may know," he said carefully.

Success moments away, Griff laughed. "That is one reason I come to you with my plan."

Without asking the other reason, Emile said, "We raised one hundred and ten thousand dollars at our annual dinner, and bought one hundred computers for the schools, which will be shipped next week. With your generosity, another fifteen hundred or more could be in place by the year's end. Think of what such technology can do for the children!"

When Griff did not respond, Emile changed his tack, "You could fashion your own project."

This was the opening Griff waited for. He offered Emile a cookie, which he took.

Griff lobbed his final pitch. "I trust you do not object if some of my donation is given to those that can best help you."

Emile stopped chewing. "Who do you have in mind?"

Griff named the man in Lebanon who was ARC's top financier. Trenton had told Griff that Emile had placed one call to this man, and he hoped to uncover their relationship.

Griff silently observed Emile's reaction to the two million within his reach. Emile hesitated, pursed his lips, tapped a finger on his knee. Griff longed to know his mental calculations, so he could rebut arguments against his plan.

Emile said, "You could give some to us, some to your friend, without involving me."

Griff replied, "I considered that. Helpers should get credit for the whole contribution. You do not have to tell your board everything. My way, we both win."

Emile shook his groomed head, began closing his computer program. "Mr. Wadi, if the price of doing business with you is to be publicly associated with the man whose name I will not mention, I must decline. Surely you know he is a Hezbollah sympathizer on the State Department's list of terror organizations. It is illegal to give money to him or to Hezbollah"

His eyebrow arched, Griff exclaimed, "He has no official ties to Hezbollah."

Emile's hand hovered above his computer. Griff could tell that Emile wanted the money. If he took it, Griff would have proof he was willing to aid a terrorist. But Griff miscalculated.

The Helpers International CEO turned off his laptop, folded it closed, and placed it into a leather case. "I cannot take that chance. Neither should you." He did not shake Griff's hand.

What more could Griff do? He walked him to the door and said, "Give it some thought. Let me know if you change your mind."

The door closed with a snap. Before Griff could mourn Emile's rejection, the undercover phone rang. It was Eva. She sounded frustrated and out of breath.

"Griff, you didn't return my call. Trenton learned Emile made two other calls, one on his cell and one on his direct line, to the same number in Lebanon. The calls were to an operative in Hezbollah! I'm glad I caught you before your meeting with Emile. He must be due any minute."

Not one to perspire in difficult circumstances, Griff had flecks of moisture on his brow. He wiped it off with his hand. "Slow down. Was I supposed to call you?"

"I left a message on the undercover answering machine an hour ago."

"I couldn't check. The FBI agents never showed. Emile arrived early. He just left."

"What happened?"

In no mood to recount his failure, he had to tell her something. "He may have called those numbers in Lebanon, but Eva, he gave *no* indication of any ties to terrorism. Stared me in the face and refused two million dollars if any of it went to Hezbollah. Warned me against them. Said it was illegal. I got nothing."

Eva sighed. "For that amount of money, he may have second thoughts. Bring the recording to our meeting with Dan on Friday. Maybe he'll approve keeping the case open."

"Don't forget. I get in at nine tonight."

Eva sighed. "I'm supposed to take Andy and Kaley to a party at church."

"Send Trenton."

"You don't mind?"

Griff said, "Just make sure he has my flight number."

As Griff retrieved the memory card, he pondered, but only a moment, what he might have done if he had known about Emile's phone calls. Maybe the recording would show something incriminating, but he doubted it. Emile Jubayl was as good as free.

Friday noon, as Eva took off her raincoat she saw a photo of Dan's baby on his credenza. Even with his eyes closed, he was beautiful. She was looking forward to seeing Dr. Cole next week.

"Who wants a sandwich? The deli's on the line, " Dan asked.

"Turkey on whole wheat." Griff patted his stomach. "Got to watch my weight."

Dan gave that order, then looked at Eva and Trenton.

"A toasted bagel, I guess," Eva said finally. With decisions about Emile Jubayl minutes away, she had no appetite. Did Dan do nothing but eat?

"Trenton, this may take awhile. You should nourish your brain," Dan quipped.

Trenton looked as frustrated as Eva felt by the delay in getting their meeting started. "Pork barbecue with chips."

Dan smiled. "A happy stomach does more to stimulate the brain than an empty one."

Trenton rolled his eyes and stalked over to stare out the window. As Dan and Griff talked about the Redskins' loss in overtime, Eva engaged in an internal debate. The evidence did not prove Emile was guilty beyond a reasonable doubt, the standard for a conviction. There were a lot of dots, and the connections were hazy.

The sandwiches arrived and, for a few minutes, they ate in silence. Eva rechecked her mental scorecard of evidence. Dan was the first to finish.

He said, "Griff, let's play the recording from yesterday. I understand you didn't get much."

Griff removed a copy of the memory card from a plastic envelope. The original was stored in the office vault.

Without enthusiasm, he said, "Perhaps you will see something we can use."

They watched the meeting on a small television in Dan's bookcase. At the end of eight minutes, Trenton said, "He played you like a fiddle."

Eva glanced at Griff, who just shrugged.

"Emile is a smart fellow," Dan said. "He wavered by the edge, but never went over. I saw a man tempted by two million, who skillfully rebuffed attempts to link the donation to Hezbollah."

Eva launched her wrapper into the wastebasket. "Any humanitarian organization who helps people would want two million."

Dan replied, "You're right. Griff, tell us your impressions from sitting face to face."

His sandwich mostly uneaten, Griff said, "Emile is an enigma. He's polished like a stone, but has questionable contacts. You saw how deftly he questioned me about activists in the Detroit area."

"You couldn't know every name he might throw at you," Eva said.

Griff shook his head. "I should have done more homework. It's impossible to fake something like that. The FBI in Detroit claimed they got the date wrong. If they had briefed me more—" Griff swallowed further complaints. "Emile may have suspected I wasn't the real deal. Who knows, he may believe I'm a government agent."

Trenton weighed in. "I think you left the door open. He may call tomorrow and accept. We should wait to see what happens."

Dan asked, "Has anyone reviewed his calls on the pen register since yesterday?"

Trenton had. "One on his cell to his wife. Nothing unusual on the home or business lines that we can tell. He made several calls to Detroit before Griff's meeting. We're checking those."

Dan clasped his hands. "What do you want to do, Eva?"

Regret welled within her. It was the right thing to do.

Eva replied, "Assuming no fireworks from these latest calls, justice dictates we close the case. We do not have enough to keep these resources in place for a man who's only *suspected* of being a suspect. We should concentrate on firming up our cases against Farouk. His indictment for aiding terrorism must go to trial in less than seventy days."

Trenton objected. "Maybe we don't have enough evidence to arrest Emile for financing terrorism. But his son was mixed up in the bombing at State. Emile has some kind of relationship with the terrorists he's calling. My informant heard him speak in Arabic and say things were at a crisis and he should have never left Lebanon." Trenton emphasized his point with his hands in the air. "We need more time!"

Dan aimed at the wastebasket behind him and propelled his wrapper with a hook shot. He missed. "Trenton, you'll learn that rules of evidence require the government to provide defense attorneys with any exculpatory evidence. If we pursue Emile, the defense will use Griff's recording and argue to a jury the government enticed Emile to violate the law when he had no such intent."

Eva agreed. She once had the entrapment defense successfully used against her by Harlan Scribbs. They had to be careful. "We shut down the pen registers immediately. Trenton, you take care of it. If Emile approaches Griff, we can apply for a new court order to resume them. As of today, we administratively close the case."

Without waiting for Eva or Griff, Trenton left. The door banged behind him.

Trenton did not go to the FIG office to shut down the recording devices nor did he notify the court. He first had to resuscitate Emile's case, and he needed his dad's help. Disdain for Eva fueled Trenton's speed along the Beltway to Annapolis. His boss was never supportive, always boasting about her superior federal system.

His cell phone rang. The phone to his ear, he said, "Deputy Nash."

A woman's soft voice said, "I have something to tell you."

It was Hannah! "No lectures on religion, I hope." He wanted to say it was great she called.

She laughed nervously. "First, I'm sorry for saying you failed to produce evidence. That was harsh. I did not mean to be."

Trenton had not forgotten what she said. "If you say so."

Hannah was silent for a moment, then added, "I thought you should know, Mr. Jubayl disappeared. He's been gone for days. No one knows where he is."

Trenton tried to steer around a van that pulled out in front of him. He dropped the cell phone. When the way was clear, he picked it up and said, "Sorry. I'm driving."

"I'll hang up then. You shouldn't drive and talk on a cell phone. It's dangerous."

"I'll pull over," he said, but kept driving. Trenton knew Jubayl was in Detroit on Monday, but he could not admit that to Hannah. He tried to ease her mind, "Maybe he went to Lebanon. You said he travels there often."

Hannah replied, "That's possible, but I'm worried. It's not like him to leave without an explanation. What if he has been kidnapped for ransom? That happened recently to several missionaries, you know."

A note of fear in her voice moved him to say, "Hannah, if he was kidnapped, someone would have contacted Helpers requesting money. I'll check with my sources at the State Department and the FBI. What about his wife and George?"

Hannah sighed. "I called his home, spoke to George. He was—ah—secretive. Will you let me know if you find out anything? My mom and I are afraid something is wrong."

"Hannah." Trenton stopped. What did he want to say? Smart and compassionate, she was unlike any woman he had ever met. She had already told him, in so many words, she wanted nothing to do with him. And yet she had called him. Still, it might be better to keep his personal interest in her below the radar, at least for now.

He assured her, "If I find out anything that I can tell you, I will." On an impulse, he added, "Can I call you, even if I don't?"

Without hesitating, she said, "Yes." Then, "Someone is paging me at work. Goodbye."

Trenton believed Emile was safe and busy secreting money to terrorists with no one at Helpers the wiser. He almost called Eva, but he'd reached Annapolis. His dad's opinion meant more to him than hers.

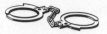

EIGHTEEN

"It feels good to get away for a day, even if it is Richmond." Eva stretched her legs forward.

Scott drove away from her parents' brick ranch home. It was Saturday night, and Scott had surprised her with an overnight trip. He reached over and squeezed her hand.

"I agree with your father. You have not looked this relaxed in awhile. Andy and Kaley will have a good time with your folks."

Eva grinned. "And the kitty, Zak. Making caramel apples does sound like fun."

Scott slowed the van. "Should I turn around?"

"Don't you dare. I want to enjoy dinner with my husband, alone."

Scott accelerated and Eva rested her head against the seat back, glad she left her cell phone at her parents.

"Where are you taking me?" she asked, her eyes shut.

"Another surprise."

"I like it when you take charge."

Silence flowered between them like a fragrant rose. Twenty minutes later, Scott pulled the van into a restaurant parking lot.

Eva's eyes flew open. "Scott, I love it here!"

Scott had taken Eva to the Naples Restaurant when they visited Richmond during the year they dated, and they had saved it for special occasions ever since. The authentic Italian atmosphere reminded them of being in Florence on their European honeymoon. Within minutes, they were ensconced in a corner booth with a red-and-white checkered tablecloth. The waiter brought a large antipasto salad, with olives and mozzarella cheese.

"Save room, Eva Marie. This is our first course. Chicken oregano with pasta, garlic bread, and tiramisu are still to come."

Eva's laughter rang true. When Scott laughed, too, Eva realized such happy sounds had been absent from their home for some time. They munched on salad and talked about the children. When Eva set down her fork, Scott held out a wrapped box with a silver bow.

Ever since she was small, Eva poked and prodded her presents to guess what they were. "A DVD?"

"Open it," was all he said.

Eva tore off the silver wrap. Inside was a smaller box in gold paper. She ripped off the paper to find a black velvet box.

A playful look on her face, she said, "Scott. What did you do?" But, she didn't wait for him to tell. She snapped open the lid. The sight of a 24-carat gold heart-shaped locket brought tears to her eyes.

"Happy anniversary, honey. I love you." Scott's smile deepened the lines beginning to etch around his eyes. "The heart opens."

Sadness tugged at her own heart. She had forgotten that it was their special day. Her fingers trembled as she pressed open a little spring. The heart popped open. Inside was a photo of her and Scott. It was so small only their faces showed. Eva remembered where the photo had been taken, by the old church at Maria Alm, tucked between the Steinerne Meer and the Scheifer Alps in Austria. They spent a wonderful week in the shadows of the towering mountains, startling beauty all around them. It felt like heaven brought to earth. Scott helped her fasten the necklace, which sparkled against her black sweater.

"Your gift is beautiful." Eva looked into his eyes. "I treasure the love that goes with it." She swallowed. "Scott, I need you to know something. Work has really kept me busy, but yesterday a great burden was lifted. A complex case closed against someone at church."

A puzzled look fell across Scott's face.

Eva waved a hand. "Forget I said that. Even though I didn't get you a present, I want to give you and the kids more of my time." She missed their walks after dinner and long talks before bed. Maybe he did, too, and his gift was meant to remind her of more carefree days. Eva searched his face in the candle glow and saw contentment.

Scott pressed her hand gently in his. "I don't want you to put more pressure on yourself."

Eva was about to tell him she had rescheduled the appointment with the baby doctor when the waiter set sizzling plates in front of them. An aroma of fresh garlic and spices hovered between them.

She whispered, "I love you, Scott. I get scared when I realize how much."

"I always knew you were a scaredy-cat, deep down."

"Ooh, that hurts." Eva returned Scott's indulgent smile.

Savoring the flavors of her dinner and the time alone with Scott, Eva knew something needed to change. How she longed for more family time. Her high-powered job demanded constant feeding, like a newborn. Scott broke off a chunk of bread and, after buttering it, handed it to her. His obvious happiness kept her from saying what she was feeling. She'd keep the conversation on the lighter tone he introduced, and not rehash things that caused them stress.

Eva tried to pay attention as Scott recounted the absurdity of politics inside the Pentagon. Prompted by Scott's clever packaging of her gift, a burr chafed at her mind. Was Emile cleverly hiding his real actions? Eva picked at her favorite dessert, her heart laden with doubt. Perhaps Emile was guilty, and she was wrong to close the case.

By Monday morning, Eva had resolved the question. Emile's case was closed. One step remained for her to know it was final. Still, she had misgivings about writing the letter. She touched the keyboard, her monitor sprang to life, and she typed to the local telephone company:

Dear Director of Security:

Re: Emile and Sari Jubayl

To avoid compromising an ongoing investigation, in an earlier letter I asked you to keep confidential that there was a subpoena for this customer's home telephone records. Our case is closed. You are free to follow your company policy concerning these matters.

Eva typed her name and title at the bottom. She spellchecked the letter, printed it on ICE letterhead, then typed an identical letter for Emile's direct telephone number at Helpers International. While Eva was required to send these letters, she hoped the phone company would not notify the Jubayls.

She breathed deeply, then blew the air out slowly. Last night she dreamed of Sari Jubayl in a hospital bed, her pale features made all the

more stark by deep, black eyes. Sari lifted up an arm with an intrave-
nous needle and cried out for Eva to help her. Eva was whisked away
to another room and could not find Sari again.

When she woke this morning, she felt tired. Dream or no dream,
she was the lead investigator in a case against the Jubayls. Even if Sari
wasn't involved in illegal activity, Eva could not call her to chat about
her anti-American son and peculiar husband. There was no way for
Eva to counsel Sari.

She signed her name to both letters, then called Wanda on the
intercom. "I have letters for the afternoon mail."

A few minutes later, Wanda breezed into Eva's office, smelling like
smoke from her most recent break, and said excitedly, "Trenton just
left in a hurry. What's up?"

Eva had no idea and told Wanda as much, but Wanda persisted.

"A young woman called. He shot out of here like a rabbit."

Eva searched in her side drawer for a peppermint. There were
none. Maybe Grandpa would pick up some on his next trip to the
Netherlands. Eva looked up. Wanda was staring at her.

Eva pushed her bangs out of her eyes. "Griff in yet?"

Wanda shrugged. "I've seen him once since he got back from
Detroit." She picked up the mail in Eva's OUT basket and left Eva
alone.

Eva slumped back in her chair. Wanda had a point. She and her
team needed to regroup. Like a coach after a weekend loss, it was her
job to rally them to go after ARC's money. How did she move forward, now that their case was in pieces like a shaken puzzle?

She'd do what she always did: make a list. Down one side, she
penned in FIG's current cases. Next to each, she noted the status.
When finished, she realized Emile's was only one case. Several FIG
officers were tracking drug funds through sham companies and bank
accounts. And there was always Farouk. The indictments against him
had multiplied.

Eva stared at Emile's name on the list. That dream of Sari had
seemed so real. Whether from past habit or sudden desire, for the first
time since she became supervisor of FIG, she uttered a real prayer to
God. More than words, it was an upward plea for help to keep her
promises to Scott, and for Sari Jubayl. Maybe that was the reason for
her dream. She opened her eyes and sensed a feeling of calm. As her
finger touched the gold locket, Eva wondered why she had neglected
this part of her life for so long.

Later that week, outside the office building, Trenton checked his watch. It was 6:45 p.m. Everyone should be gone by now. With a swipe of his magnetic entry card, he entered the rear door. Trenton walked up the steps, punched in the code, and pushed open the FIG office door. He listened. No sounds but the electric clock buzz. He was alone, which was good; he was not up to being ribbed about Emile's case. Griff had blown the undercover meeting, and he was supposed to be a hot shot FBI agent.

He called Annapolis. "Dad, your idea worked. Ari Rosen let it slip that he'd already heard from his father."

"Mr. Rosen and I go way back," Duke said into the phone.

"Yeah. Ari mentioned his dad told stories about when you and he were partners."

Trenton cradled the receiver between his ear and shoulder, and moved the trash can closer to his desk. While his dad talked, he cleaned out his drawers. Half-listening to Duke reminisce about his years in Chicago, Trenton decided to leave his pictures on the wall until after Eva was informed.

"Ari can't wait to work with a Nash. He's going to talk to Eva tomorrow. If she agrees, in a few days, I'll transfer from FIG to the FBI Terrorism Task Force!"

"Son, that's a great place for you to serve while you finish your degree. Once you have that, with your time assigned to the FBI's task force, the FBI will be sure to accept your application to become an agent."

Trenton felt his dad's approval, even over the phone. Duke reminded Trenton that, when he worked with Ari's father, he was able to be home Friday nights. Mr. Rosen had to be home before dark for the Jewish Sabbath.

His side drawers empty, Trenton said, "Kiss Mom for me. Bye."

The transfer would be great. Perhaps he should be the one to tell Eva and not leave it up to Ari. He told himself she'd be relieved to see him go. He noticed a stack of documents on the desk corner. A note in Eva's handwriting was attached on top.

"Trenton, review these bank records delivered today as a result of the Grand Jury subpoena. When done, return to me for the closed file. Eva."

Trenton rolled his eyes. Of course, she had to underline the word "closed." From a small refrigerator in the kitchen area, he got a can of diet cola and tossed a quarter in the honor box. Back in his office, he popped it open and thumbed through Emile's personal bank statements. After awhile, the monthly tally of checks written for twelve dollars, thirty dollars, and one hundred dollars numbed his brain.

One pattern was interesting. Each month, Emile deposited three thousand dollars in his personal checking account. Probably his monthly salary. Nothing unusual there.

On the final statement for the month of October, he almost missed it. Black numbers against the white page, a deposit of two hundred and fifty thousand dollars! Trenton sat upright, his heart thudding. He knew it had been a mistake for Eva to end the investigation. Emile Jubayl smelled like trouble, and this proved it. All the other deposits were for three thousand dollars or less. Was the huge sum for ARC?

He'd convince Ari of it, no matter the time, or what, it took. With the same determination he showed when pinning an opponent in a wrestling match, Trenton returned to the first bank statement. For the next hour, he reviewed every entry on every bank statement, which he then photocopied. The copy pile went into his briefcase. He made no copy of the original October statement. He kept that one for himself.

Trenton gathered up the other originals and, with a flourish, wrote on a yellow sticky note, *For Closed File.* He stuck it on top where Eva was sure to see it, and put the bundle on her desk. If she never learned of the deposit, that was fine with him. She would just argue it meant nothing significant. Eva was competent, but she had no gift for thinking like a criminal.

Trenton was exhilarated. He was on Emile's scent. If only he had met with him undercover, he'd have convinced Emile to take the money. Tomorrow, Ari would learn of the huge deposit. Maybe then, Midge Hopper, the federal prosecutor assigned to TTF, would let him work undercover against Emile. On the way home, he would drive by Emile's house. A little surveillance never hurt.

In an eerily painted yellow hallway, Sari stood by a bank of pay phones. Phone card in her hand, she hesitated. Emile had not given her permission to tell anyone. But Thelma was her friend. Sari placed a long distance call from Rochester, Minnesota, to Columbia City, Virginia.

On the fifth ring, Thelma answered, "Hello."

Sari began to sniffle. "Thelma, I am in Minnesota."

"Sari, do you have a cold? You missed prayer meeting."

She looked around the hall, then whispered, "I have to hurry. Remember my unspoken prayer request last week?" Sari swallowed a sob.

"Honey, if that son of yours is in trouble again, let me talk to him. He needs a strong hand. He's goin' in the wrong direction. Let me turn down the radio so I can hear."

"George is at home, as far as I know." Sari wiped her nose. "Emile and I are at Mayo Clinic. They ran tests. He has prostate cancer. They're going to operate." Sari's tears flowed freely.

"You might have told me. I could have come with you," Thelma said gently.

"Emile does not want anyone to know. If word leaks out he has cancer, he is afraid it will affect donor support."

"You were right to call. Are you sleepin' and eatin'?"

When she was alone in her hotel room, she did neither. Sari reached into her purse for another tissue. If only Thelma, or George, were here at Mayo Clinic with them. It was so big and businesslike. No one here understood her fears or had any time for her.

Thelma spoke soothingly, "Promise me you'll get dinner."

Sari heard, but her mind slid down a steep hill with no hope of climbing back up again. "Maybe later. Emile is in the operating room right now!"

Sari's mind reeled. Even though she and Emile had carved out separate lives, he was her husband. What if they never had a chance to get things right? What if—?

Thelma interrupted this last disturbing thought. "God is in control, Sari."

Her legs weak under her, Sari confided, "I'm worried. Emile goes to church and claims to be a Christian. Is he ready to meet his Creator? What if he dies before he is sure?"

Thelma did not hesitate. "We'll pray, right now on the phone, and ask God to allow him to recover."

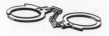

NINETEEN

Wanda held her hand over the receiver. "Collect call for Trenton, from the Alexandria City Jail." Griff's right eyebrow cascaded up his forehead. "Who is it?"

"Farouk Hamdi. I'm not supposed to accept collect calls," Wanda whispered, as if part of a conspiracy.

Griff had not seen Trenton, but he was pretty sure Eva would want someone to speak to their prior informant. "Put it through to my office." He sprinted back to his desk and grabbed the phone on the second ring. "Agent Topping. What do you want?"

In a friendly voice, Farouk said, "Thanks for taking my call. I will make it worthwhile."

"You wanted Deputy Nash. Now you're glad to talk to me?" Griff would not be easily fooled by Farouk. "After the way you abused Trenton, don't call him again. You deal with me."

"I want to tell you more about my connections. I waited to see if they knew I was arrested. The Cobra did not, but after that show at the airport, I am not so sure."

"Won't he be suspicious? You failed to show up in London for the second meeting."

Farouk cleared his throat. "I hoped Trenton would put me in touch with you."

Griff's laughter was spontaneous. Whom did this guy think he was toying with, a rookie? "Guess what, pal? After you double-crossed us, we arrested your girlfriend."

Farouk was silent at the other end.

Griff continued, "Farouk, does your lawyer know you are calling me?"

"My court-appointed lawyer has yet to see me. I *really* wanted to talk to you." His voice lowered, and Griff had to strain to hear. "One of your previous—ah—clients, is my cellmate. He tells me you are tough, but fair."

Griff said, "Just so you know, I'm the lead agent for your prosecution. Are you willing to sign a statement waiving your right to counsel?"

Farouk did not flinch. "Yeah, and I don't want my attorney to know."

This defendant had figured out more than a few angles. Griff said, "Tell me why I won't be wasting my time if I talk with you."

"My acquaintance is in the inner circle."

"Heard that one before."

Farouk lowered his voice, "I cannot say more on a jail phone. Come see me."

It was possible that a correctional officer was listening to their conversation. They were all taped. A further briefing was best done in person. "You won't get out on a bond like last time."

"Reserve judgment until you hear what I say. Can you come today?"

"Always eager to help American justice. If I see you at the jail, word will get around instantly. You have a hearing day after tomorrow, the day before Thanksgiving. Your lawyer wants to suppress the valise you dropped on Trenton's foot. Good luck."

"I haven't even seen my attorney yet."

Griff had an idea how he could meet Farouk so few people would know, and there would be no written record. "After your hearing, I'll ask a trusted U.S. Marshal to bring you to a private office in the courthouse. Sign the waiver and we'll talk."

Farouk whispered. "Mr. Topping, I'll be ready."

Griff hung up the phone and dialed Eva, who had taken Kaley on a field trip with her class to the Air and Space Museum. She answered her cell before the first ring had rung.

"You must miss this place," Griff said.

"Not at all. What's up?" she asked.

"Trenton's nemesis at the jail just called. Wants to meet me."

"I thought we were finished with him. He's just trying to avoid trial and a stiff prison term."

"It's me, hard-nosed Griff, remember? My mom says I have Winston Churchill's genes. He called me Mr. Topping. I plan to keep it that way."

"What did he want?"

Since Eva was on a cell phone, Griff disguised the facts. "He knows a guy on the inner circle, and claims he can deliver Mr. Big."

"Mr. Big?"

"You're on a cell," Griff replied. "Think the biggest Mr. Big."

"Should I come in?"

"We'll talk in the morning. Enjoy all the planes."

He hung up. Thoughts of the airplane Charles Lindberg flew across the Atlantic to Paris in 1927 led to memories of the last flight he took with his wife, Sue. Devastated by the diagnosis of ovarian cancer, they drove to Charlottesville to get away. On a whim, he rented a Cessna Skyhawk. They spent that afternoon flying high over the Blue Ridge Mountains until the sky painted itself fuchsia and gold with the setting sun. Sue died two months later. That was almost eight years ago. Why was he thinking of her now? Because he still loved her. Always would.

Early the next morning, Trenton sauntered into Eva's office. She was talking to Earl and motioned at Trenton to take a seat. She handed Earl an envelope. "Good work finding drug profits invested in the used car business."

On his way out, Earl smiled at Trenton, who did not return the gesture.

Eva eyed Trenton, who seemed to have less than his usual air of confidence. "I know Ari Rosen asked you to join his Terrorism Task Force, and that you agreed."

Trenton visibly relaxed.

"Is this because of what happened with Farouk?"

Trenton gave her a sheepish grin.

"I'm sorry to hear it."

Eva studied his firm jaw and set eyes. He had tremendous creativity, but a dose of stubbornness caused him to do things his way. Before she judged him too harshly, she realized she was also determined to succeed. Eva handed him the signed transfer papers, along with his time and attendance records.

Trenton took the forms and stood. "Before we went to London, Farouk took me by the address for Richard Salem, the guy who, uh—" He stopped abruptly.

Eva smiled, "The man who ran me over at the townhouse. What did you find out?"

"A Richard Salem owned that house, but he died a year ago. The estate is in probate. I guess the guy at Farouk's used a dead man's identity."

Another dead end. Probably the passport in the name of Salem was also false. That reminded her to get Griff back working on the name of the other passport, Drury Baptiste.

"Glad you checked." Eva rose and extended her hand. "Your father's legacy inspires you to match his career. You had a rough go with Farouk."

They shook hands and she continued, "All investigations have weak points. Your idea to send Emile a donation was great. Keep honing your instincts."

"Thanks. I learned a lot from you and Griff. And I'll be just down the hall. What's up with Farouk?"

She nearly forgot. "You need to appear at a hearing tomorrow about the valise he dropped at your feet. His lawyer is trying to keep it out of his trial."

"Can he do that?"

"We didn't have a separate search warrant for the valise."

Trenton asked, "Did we need one?"

Eva picked up Jillie's paperweight. "His attorney will argue that, because you found the valise outside, it was not covered by the warrant for the contents of his house."

She placed the paperweight in her briefcase; she was taking it home. Eva picked up her coffee cup and walked Trenton out of her office.

"We should win. The valise was always in our sight, so it remained part of the house contents. Either way, be at the federal Courthouse in Alexandria tomorrow at ten a.m."

"Think he'll plead guilty? Farouk doesn't seem like the brightest bulb."

Eva laughed. She would miss his exuberance. "As the lead agent, Griff is working with Dan Simmons. Farouk will try to make a deal. None of us has any stomach to cut him a break."

Trenton followed her to the coffee pot. "He deserves every year of prison he gets."

Eva poured a cup. "What cases will you work on with Ari?"

"Ah," Trenton twisted his transfer papers. "I should drop these off. Nothing's been assigned, yet."

Eva watched him duck out of the eating area. She downed the coffee, which made her stomach growl. Back at her desk, she rummaged in the side drawer through dried-up pens and outdated floppy disks until she found an oatmeal granola bar. She unwrapped it and took a bite. It was stale, but she ate it anyway.

Since Griff's cryptic call yesterday, her mind was stuck on how to manage Farouk. Even the chance to be with her daughter at the Air and Space Museum had lost its intrigue. It had been all she could do to keep from returning to the office before Kaley saw the Apollo 11 exhibit. Eva's mind wandered back to work. Could she reach beyond El Samoud's financiers and arrest the terrorist himself?

Thirty minutes later, Trenton slipped past Eva's office where she was meeting with Griff. He closed his office door and called Hannah at work. If she was too busy to talk, she could at least answer a question. When the receptionist put him on hold, he unloaded his top desk drawer into a large envelope and clasped it shut. Into another, he slid a photo taken with his Dad on the *Enforcer*. Duke and Trenton, GMU cap on his head, displayed record rockfish catches from the Chesapeake. In ten minutes or less, his favorite photo would have a new home.

"This is Hannah. May I help you?"

"It's me."

"Hello, me."

She recognized his voice! "Very funny. Can you talk?"

"I'm in the mail room. It's quiet, but that could change."

Trenton asked, "Is Emile back?"

"Yes, a few days ago. He was on a vacation with his wife. I meant to call, but it's been so busy. It was silly of me to send out an alarm."

He hesitated, then said, "I enjoy talking to you." When she said nothing, Trenton moved on. "Has he bought any new items, besides expensive vacations?"

Hannah forced a tiny laugh. "A new phone system was installed a few months ago. Yesterday, a new copy machine was delivered. I'm learning how to operate it, but it's twice as fast—"

Trenton reigned her in. "Forget the machine. Find out where Emile went on his so-called vacation. Let me know if he shows up in a new car."

Hannah sighed. "All right. When is this going to end? I told you nothing is wrong."

Trenton snickered. "Right. Remember, you called me in a panic because your boss mysteriously disappeared. Why didn't he tell the staff he was taking a vacation?"

That question silenced her. It was a natural thing to tell coworkers about a vacation destination, yet Emile kept it secret for some reason.

Trenton's next question proved easier to answer. "Want to meet at GMU tomorrow for our special coffee?"

"Hmm," she said. "I work tomorrow morning. Then it's my turn to buy groceries, and I have to be at church by seven to lead a Bible study for teen girls."

Trenton ignored her reference to her religion and said, "I testify tomorrow on a big case. I could leave work early and meet you at five." He held his breath. Would she come?

Hannah relented. "I'll wait for you at the Commons. I have to deliver the mail now. See you tomorrow, Trenton."

This time, she didn't call him Deputy Nash! He hung up the phone, feeling terrific. Things were finally going his way.

Emile survived his surgery and the flight home. Now all he had to do was survive Sari's fussing over him. She had already brought him the mail and a cup of tea.

"Want some honey?" she asked.

He snarled, "No."

She dribbled some in. "I took out the catalogues. Remember, the doctor said to rest."

"Sari, enough. I can take care of myself." At the pained look on her face, he softened his tone, "Thanks for the tea. I want to finish these bills."

Sari left him alone in his den. Emile gently lowered himself to the chair and felt a stab of pain. For more than forty years, he refused to put foreign substances into his system except for an occasional aspirin. He was not about to break that rule now. He set aside a recently mailed solicitation from Helpers International to admire later.

The telephone bill was due. Tomorrow, he would set up an automatic bill pay option at the bank. He had waited long enough to get with the modern era. What was the other letter from the phone company? Thinking it was an advertisement for the new Internet broadband, Emile almost threw it away, then slit it open with a knife.

Addressed to him, it was from the regional Director for Security. Emile's eyes consumed the brief paragraph. Hands shaking, he called the number listed. Emile explained to the woman who answered that he received a letter that said to call if he had questions. He had questions.

"I'll see if he will take your call."

Elevator music played in his ear. Emile was surprised when the director came on the phone.

"Why were my home telephone records subpoenaed? What about my cell phone and business records?"

"Sir, I have limited information. Such letters are usually sent after an arrest."

Anger boiled within him. "I'm not a criminal," he snapped.

"I don't have to take this abuse. I can tell you nothing more."

"It's abuse for a customer to ask who looked through his personal phone records? This is a breach of my privacy."

The director replied, "We sent the letter because we felt you had a right to know. If you have concerns about privacy rights, talk to a lawyer. If we comply with a court-ordered subpoena, we violate no laws."

Unsatisfied, Emile asked, "Which federal agency got my records?"

"I have nothing more to tell you. Call your lawyer. Good day."

The phone connection went dead. A lawyer? Was he about to be arrested? Helpers International had a tax attorney who handled corporate matters. He was a nice guy, but no way Emile was putting his life in that lawyer's hands.

Sari came into his den carrying a pot. "Want more tea?"

Emile did not answer. His bottom was sore. With her hair pulled on top of her head, Sari looked like a character from a bad comedy. How could he tell her about a court subpoena? She'd dissolve on the spot.

Sari set down the teapot and looked at Emile. "Is something wrong?"

Emile shook his head. "I am tired and am going to lie down." This was true, and she would believe it. Ever since his surgery, she was consumed with his health. He did not intend to die, yet. He had too many children to help.

The phone company's letter clutched in his hand, Emile glanced over his shoulder. Good. Sari was not following. He went to the first floor bathroom and locked the door. With a small pair of scissors from the medicine cabinet, Emile cut the phone company letter into pieces and threw them into the toilet bowl. The particles spun from sight. The Security Director had said, "These letters are sent after an arrest."

Of course. Their records were searched because of George's arrest. He still lived at home, used the phone. Emile put back the scissors, then walked slowly upstairs. In the master bedroom, he removed a package from a temporary hiding spot. After a short search, he found another place to secrete it. He'd never tell Sari it was there.

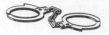

TWENTY

Trenton set the fishing photo on a shelf behind his desk. His new office was a cubicle with soft walls. He'd have less privacy here. Into the middle drawer he emptied pens, clips, and paper. Ari Rosen, Supervisor of the FBI's Terrorism Task Force, walked in.

He said, "Since you worked for Eva, I assume you know the ropes. She is one of ICE's brightest stars.

Trenton nodded. He really wanted to talk about Emile's large deposit.

Thankfully, Ari switched from praising Eva to business. "Besides Helpers International, you have two other cases. I point you in the right direction, then you're on your own."

Ari set two files on the desk, then gestured to a photo of John Wayne in a cowboy hat. "My father had a picture of the Duke in his office, when our fathers were partners. That's how your dad got his nickname. My father thought an FBI agent would have more respect being called Duke than Harold."

Trenton laughed. After Mr. Rosen christened his dad with that name, it stuck all these years. It was as if Harold Nash never existed.

"My informant says Emile bought lots of new equipment and lives pretty high for a CEO of a nonprofit organization. I'm sure that $250,000 deposit is destined for ARC cells around the world. It could be from a terrorist group overseas."

Ari's fingers ran through his black hair. "I thought it went into a joint account with his wife."

Trenton did not see the relevance. "She doesn't work."

Ari replied, "It *is* curious. Why would he put it in their personal account if he uses Helpers International to launder money?"

"I'll find his reasons."

"Do a trash pull," Ari suggested.

Trenton was unsure he liked the sound of whatever Ari had in mind.

"Is that legal?"

"What do they teach you at Jefferson County? The Courts have ruled garbage placed at the side of the street is abandoned property. You can search his trash without a warrant." Ari showed a lot of teeth when he smiled.

Trenton was amazed. He had never heard of this before. "You mean, I can go to Helpers at night, take away their garbage, and won't get into trouble?"

Twirling a pen in his fingers, Ari nodded. "That's roughly the idea. Try his home first. Helpers probably uses industrial dumpsters. You'd need a truck to haul it away and spend days pouring over shipping and receiving records, which is not what we focus on here."

"How should I do it then?"

"When you pull his trash, the trick is to search for evidence of his habits, his sympathies. A scrap of paper might reveal a name that connects him to ARC. What does he read? Where does he shop? Then, follow up every lead. Get the picture?"

Trenton did. He liked Ari and was glad to be working for him now, thanks to Duke. He replied, "I'll find out when the trash is collected, and go the night before. Maybe I'll get lucky."

"Did Emile deposit cash or a check into that account?"

"I am not sure, yet. Probably not cash, for fear of raising suspicion."

Ari agreed. "If it was a check, we'll need a grand jury subpoena to get a copy of it."

Trenton asked, "Couldn't we get around that?" Eva's Grand Jury might know by now she had closed Emile's case.

"I suppose we could use an administrative subpoena signed by me." Ari paused. "Sometimes, the bank's attorney challenges those."

Trenton wished he knew more about the federal system. Going to law school flickered across his mind. The FBI recruiter said a law degree would give him a leg up in getting hired.

Ari shook his head. "I don't like to set bad precedent. I'll ask Midge Hopper to present the matter to a new Grand Jury being sworn in next week. You'll need to meet the AUSA sometime. She's not as picky as Dan is about how we handle our investigations."

Trenton relished the idea of more freedom to target Emile. "I'm on my way to testify at a hearing on one of my old cases. Then, I'll get right on it."

Ari left, and Trenton retrieved his file on the raid at Farouk's. He had gone over his report last night and was ready to testify. If he saw Eva, so be it, but he would not tell her that he and Ari were working on Emile. With Ari's new ideas, together they would nail Emile.

Griff had been up since before sunrise. Used to living alone, his morning routine was perfected. This morning was no different. He ran two miles in the cold to perk up his appetite. The scrambled eggs and toast he fixed would carry him all day. With the hearing and interview with Farouk, he'd have no time to eat again today.

He arrived at the office before anyone else and fired up his computer. Finished typing, Griff hit the print command. The printer worked its magic. He snatched the attorney waiver form for Farouk to sign, tucked it into a pocket of his leather jacket, and grabbed the keys for his G-car. On the way out, he passed by Earl, hunched over his keyboard.

Griff zipped up his jacket and said to him, "If anything bubbles up, you're in charge. I'm on my way to the federal Courthouse." He did not say Eva was joining him. They decided it was better to keep it to themselves.

"Where's Eva? Got a new case?" Earl typed one finger at a time.

Griff laughed. His high school English teacher had predicted that learning to type would be beneficial. He was glad he believed her.

His reputation for being tight-lipped intact, Griff replied, "If you need me, leave a message on my cell."

Earl never stopped hunting and pecking. "Yeah, right."

Whatever Earl meant, Griff was determined not to tell him about Farouk. Not until he was certain the slippery fellow delivered something solid on ARC. While the terror group had not set off recent bombings, Griff feared a sneak attack. ARC hid like a tiger in the weeds by a waterhole; when its prey was convinced there was no danger and came to drink, ARC sprang with horrific violence.

Griff slid behind the wheel and turned on the radio. The meteorologist warned of heavy rains. A possible Nor'easter over Thanksgiving. Winds were already gusting. Two years ago, a storm shut down the whole East Coast for days. Another huge one would really mess up things. Today, he and Eva would squeeze information from the ARC convert. On Friday, they were meeting with Brewster Miles, who was in town, and Griff didn't breach security to ask why.

They had important things to talk over with Brewster, like if Farouk went to trial, would the Brits make Camille available to testify against him? Nothing appeared in the British papers about her arrest. Griff had checked. There was also nothing new about Ambassador Cook. It was as if, after his daring escape, he just disappeared.

Griff turned up the heat in the car and formulated a plan to get information from Farouk. After Trenton managed to trash the case, they needed a break. It was wearing on the group, especially Eva. With Trenton working with Ari, Griff could focus like a laser beam on turning Farouk into a useful informant. No other commitments distracted him from work. He loved baseball, but the World Series was long over.

Since Sue died, he didn't fly much anymore either. Griff kept up his license, but that was all. No one at home to worry about, not even a dog. That was the way he wanted it. He would never marry again. When friends arranged for him to meet someone, Griff dated occasionally. It never took, except for Jillie. But enough of that. He had to keep his eyes on the ball. Griff turned into the parking lot and grabbed the ticket.

Emile sat with his back to the window. Outside, winds blew thirty-five miles per hour with gusts up to fifty, but he was oblivious. All he could think of was that the criminal lawyer had not returned his call. He had to ask him about those subpoenas before the long Thanksgiving weekend.

He called the law firm again, told the receptionist, "It's important." Emile listened, then replied, "Have Mr. Scribbs call me at home in an hour."

Replacing the receiver in the cradle, he wrote on his calendar, "Follow up with lawyer. Fly Lebanon next week—Urgent." His briefcase in hand, he opened his door. Hannah was about to knock. Her other arm was folded around papers.

She dropped her hand. "I have my mom's report, and letters from volunteers. Should I put them on your desk?"

"Fine, Hannah. Then go home, which is where I'm headed. A Nor'easter is coming. We're closing now for the holiday weekend." That should give him time to consult with Harlan Scribbs, his new criminal attorney.

"Thanks, Mr. Jubayl. "

She stepped around him. Emile watched Hannah set the reports on his desk next to his calendar. Her head turned slightly. Was she looking at what he wrote? He'd have to be more careful.

"Coming, Hannah?" he asked.

In the U.S. Marshal's conference room, Farouk sat in a metal chair, hands cuffed behind his back. Eva and Griff reversed roles. She played nice, while he pressed hard.

"Mrs. Montanna and Mr. Topping, give me a chance to prove I am a loyal American and not a terrorist."

Eva easily dismissed Farouk's declaration of patriotism. They had just listened to his tale of a connection to a Frenchman named Jacques, El Samoud's mechanic and captain of ARC's seagoing vessel, which gave Farouk an inside track to the terrorist.

Griff sat across from Farouk, arms folded. "You and I both know what you are. Skip the soap opera. What we want is corroboration. Convince us you know Jacques and that he can help us arrest El Samoud."

"Agent Topping, let me think."

Farouk acted as if he forgot Eva was there, so she waited, willing herself not to be duped by him again. Cleanshaven and sporting a haircut, he actually looked human. If he wore a suit rather than the orange jumper, he could pass for a banker, or with his clipped accent, a British news anchor.

Griff was not so patient. "While you plan your next scam, let me remind you of your last one. When we arrested you in your town-house, you faked not speaking English. Now you sound like a regular radio announcer. You pretended to know Cobra, El Samoud's second-in-command. We know that came to nothing."

Farouk interrupted, "If Cobra finds out I am talking to you, I am a dead man. As sure as these handcuffs are cutting into my wrists. Can't you loosen them or take them off?"

"I wasn't finished. You smuggled diamonds under Trenton's nose. With that track record, I find it difficult to believe you are the key to arresting El Samoud. "

"I know the Cobra!" Farouk hissed. Using the only means available to emphasize his point, he kicked the table leg with his unshackled foot. "His contact in London passed me the note with the arrange-ments to meet him. If you're so smart, you know that a short fat man wearing a turban came in behind me."

In response to Farouk's outburst, Griff said cooly, "One more time, bud, and you'll be kicking yourself in your cell, alone."

Farouk nodded his head. "I tested Trenton. Now, I'm in a worse mess." He licked his dried lips before saying, "You know I passed funds to ARC. But I am not of ARC's mindset."

Eva smothered a laugh. Griff was so much better at this than she was. Farouk had called to meet with Griff without the knowledge of his attorney. That morning, his attorney's motion to suppress evidence taken from the valise was denied. His lawyer was appealing the ruling, and Eva wanted to talk to Farouk before the appeal was heard. With analysis of Farouk's software taking longer than expected, they could not risk a weak case going to the jury.

She spoke for the first time. "We believe you."

He licked his lips, again. "Mrs. Montanna, thank you for saying that. I have wanted to tell you how I kept twenty-five percent of the funds moved for ARC. The Cobra knew it and accepted my fee because of my deep embed in the American culture. He kept a share, too, which he hides in a Swiss bank account. I am not sure if El Samoud knows this."

"Do you have those bank account numbers? Where do you stash your money?" Griff asked.

Farouk looked right past him and over to Eva. "May I tell you about Camille?"

Eva nodded and said, "Please. I want to hear everything."

"She grew up in a French community sympathetic to ARC's cause. It is all she knows. Her stolen gems are a small part of their funding. I helped her," he lowered his eyes, "because of my affection for her." Farouk said no more.

"Go on," Eva replied.

Farouk sat there, swaying on the metal chair.

"Are you all right?" she asked.

Farouk shook his head. "I feel dizzy. My sugar level must be low. Do you have gum?"

"No, but I might have candy." She reached into her jacket pocket and found a couple peppermints.

She handed one to Griff, who said, "Hold out your tongue." Griff put the white candy on Farouk's tongue. "Chew it in front of us."

Farouk did as he was told. If he was diabetic that might be one reason he wanted out of jail. It was hard to regulate sugar levels in prison. Eva filed away the tidbit to use later if Farouk proved difficult.

At length, Farouk sat up straighter, the candy having the desired effect. "I can get you to Jacques. He travels with El Samoud wherever he goes."

Griff replied, "Let's say I believe you. Where are they now?"

"I missed the second meeting, remember? But I can find out."

"Don't go there today, Farouk," Griff said calmly.

"I am more useful outside."

Griff's eyes narrowed. "Being more useful outside is what got you back inside. And we need proof of Jacques beyond your say so."

Farouk swallowed loudly. "You must not have found the secret hiding place in my valise."

Griff's eyebrow shot up, but neither he nor Eva said a word.

"In the bottom of the valise, a satin fabric has a small spot of glue. Lift it up. You'll find the address in Paris where Jacques lived. His cell phone number, too. It may be changed by now. He could be in Yemen or Egypt."

Eva let Griff continue the questions. "Jacques could be anyone. Can you prove he is in El Samoud's inner circle?"

"Two other names are on the paper. Camille's number was still good when I was in London with Trenton. If she is in jail as you say, you will get her voicemail. The other name is one I have not mentioned. Zayed is El Samoud's leader of the New York cell; he's my main contact."

Eva recognized Zayed as the man who got Ambassador Cook out of Lebanon. MI-5 had him in custody. At last, Farouk might be nearing the truth.

"We want to hear everything you know about Zayed and the guy hiding in your closet. Turns out, he was not Richard Salem. That was a fake name. Was he Drury Baptiste or is that a phony name too?"

Farouk was silent for some time, then wiped his mouth on his sleeve. "If I tell you want you want to know, what will you do for me?"

Griff said, "It's too soon to promise leniency. We'll check your valise. If your info pans out, in the next couple days, we'll arrange for you to be brought here. Then, Agent Montanna and I will debrief you thoroughly. No secrets. If you hold back so much as the name of your grandmother, no deals."

Farouk looked at Eva, who nodded in agreement. He tossed out a final test. "You could make up something and ditch me on purpose."

Griff was not buying it. "You make us sound like you. We keep our word. Besides, you'll take a polygraph. If you pass, the U.S. Attorney will draw up an agreement stating what you can expect by cooperating. Before we leave today, you'll write out everything you tell us."

Griff set a yellow legal pad and pen in front of Farouk.

Farouk stared at the pad, then croaked in a half-whisper, "I have more to tell you, but it's so secret, only a few people in the world are privy to it."

After their meeting with Farouk, Eva and Griff went back to the FIG office and removed the valise from the vault. On the conference table in Eva's office, Griff dismantled it. Inside they found the slips of paper under the lining, just as Farouk said they would.

Griff slid some slips of paper toward Eva. "What do you think of Farouk's lastest tale and these new records?"

Eva ran her fingers across one sheet of paper. She smiled. "I think Farouk sealed the lid on his coffin by admitting how he helped finance ARC and skimmed the money off the top. Now, if his attorney wins the appeal, Farouk's own words," she tapped the yellow legal sheet, "will be used against him at any trial."

Griff nodded in agreement. "He finally gave us a better understanding of ARC's structure and pointed us to El Samoud's ship captain."

Eva stood. "I know it's the Thanksgiving holiday, but this is much too important. I'm going to try to reach the Assistant Director for Homeland Security and have him start searching for Drury Baptiste. Farouk claimed he did not know his exact position, but we'll find him." She shook her heaad. "If it's true he even has a source inside."

Griff followed her out of the conference room and stopped by his office door. "Do you mind if I stop to see Brewster at his hotel and give him a heads-up before we meet with him on Friday?

"Please do. He'll want to know what Farouk told us about Jacques and Camille. We need all the help we can get."

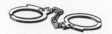

TWENTY ONE

In the gale blowing in off the Chesapeake, Trenton checked the lines holding the *Enforcer* as she bobbed at her mooring like a duck decoy during hunting season. She seemed secure, but with the rain pelting his face, he wasn't certain. In the growing darkness, he felt his way to the other side.

"Dad has impeccable timing," Trenton grumbled.

Not even a sea bird could be heard in the roar. He was watching the last quarter of the annual Detroit Lions Thanksgiving Day game when Duke called from Orlando. The weather forecast was for high winds in Annapolis. Would Trenton check the boat and condo?

Back in the warmth of his car, Trenton blew a sigh. The least he could do for Duke was to ensure that his boat survived the Nor'easter. He drove out of the complex. When he reached the highway to take him back to Virginia, he turned on the radio. He'd drive past Emile's house, if for no other reason than to justify driving his G-car on what Ari would say was personal business.

As Trenton cruised west along Route 50, he remembered with pleasure having coffee yesterday with Hannah. They didn't argue, but she told him nothing new about Emile. His headlights caught the silhouette of a Maryland State Police car behind low bushes at the roadside. He checked his speedometer. Seventy-three in a fifty-five zone. Not good. In the rearview mirror, his eyes met a blast of headlights. The trooper fell in behind him, red and white lights flashing. Yup. He'd been clocked on radar. From his early years of working patrol, Trenton knew what to do. He reached for his federal radio and dialed in the shared Maryland State Police channel.

In the microphone, he stated his car number, which identified him as a federal Task Force vehicle, then, "Calling the MSP car that just pulled out of the bushes on Route 50."

The worst thing he could do was slow down. No response to his call. The lights grew closer in his mirror. He repeated his broadcast, and the speaker mounted under his dash board crackled to life.

"I do not recognize your call sign," said a female officer.

Trenton keyed his microphone. "I'm a federal Task Force car, ahead of you in a metallic blue Grand Am. Sorry I lured you out of your hiding spot."

"Tap your brake lights twice so I'll know it's you," she replied.

Trenton did. "I would stop but I'm surveilling a suspect in the second car ahead of me."

He was not trailing a second car, but she did not need to know that.

Her voice adopted an official tone. "10-4 on that." She paused briefly. "I can stop the car on a pretext and get identification. I might even get probable cause to search the car for you."

Trenton had to think of something to keep her from interfering with his getting home. "Thanks for the offer. We already know who he is, but not where he's going. That's why I don't dare stop."

The flashing lights in his rearview mirror went out and the officer responded, "10-4. Hope it goes well. You have a good night."

Trenton relaxed in his seat before keying his Mic. "10-4, you have a good one, too." He laid the microphone on the seat next to him and returned to his music as he drove to Emile's house. He wanted to check out his neighborhood one more time before Monday night.

Eva and Griff arrived at the Crab Shack a little before one. As they got out of Eva's car, she said to Griff, "I should have mentioned it on the drive here, but we were so focused on Farouk, I forgot. Lou called me at home this morning. He put in his resignation and is going back to Congress to work for a Senator who oversees Homeland Security. Said it would be easier on his back. He did not mention if Wanda is going with him."

Griff opened the door for her and quipped, "But we can hope."

Inside, Brewster was waiting for them by the large saltwater fish tank in the lobby.

As they shook hands in greeting, Eva said, "We have a lot to tell you since we last talked. Griff came to see you at the hotel Wednesday night, but you were out. We thought it best not to discuss things on the phone."

The hostess took them back to a rear table, near the outside deck, which was filled with diners in the summer months. Eva had never been to this restaurant and thought the view over the bay was spectacular. She sat in a side chair so that Brewster could have the best view of the water. A server dressed in black slacks and a crisp white shirt, her brown hair pulled back neatly, took their drink and food orders, which arrived altogether in minutes.

The Crab Shack was used to a busy lunch crowd, and today was no exception. There was no need for the three agents to worry about being overheard. The storm had spent its fury overnight, and the restaurant was bustling with customers the Friday after Thanksgiving. But they would be careful, just in case.

"We don't have soft shell crab like this in London. I do know of a pub that serves great fish and chips. Eva, how about a trip across the Atlantic soon?" Brewster bit into his crab sandwich.

Eva slathered mayo on her lobster roll and tested it. "Our plans are up in the air, so to speak."

Griff laughed. His plate was empty except for a dill pickle, which he never ate. He lowered his voice from habit. "Our diamond smuggler knows a contact, a Frenchie by the name of—" Griff stopped speaking as the server poured diet cola into his glass. "You forgot my lime," he said.

"Oh," she giggled and disappeared.

"Jacques. He is Camille's brother." Griff finished.

Brewster frowned as he chewed the last of his sandwich before saying, "Camille said nothing about a brother. She is extremely uncooperative. We're holding her under a provision of our new terrorism laws. She's not been allowed to communicate with anyone. We do know that ARC has a terror cell in Paris, begun after September 11, that carries on work begun by al Qaeda."

"Did you find evidence in her apartment linking her to Farouk or Emile?" asked Eva.

Brewster wiped his mouth with a blue paper napkin. "A search of her computer revealed websites sympathetic to ARC. But no bank records. Farouk must have transferred the proceeds from the diamonds directly into ARC accounts."

Eva gripped her cup. "We have a new lead. In Farouk's valise, we found numbers, maybe to Cobra's bank."

"I would like to see those," Brewster said.

"We'll get them to you before you leave town," Eva said.

Brewster looked around the room and said quietly, "Zayed is beginning to talk, but he's being cheeky."

The server returned with a large dish of sliced limes. "Is that enough?"

"Plenty." Griff waved her away.

She smiled at him and cleared their plates. "Want dessert? Homemade peach cobbler."

"We're good for now," Griff interrupted.

Brewster added, "Except for my tea. With extra cream."

As the server left, Eva leaned toward Brewster and whispered, "Farouk admitted his cell leader was Zayed, and that Farouk told him he had a highly placed source at Homeland Security."

Startled, Brewster clinked down his cup.

Their server was back with more hot water for Brewster, coffee for Eva, and a small plate of the cobbler for them to sample. "I'll bring you each a big piece. Just flag me down."

Griff said, "Nothing more," and was about to add, "Leave us alone," when she left.

Alone again, Brewster hissed, "Zayed did not mention that. What else did your man say?"

The server was back. "May I bring more cobbler?"

Griff barked, "Not now."

She shrugged and stalked off to the kitchen.

Eva said, "We should have met in our office."

Griff told Brewster, "Farouk wants a deal where we dismiss the case against him, so he can go into the witness protection program with Camille."

"Did you agree to that?"

Eva set down her coffee cup forcefully. "Not yet. We found Farouk's source at Homeland Security." She lowered her voice and said, "Drury Baptiste was not so highly placed."

Griff laughed, "He's a mail clerk."

"That may be, but we've reassigned him to washing cars in the motor pool until we can figure out what he was up to, and if he compromised sensitive documents from the mail room."

"When we're ready to make our cases public, we'll charge Drury Baptiste with assaulting a federal agent, and Farouk will have to testify," Griff said, then added, "We found Zayed's name in Farouk's valise."

The Brit ignored his tea. "Zayed hinted he knows El Samoud's new headquarters. Before his memory crystallizes, he's demanding your government's fifty-million-dollar reward."

"Farouk wants a piece of that, too. Is that why you wanted to meet? For me to give you that promise?" Eva suddenly felt tired. She drained her coffee, but did not dare call back their server.

"Sort of." Brewster nestled his cup into the saucer. "MI-5 wants me to turn Zayed over to you. It is best if our participation stays in the background. We do not have a death penalty." He looked at them both. "El Samoud should face death for all the lives he has taken."

Eva was speechless. Here, in the Crab Shack, Brewster was handing them a witness that could lead to the biggest case of both their careers, or any agent's career. Bigger than Duke Nash's heroics on the hijacked plane. Her mind soared. Eva reminded herself that glory was nothing compared to finding El Samoud and giving him the justice he deserved.

"Do you believe Zayed can deliver Mr. Big?" Griff looked skeptical. After what happened to Trenton in London, he had a right to be.

Brewster poured cream in his cup. "Yes. So does MI-5. I question, however, how old is his information and if you can act on it without tipping El Samoud."

Eva let Brewster's offer percolate through her mind. But, with his track record, could Farouk deliver Jacques?

Brewster said, "One of our female agents is talking to Camille, trying to get her to open up. What you told me about Jacques confirms her connection to ARC is familial. Her father was one of El Samoud's top people."

"Was? I didn't know you could leave the organization and live." Eva's eyes burned, and so did her throat. A bad sign after all that rain.

Brewster grunted. "He didn't leave, and he didn't live. What was left of him was found in the remains of a building bombed outside Paris. The French think he was making bombs when something went wrong." Brewster raised his cup halfway to his mouth and stopped. "Our agency is convinced Camille will not cooperate. You may have found a way around her."

"Because of Jacques?" Griff glared at the server, who turned away.

Brewster nodded. "MI-5 suspects that Camille is engaged to Farouk, which makes him a key player. By working with Zayed and Farouk, without them knowing it, you may reach in and grab El Samoud from his hideaway."

Griff grinned. "I believe we found the mystery woman who left Farouk's in the cab."

Eva got to the heart of the discussion. "How do you propose turning over Zayed?"

Brewster smiled. "I came to the States for that very reason. When my superiors learned Admiral Topping was Griff's grandfather," he chuckled, "they made quite a ruckus. You and Eva are to fly to London. Zayed is in a safehouse on the coast." Brewster's eyes twinkled. "I cannot give his exact location. However, Griff may be close enough to visit his grandmother."

It was almost noon on Sunday at Hadibu. From the bridge of ARC's vessel, the *Crescent*, Jacques de Berg's biceps pressed against the shirt sleeves that were rolled above his elbows. He watched a white-and-blue utility boat pull to the dock. Minutes later, a group of men wearing khaki shorts and tee shirts departed. El Samoud's captain knew that a scientific group was coming to study the frankincense trees on the island of Socotra. A man strong from constant physical labor, Jacques' job was to be alert to all that went on at the dock. Brown eyes, set wide in his broad face, observed an ARC guard greet and accompany the scientists to waiting taxis. When quiet again enveloped the area, Jacques lost interest in the foreigners.

He walked over to the radios and resumed testing them. The last time they were in Yemen, he tried unsuccessfully to buy new radios and navigational aids. This morning he was reduced to nursing the old ones. Over the past few days, the lowliest of ARC's members had loaded supplies and El Samoud's personal property into the ship's hold. Jacques was forbidden to ask, but he assumed they would depart soon for another secret destination.

He heard a scraping sound, metal against metal. He looked up. El Samoud and Cobra were walking onto the bridge. He had not heard their footsteps. That could be dangerous. A guard's AK-47 hung from a strap over his shoulder and rubbed against the hatch cover.

El Samoud approached Jacques and asked in Arabic through his black *isharb*, "Is everything in order?"

Jacques dipped his head, looked around at the ship, his kingdom for the last nine months, then said, "She is safe, as always."

He paused. He decided to tell El Samoud about the radios. If they failed, it could only mean trouble for him.

The Frenchman said, "We need new equipment to ensure your safety."

With bony fingers, El Samoud examined the radios himself. He nodded to his captain. "Your radio still works. Plot a course for Aden.

We leave soon. When we return you can get your equipment. Don't buy it from the Americans or British, but from the French."

Jacques replied, "Of course. Since you bought the *Crescent* from the French, I have all my dealings with them. It will be good to return to my homeland, if even for a day."

His leader's black eyes darkened. El Samoud pointed a thin finger at Jacques. His voice rose as he said, "Spare no costs in the new radio. Our next attacks must succeed. Be sure everything on this ship is in perfect working order, or I will hold you responsible."

Jacques swallowed, then nodded. He had already refurbished the engine and installed a new galley to cook lamb and goat just how El Samoud liked it. What else could he do?

El Samoud seemed satisfied, and he turned to go below the deck. Jacques' eyes lingered on the retreating form of his Supreme Leader. The rifle-toting guard followed at a discreet distance. Jacques' mission was to obey, not ask questions. Yet he wondered what awaited them in Yemen.

A strong aroma of garlic offended his nose. Jacques moved his head and saw the Cobra had stepped close. He was so near, Jacques saw wavy red lines in the whites of his eyes.

The Cobra's voice was hard. "Need I remind you to uphold the utmost secrecy?"

Jacques' neck bent downward. "I am El Samoud's loyal servant."

El Samoud's deputy chief narrowed his bloodshot eyes, "As am I. One recently tested has not been heard of."

Jacques wondered if he meant Zayed. None of them dared speak of him, yet Jacques had reached his own conclusion—Cobra had Zayed killed. Cobra walked away, and Jacques was grateful his garlic breath went with him.

He was not, however, thankful for what Cobra said over his shoulder, "If you fail, you will meet a similar fate."

Jacques's hand involuntarily rose to his neck. However Zayed had angered the Cobra, Jacques would not be so careless. He'd stay out of his way and continue to please El Samoud as he had these last five years.

Jacques put the disagreeable Cobra out of his mind and spread his navigational charts to plot the trip from Socotra to Aden, from where he would call his sister in England. When he traveled for the radios, he would fly to Paris using a false passport. From there, he would take a taxi through the Chunnel and visit Camille in London for the first time in two years. But that part of his plan he would not tell to Cobra or El Samoud.

Sunday afternoon, the doorbell pealed loudly. Sari set down her potato peeler and wiped her hands. She had to finish dinner, eat, then get Emile to the airport by five. Her watch read 2:20 p.m. In fuzzy slippers, she plodded from the kitchen to the foyer. She peeked out the door, through beveled glass. Sari recognized her neighbor, Mr. Palmer, wearing a yellow rain slicker and hat. What brought him out in the rain? She opened the door.

He handed her a colored tin. "My wife baked two batches of cookies for the grandkids. With this weather, they decided not to come. She sent me over here. They're chocolate-chip."

Emile's favorite. She could pack some for his trip. Sari set the cookies on the foyer table and said, "Thank, you. Would you like to come in?"

"No. I would get your floor wet. Is your husband around?"

"He's resting before his flight tonight."

Mr. Palmer's glasses fogged up. "With this weather, better check with the airlines for cancellations. It's the best way." He removed his glasses and put them in his pocket. "Tell him Roberta and I saw something funny last Monday night."

"What?" Sari hoped George had not woken them up when he came home late.

Mr. Palmer wiped water from his face. "We went to a concert and got back late. We already put the garbage by the street for the morning pickup, but Roberta had an extra bag of trash. About eleven o'clock, I remember it was a little after eleven—the news was on—I took that bag to the curb. I returned to the house and shut off the outside light. That's when I saw a car at the end of your driveway."

"Yes?" Sari had to get her potatoes cooking. The lamb chops were almost done, and Emile liked his lamb moist. Every neighbor knew of Mr. Palmer's propensity to tell a long story.

Excitement rang in his voice, "A man wearing a baseball cap got out and walked to your garbage caddie. He tossed your garbage into his trunk and drove away!" Mr. Palmer looked triumphant.

Sari gazed at water running down Mr. Palmer's face. "Did he take your garbage, too?"

"No, Mrs. Jubayl, he did not." He shook his head fiercely.

A garbage thief in the neighborhood? Sari thought a moment, then said, "Maybe he's homeless, living in his car. Poor man. They say some live that way in the District."

Mr. Palmer took off his rain hat and shook it. "Roberta and I never thought of that. Here I was worried it was too dark to see the license plate. Maybe she'll put a tin of cookies on top of our garbage can tomorrow night and see what happens. Tell your husband to have a safe trip."

Sari stood in the open door as Mr. Palmer jogged home in the rain. What was a homeless man doing in their neighborhood?

Sari hurried to finish dinner. They would leave in less than an hour. She handed Emile the mint jelly. "Spoon extra on your chops. They are dry."

Emile pursed his lips. "I cannot chew these. They're as tough as fried clams."

"It is not my fault. Mr. Palmer brought cookies his wife made and stayed forever to talk. Emile," she paused, "he told me a homeless man stole our garbage last Monday night."

Emile's knife landed on his plate. "What did he look like? Was he on foot?"

Surprised by the velocity of his questions, Sari looked up. "Can you imagine being so hungry as to take garbage?"

Emile was unmoved. "Did he take anyone else's garbage on the cul-de-sac?"

"Just ours." She sniffled, wiped her eyes.

Emile had heard enough. "The government is going through our trash!"

She set down her fork. "I do not understand."

Emile pushed away his half-eaten plate. "I did not want to upset you. Last week, the telephone company sent a letter. They gave our phone records to the federal government under a subpoena. I called them, but learned nothing. I contacted a criminal lawyer, who said most likely it's because of George. Where is our son, by the way?"

Her hand trembling, Sari pushed hair behind her ears. "May I read it?"

Disgusted at himself for revealing the now destroyed letter, Emile tried to keep her from overreacting. "It's gone. I told you, I don't want you to worry."

"I could call George's lawyer tomorrow." Her food looked like a congealed mass. Sari picked up her plate to scrape it in the garbage. "That is, if George gives me his name."

Emile briefly touched her hand. "The attorney I spoke with, Harlan Scribbs, used to be the federal prosecutor. He said because George was at the State Department bombing, the Feds may be investigating him for being a suspected terrorist."

Sari started to cry. Her son was not a terrorist!

"Don't. The government will see we are law-abiding people and leave us alone. When does George's case come to trial?"

Sari blew her nose into her napkin. "That's why I want to call his attorney."

Emile pressed her hand. "Leave it. I'll call Scribbs from London, have him check."

Emile went upstairs to pack. Dazed, Sari cleared the dishes. She loved her country. The government had it wrong. The longer she thought about the man who stole their garbage, the more her confusion turned to anger.

Sari slammed the dishes into the dishwasher. She thought the man was poor and needy when all the time he was spying on them. She decided there was something she could do, and it did not involve cookies. Emile was coming down the stairs. Sari did not want him to know! From the refrigerator, she removed salmon fillets she had intended to fix for Emile two days before. She unwrapped them, went to the garage, and set her plan in motion.

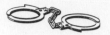

TWENTY TWO

Monday wore on with Sari preoccupied by the man rum-
maging through their garbage. Even though it was stuff she
had thrown out, it was still hers. By evening, her emotions
were like a stove turned on high. George came home and complained
the garage smelled. As he dug in the freezer for a frozen pizza, Sari
revealed nothing of her plan.

"Where's Dad this time?"

"London." Sari kept writing.

George set the oven temperature and poured himself a large glass
of milk.

"I cut up nectarines and plums, just how you like them," she said.

"He goes there a lot."

George found the fruit and put the pizza in the oven. Sari looked
up from her notepad. "Grammy's unwell. She may not live long."

A bowl of fruit in his hand, he said, "I wish he'd take me to see her
before she goes. Call me in twelve minutes. I'll be in my room."

The kitchen became quiet, like when she was home alone. She
was able to finish the letter that had bounced in her mind. It felt good
to write it down. Sari took the trash basket from beneath the kitchen
sink and carried it with the letter to the garage. The stench of unre-
frigerated fish overwhelmed her.

With her hand in a plastic bag, Sari picked up pieces of salmon fillets from yesterday, and sprinkled them in the trash bag on top of her
letter. She did not tie the kitchen bag, but rested it inside the garbage
caddie, on top of two other bags. The putrid smell made her gag. She
plugged her nose with one hand, flipped on the outside light with
the other.

Sari pressed the button to open the garage door. It did not take long to roll the caddie to the end of the driveway. The setting sun etched deep indigo streaks in the sky, but Sari's eyes searched for one thing—the Palmer's garbage can. Sure enough, a red tin sat on top. Sari shook her head. Roberta spent all that time baking cookies for a homeless man, who was actually a federal agent. Sari's anger blossomed like fungus after spring rain. Well, he could go through her stinking garbage for all she cared. She hoped he got sick from it.

Somewhere in her confused mind, a thought emerged: They were in this situation because of George. Sari quickly quashed feelings of resentment toward her son. He was going through a rough patch. His friends were weird, but he was no terrorist. If only he took an interest in Emile's work or in the youth group at church, he'd be all right.

She walked back toward the house and saw the Palmers on their front porch. Rather than admit the truth, she smiled and waved. If they wanted to believe they helped an unfortunate soul, who was she to interfere? Besides, after reading her letter, that agent would not come back again. Her words would convince him to leave George alone.

Sari turned off the outside light. Inside, the house smelled of burnt pizza. With a mitt, she pulled the shriveled mess out of the oven and threw it into the trash. George never came down. For the rest of the evening, Sari sat in the living room, shoulders slumped, where she watched the driveway. Finally, her eyelids were so heavy, they hurt.

She went upstairs to bed, but no sleep came. In the cool room, lying under a down comforter, Sari thanked God that Emile's blood tests were clear of cancer and prayed for George to find his life's purpose. A noise outside disturbed her prayer.

Sari scrambled from bed, drew aside the drape. A dark object moved by the garbage can. She strained to see who it was. The shape moved again. There, at the end of her driveway, a black dog sniffed the caddie. It was funny, but Sari did not laugh. She dropped the drape and returned to bed, with a vow to stay awake until eleven o'clock. In minutes, she was asleep.

Trenton eased his G-car past the Jubayl home. A few lights flickered in the neighborhood. No one was outside. He drove around the cul-de-sac and past several garbage caddies by the curb. A half block away he parked by a tree, its branches arched over the street light. Trenton closed his car door quietly. Before dogs barked or he was spotted by a nosy neighbor, he walked briskly to grab what he came for. Last week, he had seen a neighbor on the block. To be safe tonight, he arrived at 1:30 a.m.

The Jubayl's garbage container was perched by the end of their driveway. Trenton flipped open the top and snatched a small white plastic bag and two larger black bags. Stunned by the stink, he shut the lid. Trenton hustled to the intersection and around the corner, to where his car was parked.

At the last minute, he changed his mind and, turning left, carried the bags past several houses, and set them next to a different caddy. Once inside his car Trenton relaxed and drove to his loot. He pressed the trunk release, got out of the car, and pulled up the trunk lid. Jubayl's trash safely inside, he drove slowly out of the neighborhood.

At the office parking lot, he grabbed the three bags from the trunk and swiped his magnetic entry card at the back door. A foul smell hovered around him as he hauled the bags down the back corridor, past the entrance to his former FIG office, to his new office. Trenton plugged his nose.

No one else was in the TTF office at this early morning hour. Trenton got out a clean plastic bag, the largest he could find. To the clean bag he transferred empty yogurt containers, soiled Q-tips, and hair from hair brushes. With one bag done, he began to doubt that there was any benefit to trash pulls.

Trenton opened a white bag that wasn't fastened at the top. Thankful for latex gloves, he gingerly picked up spoiled fish fillets with one hand and plugged his nose with the other to stifle his gag reflex. Trenton moved the fish and saw a handwritten letter. It was stained, but legible.

He dropped the fish in the other bag and grabbed the letter. It might contain clues about Emile's activities, including his sudden vacation. The handwriting was small and fluid, as if written by a woman. His eyes quickly scanned the first two paragraphs.

Dear Brother in the Struggle:

Remember the time we spent together in our homeland? I want to visit again with you. I recall our discussions of struggling against the evil oppression we have known. For

so long, my struggle has been lonely, but I am now aligned
with a group of others who share the same commitment.

We meet twice a week and have agreed on a plan to ensure
ultimate victory. I met my co-laborers through another
man from my village of birth. He lives here and works at
a company that has contracts to support the U.S. military.
After he learned of my feelings of oppression, he took
me into his confidence and shared how he and some of
his associates have succeeded in frustrating our common
enemy.

Trenton couldn't believe his eyes. Emile's wife must be involved,
too. He could use this letter to get a search warrant for their home. As
he continued to read, Trenton grew confused.

He and the others explained no matter how much they
prayed to their god, they never felt free. As created beings,
we attempt to please God. Because we are sinful and he is
holy, we are separated. This was shown to me in the Bible.

Jehovah God reached down to us, through his son, Jesus
Christ and I accept God's gift. Some Americans, even
those raised in Christian families and churches, fail to
understand God's plan. The man who wears a baseball cap,
steals people's garbage, and reads their intimate mail, needs
to know this plan, too.

Trenton dropped the "gotcha" missive. Surrounded by bags of
garbage and stink, he reread the last sentence. The Jubayls must have
seen him grab the garbage last week! He read the letter a few more
times. With one swift movement, he tore off the bottom half and
tossed it into the discard garbage bag.

On impulse, Trenton took the top half and made a photo copy. He
initialed and dated the original, then put it in a sealed evidence envelope. In the rest of the garbage, he found a travel agency printout for a
flight to and from London that left on Sunday. That and the letter. His

search over, Trenton locked the evidence envelope in his desk, carried the trash outside, and placed it in the office dumpster.

Sari was alone in a field. Her fingers clutched the scrap of paper written in French. No, she would not deliver it. The militants would have to kill her. The helicopter drew near. Crouched between broken bricks and glass, Sari covered her head in the tall weeds. The whirling blades grew closer until the machine was directly overhead, about to come down on her. She could not run or scream. She was helpless, her heart about to burst.

Sari awoke, startled. The blankets were wrapped around her waist. Sweat glistened on her forehead. She had not dreamed of it for years, had even begun to believe that the horrors of the Lebanese Civil War were being gradually erased. She was wrong. The savage memories were as real today as they were the day she delivered the message. And the deaths she caused never left her.

Sari sipped water from a glass next to her bed. It tasted warm. She put on her bathrobe and turned on the light. The house was still. Her mind fast-forwarded to life in Virginia. Thoughts of the garbage man took over. She had to find out. Downstairs, she threw a wind breaker over her shoulders. The sun was not up yet, but burgeoning gray light helped her see to walk to the end of the drive. Had he come?

She opened the caddie. Empty blackness stared back. Her eyes flew to the Palmer's can. There on the top, she saw the same red tin of cookies. Sari's knees felt weak. The garbage raider had stolen their garbage and left the cookies behind.

Their regular garbage collector might find the cookies a nice treat. She let them be. Sari dragged her caddie back to the garage, confident the letter would stop whoever was harassing them. He should go after the ones who posed a real threat to the country.

A cup of tea would taste good. Sari plugged in the teapot and waited for the water to boil. Numbness settled over her as she leaned on the counter. Her eyes drifted to her Bible on the kitchen table, where she had left it two days before. Sari picked it up and opened it at the lace marker Thelma had given her.

The words in Proverbs shot straight through her. "Trust in the Lord with all your heart and lean not on your own understanding. In all ways, acknowledge Him and He will make your paths straight." Sari had not trusted: She'd gone her own way!

Early that evening, Eva scrunched a black velvet hat on her head. Scott and Andy were building a toy boat in the basement. She was about to take Kaley and the kitty to the vet. Or so she thought.

"Mommy," Kaley announced, out of breath, "Zak's under my bed."

She smoothed her daughter's hair, which crackled with static. "He is afraid because last time he got a shot. Mommy will coax him. Get your coat. We're late."

Eva climbed the stairs two at a time. Under Kaley's bed, Zak was huddled in the middle of the floor. When she reached toward the 6-month-old cat, her cell phone jangled on her belt. Zak swiped at the noise with front claws and found Eva's hand. Blood bubbled from a long scratch across the top of her hand.

She muttered, "What a mess." Then, "Hello."

"You have guests?" Griff asked.

"No. I am tracking a wild animal. What is it?"

"Don't let me interfere with your safari. Kat called for you and got me instead."

"You're a riot. The cat didn't call, he's hiding. And I don't have time to talk about it."

Griff said, "I'm talking about a female Kat. Remember, the nosy lady with the camera we met at Farouk's condo, the one who keeps calling you?"

Kaley skipped into the hall. "Mommy, I have on my coat. Where is Zak?"

"Griff, I am being paged. What's up?"

"Kat says to tell you she is working on a TV special about money laundering in Northern Virginia. She wants to know if our guy is a criminal or a terrorist."

The kitty wailed from under the bed. Eva moved to the hall bathroom and found a tissue to press on her wound.

"Ouch. Anything else?" Eva asked.

"She could compromise our case."

"I'll call her tomorrow and ask her to hold off. Think she'll buy it?"

Griff cleared his throat. "Maybe. She's an aggressive type. You should know, about an hour ago, I received a secure e-mail from our English friend. He wants us there ASAP."

"I'll make it work. Somehow."

Eva hung up and went to look for a broom. She could go to London if Scott went to work late and came home early by using vacation time. Camille might be the missing piece to the ARC puzzle. And Eva was not about to let Mary Katherine Kowicki, Channel 14's "Kat," intrude into her case.

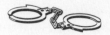

TWENTY THREE

The next morning, as Eva entered the rear door to her building, her mind lingered on the agency head meeting she just left. Ari Rosen had bragged that his group was on the cusp of getting a major terrorist. The door open, Eva recoiled. What was that awful smell? It reminded her of an alley behind a fish market. She plugged her nose. Robbie rushed down the stairs.

Eva released her nose long enough to ask, "Whew, what happened?"

"Some TTF Agent did a trash pull. Their secretary told me even the copier reeks. She calls it the 'stinker case.' We're looking for excuses to work outside the office."

Robbie ran out the door into the cool fresh air. Eva hurried past Wanda typing at her desk. Maybe she could take work home. In her office, she glanced down at Robbie's report of what he found in Farouk's computer. Perhaps, if she concentrated on work, she'd be like Wanda—oblivious to the stench.

Midday, Eva's phone rang. It was Griff.

Eva said, "I called your Kat and told her Farouk's a small fish."

"She's not *my* Kat."

"I promised her a heads up in the future if she'd hold off."

Griff asked, "You trust the media?"

Eva sighed. "For now, we have no choice."

"I just talked to the Director for Homeland Security Internal Affairs. Because Drury Baptiste's application for a passport in the name of Richard Salem was false, he's no longer in the motor pool. He's been fired."

"Did they agree to hold off arresting him?" Eva asked.

"Yup. The Director knows once Baptiste is charged with the falsified passport application and with assaulting you, Farouk will be a witness, and we'll have to turn over his statements."

"When does Brewster want us there?"

Griff replied, "Next Monday. He arranged for us to meet two friends and thinks you may succeed with the uncooperative female."

Unsure why Brewster thought Camille would talk with her, Eva turned a page on her calendar. She had not talked to Scott about next week. She had to testify before the Grand Jury, but she could send Robbie. And her mom could take Kaley to the dentist.

Eva said, "Have Brewster send a written request from MI-5. That should convince Headquarters that the British government needs both of us."

"He's sending a full dossier via the encryption system. It should be available in today's distribution."

Eva penciled London on her calendar. "I feel like a right fielder with no glove. You and I need to plan strategy. I'll get Wanda working on our flights."

"I can't find my official passport. Maybe you'll have to fly to London without me."

Eva hesitated. Was Griff joking? She did not bite. "The State Department can always rush a new one." Hers was in their safe deposit box. She'd better pick it up on the way home.

When Eva hung up the phone, the stink no longer penetrated her conscience. She pictured Camille in a damp British cell where Eva gained her confidence and learned everything about ARC's Paris connections.

Eva tapped a DVD against her fingers and said in a Scottish accent, "Come on laddie." Scott did not look up. She walked over to where he sat behind his desk.

"The online review says it's a great romantic comedy."

Scott looked over his gunmetal glasses, perched at the end of his nose. "I have a press release to finish. Secretary Cabrini leaves Thursday for the Central Asian Conference."

Eva fingered the hair on his forehead. "There is never enough time to be together." She cleared her throat. "I was waiting until after the movie to tell you this. One of my cases involves securing our country against terrorists."

Scott removed off his glasses. "Eva, out with it. I have lots to do."

Surprised by Scott's biting tone, which he rarely used, she snapped, "If you're going to be that way, maybe I'll wait."

He grabbed her hand, but his voice had an edge. "Sorry. With the appropriation bill logjammed in Congress, the pressure is on. We're managing under a supplemental budget bill. I have time for my best friend. What's eating you?"

Eva always dove head first into cold water—to get the shock out of the way. With the same tenacity, she said, "I leave Monday with Griff for London. We meet two MI-5 contacts. So much is a stake, Scott, I must see to it personally."

Her husband's eyes were mirrors to his emotions. Tonight they flickered with unhappiness. He released her hand. "When did you find out? When will you be back?"

Eva ignored the first question, and replied, "I'll be gone four days."

Her husband stared at his glasses between his fingers. She broke the silence. "I'm prohibited from saying more, but this may be the biggest case of my career."

Scott replied, "Remember our anniversary dinner a few weeks ago? You promised to spend more time with us. I see where I count in the equation."

It was rare for Scott to speak so harshly. Unsure how to respond, her mind framed two options. She could hold him and say she was sorry, or defend herself. She chose the latter.

"Why are you so ornery tonight? You knew I was a perfectionist when you married me."

Scott returned his glasses to his face. "My job is demanding, too. I seem to always draw the short straw. The Secretary asked me to go along on a strategic trip to confer with our allies on the war against terror."

Eva sat on the extra chair. "You never mentioned this trip."

"I found out yesterday. Last night, you were busy with the vet. This morning, I left before you. Tonight, I didn't bring it up in front of the kids in case we had issues. Besides," Scott laughed with true feeling, "I was going to tell *you* after the movie."

Eva sat on his lap, leaned her head on his shoulder. "I guess we're fortunate a scheduling fiasco has not happened before now."

Scott wound his arms around her. "You leave Monday, and I'm not due back till Wednesday." He looked over the top of her head to his desk clock. Scott had to finish his press release, then transmit a copy to the SecDef by nine.

Eva thought a moment. "Maybe Grandpa could come until you get back on Wednesday. I'll call him now. Then can we watch the movie?" She kissed him lightly on the lips. "I saw our baby specialist and have another appointment when I get back." Her white teeth shone when she smiled.

That should have made him happy. Eva was surprised by his flat tone when he said, "Glad to hear it. In the future, I promise not to set you up to be in a good mood for bad news."

Did he think she brought up a baby to put him in a good mood? She'd never do that. But to defend herself now would fuel an argument. Eva nodded and walked down the hall. In the kitchen, she poured popcorn kernels into a microwave bowl. Scott was right; they had both tried to manipulate the other. Their motives were valid, but their tactics backfired.

Maybe she should prepare Scott. If her London trip was a success, she might have to fly back there, or even farther away. She should also ask the doctor if such constant travel could affect a future pregnancy. Eva punched in Marty's number and saw a gray blur out of the corner of her eye. She turned her head. Zak clawed his way up the dining room drapes. After she reached her grandpa, maybe she'd call her mother. The kitty needed a new home.

On the following Monday, December 5, Trenton held the white board so Ari could see from behind his desk. With his other hand, Trenton drew blue lines from the Jubayls' names to various acts of terrorism.

"George is involved with more than a protest at the State Department, but I can't prove it. His case goes to trial in two months. By then, we should have nabbed both his parents."

Trenton drew a heavy line under the words, *Letter supporting militants.* Ari held up the transparent evidence envelope to the fluorescent ceiling light.

He said, "It looks torn. The edge is jagged on the bottom."

Trenton did not flinch but gave his rehearsed reply, "I saw that, too." Technically, that was true and not a lie. He redirected his boss's attention. "It sounds like George wrote it, but it looks like a woman's handwriting."

Ari plunged his hand into his thick hair. "George must have signed papers when he got out on bond. Get a copy from Pretrial Services and compare the handwriting." Ari checked his watch. "Game time in thirty minutes. Can we count on you to play?"

Trenton shook his head. "I'm a great catcher. Not much for volleyball. Next spring, count me in on a softball matchup."

"We could use you."

Trenton pointed to the $250,000 deposit under Emile's name.
"Emile hasn't made large withdrawals, except a five-thousand-dollar
check to GMU, which I presume is for George's tuition. I am waiting for a call back from the registrar. He wrote nine checks for $1000,
each to a different charity. A local church, drug rehab, homeless shelter,
that kind of thing."

Ari swiveled his chair. "Really? Give me a list. There may be more
to it. Small amounts capture little attention. Yet, it is near the end of
the year. Maybe he is piling up tax deductions."

Trenton's arm ached, and he set down the board. "I will have the
list to you tomorrow."

Ari rose. "You're an asset to our team. We almost have enough evidence for a search warrant for Jubayl's home. That letter you found in
the trash is key," Ari waved his hand across his face, "even if it did smell
up the office. We need a bit more to make our affidavit airtight."

As Ari slipped into his jacket and ball cap, he reminded Trenton
about the volleyball game and left the office. With his new boss close
to approving the search warrant, Trenton took the hint. He went to
the gym and watched a little volleyball to be friendly.

But, an hour later, relaxation was as far from his mind as playing
volleyball. Unable to focus on TTF's game against the U.S. Marshals,
Trenton scooped up his thermal mug of Brazilian coffee. He eased
down the bleacher seats and left the school building. In high school
and college, he excelled at wrestling. Now, Trenton had no time for
sports. On the way back to the office, his headlights shone on tiny
snowflakes that fell like confetti.

With Ari's challenge of needing more for a search warrant, Trenton knew the time was ripe to contact his "go-to" snitch. Already in
his brief career, he had learned the value of what Duke referred to as
hip pocket informants. Federal agents and police officers used confidential informants, better known as "snitches." These men and wom-
en were of proven reliability, fingerprinted, and photographed. They
were paid cash rewards for credible information, or received reduced
sentences. The key was, they could be interrogated by supervisors, or
even judges, to prove their reliability.

Then, there was the hip pocket informant. While his or her information was equally reliable, the agent or officer agreed to never

reveal their identity, even if it meant dismissing charges against a defendant, or going to jail for refusing to identify the source. Sometimes
the hip pocket informant was a family member. Or a gang member,
prostitute, jilted lover, or an important public official. Or sometimes, a
travel agent. Tonight, Trenton would use his hip pocket informant. He
swiped his card, opened the building door and ran up the steps two
at a time, carrying a bag of burgers and a filled coffee mug. He would
get probable cause, if it took him all night. But first he had to find the
phone number for the local Fox news channel.

At nine that night, alone in his office at Helpers International, Emile
drew the blinds. He turned on his computer, but grief made him
briefly put his face in his hands. The call from his mother's doctor in
London rocked him worse than his own cancer. He should call his
cousin, Duma, who was like the brother he lost. But, it was too hard
to speak of it. Emile lifted his head. He was connected online.

Thankful that he had visited his mother the week before and that
she had recognized him, Emile regretted he let her talk about changing her will. As Emile fed her chicken broth, she looked so small, so
frail. Now, his mother was dead. Emile forced his hands to the keyboard. He had to write and go home.

> Dear Duma,
>
> Sadness fills my heart. My mother, your Aunt Aida, is
> gone. When I saw her last week, she whispered she was
> going to see Jesus. She was so sure he was real. A solicitor
> is handling her estate, but I am the joint owner on all
> her accounts. Before she died, she requested you receive
> $50,000. She wanted you to have pictures of the family
> and Grandfather's watch as well. I need to call my travel
> agent but plan to fly to Lebanon tomorrow, where her
> body is being shipped.
>
> Emile

These days, sleep did not come easy. Tonight was no different. Emile
turned on his side, and checked the clock radio on the nightstand. Sari
was asleep, and he did not want to wake her. It was eleven-thirty in

Virginia. In Lebanon, Duma would be up, preparing to go to the bank. Emile put on a silk robe and walked quietly to his den.

His desk was exactly as he always left it. No papers were in sight. From the side drawer, which Emile unlocked, he drew out his ticket itinerary and dialed his cousin's number in Beirut.

Duma's voice said in French, "I am not here to speak to you. Leave a message."

Emile's mind calculated what he should say on the machine. "Duma, I forgot to mention some things in my e-mail. My ticket is confirmed. I leave this morning, eleven my time. With a layover in London, I arrive in Beirut the next day. It is the only flight on which I could get two seats. You will finally meet George; he's coming along. I am bringing part of the valuables I wrote about."

He paused to find the precise words, then added, "Be ready to take me to Bint Jubayl and, by the time I leave Lebanon, you will have the funds I wrote you about."

Emile hung up the phone. The last time he was in Beirut, Duma wanted to show him several new projects, but he had declined. After decades of war, the city was rebuilding itself. This time, Emile would send George home after the funeral and delay going to Egypt and Jordan to check on Helpers' programs. Then, he and Duma could visit the village where they were born, north of the Israeli border. He had not been to Claude's grave in years. It would be good to tell his brother all that he was doing in his name.

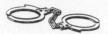

TWENTY FOUR

I t was Tuesday morning in London. Eva sat in Brewster's cluttered office, which was as drab as her own. She and Griff had flown all night and arrived at Heathrow by ten. Brewster picked them up and brought them straight to MI-5. She was bone tired, having slept a mere forty minutes on the flight. And, she was hungry. They were briefing Brewster on their last meeting with Farouk.

Brewster waved an empty pipe in the air and explained, "I promised my wife I would not smoke again."

Eva pulled her mind from her growling stomach and asked, "When do we meet Zayed and Camille?"

The MI-5 agent cradled his pipe. "I will get to that. Yesterday, Zayed confided two critical pieces of information."

To stay awake, Eva popped out of her chair. Brewster shot her a surprised look and she apologized. "I concentrate better standing."

With a slight nod, Brewster continued, "When El Samoud's head scarf slipped, Zayed glimpsed the right side of his face. He drew a picture of a nose, like this." He showed them a rough pencil drawing that looked vaguely like one of Eva's stick figures. "Zayed memorized the words that will trigger ARC's next attack."

Brewster read from a sheet of paper. "At ARC's last meeting, El Samoud told six cell leaders to act when they heard the words 'Destroy the Satans of the world' being broadcast."

Eva paced over to a window shrouded in blinds. "Did Zayed say when and where this attack will take place?"

The Brit tapped the unfilled pipe bowl into his palm. "No. We'll keep plying him with hot showers and his favorite foods to see if his memory improves. You will both meet him tomorrow."

Griff picked up where Brewster left off. "Farouk said Zayed fits into American life with ease. So you may be on the right track there. Apparently, he's not the type to enjoy cave dwelling."

Eva said, "Remember Farouk's list of account numbers? We're still tracking them, but I think we are closer to finding their location."

Brewster set down his pipe. "We found an account for Farouk Hamdi at Reni Jubayl's bank."

Eva came back and sat across from Griff. "He may avoid jail, but his profits are another thing. How much money is in it?"

"A quarter of a million U.S. dollars."

Griff let out a low whistle. "We should seize it before he can move it."

Brewster assured them MI-5 had taken steps so Farouk couldn't withdraw the money.

For most of the flight, Eva had thought about her upcoming interview with Camille, which was one reason she hadn't slept. She asked Brewster, "What did Camille say after you told her we know about her brother Jacques?"

"We saved that for you to bring up when you meet her."

Griff added, "Camille told Farouk that even though her brother travels with El Samoud, she has regular contact with him. I'm sure Eva will find out when she last heard from him."

Eva tried to stifle a yawn, without success. If she could grab a few hours of sleep, she'd think more clearly. Even a long, hot shower would help.

Brewster suddenly scowled. "When we searched Camille's flat several weeks ago, we found a digital answering device, which we downloaded. Our men left it in the flat. We should check it again to see if any new messages have come in." He picked up his pipe. "I'll work on getting permission to reenter her flat."

A memory crept into Eva's tired mind. "What about Jacques's cell phone that we gave you? If Jacques is still using it, we could try to convince Camille to phone him for us."

Griff said, "Don't get your hopes up."

Brewster picked up the telephone but waited to punch in the numbers until after his guests left. "You're staying at a safe house nearby. Get a few hours rest. The icebox is stocked with coddled cream, jam, and scones. My assistant will drive you over. We'll reconnect, say," he checked his watch, which read just past noon, "in four hours."

Eva held out her hand. "When do I meet Camille?"

Brewster said, "We'll know that after I check her phone messages at the flat."

"Empty your pockets. You must have metal in them," the TSA screener told George.

In line behind his son, Emile was having second thoughts about bringing George along. His son's long hair and diamond earring captured too much attention.

"I emptied my pockets. It must be my tongue stud." George stuck out his tongue so the officer could see the silver metal ball.

The officer waved an electronic wand over George's face. It beeped. He signaled George through the magnetometer. From the conveyor belt, George retrieved his shoes and carry-on bag. Emile placed his gold watch, change, handheld computer, and shoes into a plastic basket. The magnetometer still beeped when he passed through. The screener ran the wand around Emile's frame. Pronounced "clean," he walked through the security gate. Emile put on his shoes and grabbed his bag. George was distracted by two teens chanting a hip hop song.

Emile steered him by the arm toward their gate. "Our plane leaves in thirty minutes. We still have to take the people mover to the plane."

George grinned at his father, lights reflecting off his tongue as he talked. "Did Mom tell you I had it pierced while you were in London?"

Emile ignored the question, slung his trench coat over his rolling bag, and walked quickly, unconcerned that George had a hard time keeping up with him.

Thirty minutes later, sitting in the middle seats in the middle row of a 747 flying to London, George complained, "It's hot in here."

Emile reached up to open the air nozzle above them. "That should help. Take off that hideous sweat shirt. Don't you have any nice looking sweaters?"

George rarely followed his fathers' requests. On this day, he stayed true to form. He put a heavy metal CD in his portable player and snapped on a set of head phones. Glad for the silence, Emile ignored George's snub. He should have insisted George stay home. Emile heard flight attendants secure the doors and begin their pre-flight preparations. He paid no attention to how to wear a seat belt or what to do if oxygen was needed. The familiar sound of the people mover backing away from the aircraft gave him relief. Takeoff was imminent.

Five minutes passed. Still, they sat in place. Emile checked his PDA, then looked around. The plane was behind schedule. Five minutes became eight minutes, then ten. A sprig of irritation grew within the punctual CEO. Then he felt a nudge from a people mover again and heard the doors being unlatched. The pilot must be letting on a late passenger.

In exasperation, Emile looked up the aisle. Two male flight attendants, with sour expressions, walked briskly from the front of the plane. Several male passengers followed the attendants down the aisle. While other passengers fidgeted in their seats, Emile put away his PDA, sure they'd depart any minute.

A thin flight attendant with red sideburns leaned into their row and asked frostily, "Are you Emile and George Jubayl?"

Emile nodded. George sat with his head scrunched on his shoulder, listening to the wild beat of drums.

"Please come with me," he ordered.

"Are we in the wrong seats?"

"Sir, come with me."

Emile grabbed George's headphone and hissed in his ear, "What troubles have you gotten us into now? We're going to miss our London connection to Beirut."

"Now, please." The attendant stepped back to allow Emile and George to exit their seats.

"These are our seats, I can find our tickets, " Emile replied. He usually flew first-class, but because George was with him, he purchased coach tickets. What a mistake.

"We can talk up front." The attendant pressed Emile's shoulder, giving him no choice but to comply.

Emile stepped over two passengers while holding onto the seat backs in front of him. As he stepped into the aisle, he was tightly enveloped by men in suits, like husks around an ear of corn. Emile tried to figure out what was going on. Did they find something weird in George's luggage? Had they searched his own bags and found the jewelry for Duma? One of the people he had assumed were passengers removed the Jubayls' carry-on luggage from the overhead bins.

Emile pushed toward them. "Hey, those are our bags. Put yours somewhere else." He soon learned they were not passengers.

A man with thick black hair reached into his suit coat and pulled out a leather credential case, which he flipped open and shut. "Federal agents. You better cooperate." He did not mention what would happen if they did not.

At the words "federal agents," George protested in a loud voice, "Leave me alone. I've done nothing wrong."

At the disturbance, some passengers half-stood and looked around. The attendant tried to calm them. "The flight leaves soon. Please take your seats."

Ari Rosen grabbed George's shoulder, squeezed the soft area near his neck. "Move along, and no one will get hurt. We'll explain after we exit the plane." Ari swiped George's backpack off his shoulder. "This looks heavy. I'll carry it for you."

Another agent took the PDA that had frozen in Emile's grip. He gave it up without a struggle. Sweat pooled on his forehead. As they boarded the people mover, agents swarmed around them. The giant mover lowered itself from the plane's door and maneuvered back to the terminal, where Emile and George were hustled to government cars.

On the way from Dulles Airport, Emile said nothing, but his brain was on overdrive. He wished George would quit making unhelpful comments so he could think of a way out of this mess. Was Harlan Scribbs' number in his computer? He would call him as soon as he arrived at wherever these agents were taking him.

Never in ten million years could Sari have foreseen the events of this day. Emile and George had left for the airport. She cleared dishes from the kitchen table, thankful for the quiet. Because George slept late, neither he nor his father ate their eggs and toast. Being around Emile and George together was barely tolerable. Each had little understanding of the other, and no patience for the other's strengths, which they each saw as weakness.

The dishwasher set on the scrub cycle, Sari hastened up the stairs for the laundry. On the way, she passed her Bible on the small table, waiting for her to come and open her heart. This morning there had been no time for her to sit in her favorite chair with her Bible on her lap to see what God showed her for that day. Sari tucked the plastic laundry basket under her arm and headed downstairs. An inner voice prompted her to stop and connect with God right then, but her mind told her she'd have more time in a few minutes.

In the first floor laundry room, she dropped a load of towels into the machine. As it filled with soap and water, she shoved them to the bottom, her arms wet to the elbows. With the wash machine and dishwasher running, she did not hear the loud knocks at her front door.

In the kitchen, she was pouring coffee into her mug, when a terrible sound of crashing wood and glass reached her ears. Fear buzzed through her like electricity. The cup slipped from her fingers and dropped to the floor, where it shattered into small, sharp pieces. Someone was breaking into her house! Sari grabbed the cordless phone to call 911, but her fingers refused to find the numbers. At the sound of more breaking glass, her fear found a voice. She screamed.

Several men, wearing black pants and jackets, rushed into the kitchen. They yelled, "Federal agents! We have a search warrant."

Her panic was so great, she stood rooted to the kitchen floor, like a hiker facing a grizzly bear in the wild. Shards of broken glass lay at her feet.

"Down on the floor," one of them commanded.

If she moved, she would be cut. "I can't!"

Several agents lifted guns to her face. "Now!"

Sari's courage left her. Her mind a blank, she collapsed, unaware her hand slipped onto a sharp piece of glass, slicing her finger.

Ten minutes later, Sari struggled to tuck her bare feet under her legs without falling off the sofa. An agent had pressed a paper towel against her wound. Now, her arms were held behind her back by metal handcuffs that bound her wrists. Clad only in cotton work pants and top, Sari was cold. Her leather slippers had fallen off somewhere between the living room and the kitchen, where they cuffed her. If only she could turn up the heat. She always kept it low while cleaning.

Since George's arrest, their phone records were taken and a federal agent snooped through their garbage. Now, those same agents were violating their home. They emptied drawers and tossed cushions on the floor. Sari shut her eyes to the thumping upstairs. She had nothing to hide, but the thought of strangers rifling through her underwear drawer brought feelings of desperation. Her heart wrenched with pain. God's words in the Bible, "I will never leave or forsake you," drifted in and out of her tortured mind. If only she could cover her face with her hands and sob.

Was her palm leaking blood onto the sofa? Her hands were numb, so she could not tell. Her eyes stayed closed to the intruders who marched like warrior ants through her house. Sari pressed her face against the back of the sofa, not caring if her tears stained the red-flowered fabric. She wished she'd never come to America. The sound of a woman's voice pierced her sorrow.

"Mrs. Jubayl, I am Special Agent Hollings. I need to explain some things to you."

Sari nodded her head but neither lifted it nor looked at the agent.

"A U.S. District Judge authorized the FBI Terrorism Task Force to search your home. He decided we had sufficient evidence linking you, your son, and your husband to aiding prohibited terrorist groups."

Sari moaned. "It's not true! I love America!"

Agent Hollings tapped her arm. "You are not free to leave. Before we question you, I must read your rights: You have a right to remain silent. Anything you tell me can be used against you in a court of law. You have a right to have an attorney present when talking to me. Understand?"

Sari moved her head to look at the agent. Tears flowed down her face. *They think we are criminals, just like on television.*

"Mrs. Jubayl, do you understand what I said?"

Sari whispered, "Yes."

"We can take records, hard drives, software, cash, and evidence of aiding terrorists. I do not like to see you handcuffed, but it is for your safety as well as ours. In the search area, things can be dangerous," she said gently.

Sari licked salt from around her lips. With concerned brown eyes, the agent looked like Thelma's daughter. This gave Sari courage to ask, "Are you arresting me?"

"Let me get you a tissue. I'll be right back."

Hollings returned in a moment and asked, "May I?"

Sari allowed the agent to wipe off her face.

"The special agent in charge of this raid is upstairs, and he decides if anyone is arrested."

Sari was confused. "You are a special agent and the man upstairs is a special agent, but you said others were just agents. Why were special agents sent here? Am I a greater threat?"

"Officially, we are all special agents, but we shorten our titles to agents. Like shortening a Chevrolet to a Chevy. Let me get you some water."

As Sari's eyes followed her to the kitchen, she felt hope return. Special Agent Hollings was nice. Maybe she could convince her to take off the handcuffs.

As Hollings walked in, Trenton pulled a note pad from a kitchen drawer. He examined it, then placed the ivory tablet into an evidence envelope.

"Seizing empty note pads now, are we?" Hollings ran water in a glass.

Trenton scowled at the uninformed question. "It's the same paper the stinking terrorist note was written on." He nodded toward the living room and asked, "Is she saying anything?"

Hollings turned off the water. "She probably won't. I gave her a Miranda warning."

Trenton bristled. This agent graduated from basic training a month ago. What did she know? "That wasn't necessary. She's not under arrest."

Hollings shook her head. "I guess you're still learning the federal ropes. She's not free to leave, so the warnings are necessary."

Thud-thud-thud. Sounds of helicopter blades shook the house. Hollings stepped to the window and peered out. "A TV remote truck is across the street. How did they find out?"

Delighted, Trenton walked to the rear yard and watched a TV copter circle above the house. He retreated under the roof overhang where he dialed his cell phone.

"Dad, are you there? Pick up! When you get home, turn on Fox. I'm executing a search warrant on my big case."

At Helper's International, Hannah knew nothing about the search warrant being executed at Emile's home. She was typing donor addresses into the computer at a temporary station outside Emile's office when loud voices startled her. She got up and looked down the hall. Men and women wearing jackets with a TTF logo on the front and back swarmed past the receptionist and entered the executive office suite.

A tall agent with Hispanic features announced, "We are federal agents with a search warrant. Please stop what you are doing."

Hannah's hands froze over her keyboard. Her first instinct was to call Trenton on his cell phone. She reached for the phone. The tall agent stopped her. "No calls until I say so. Step away from the computer."

Trenton had been telling her that Helpers International supported terrorists, but she had not believed him! Hannah complied with the agent's order and went to find her mother. More agents streamed past carrying folded cardboard boxes. Hannah stopped outside Emile's office and peered around the door jamb. A female agent was unplugging his computer and putting it in a box. Another emptied the contents of his desk drawers into a black trash bag.

Her body felt like jelly. She walked the halls but couldn't find her mother anywhere. Was she at lunch? Hannah and her mother lived and worked together, but Hannah's life was so busy that she never realized until that moment how much she relied on her Mom. On the way to the lunchroom, Hannah passed the accounting office, where several agents talked with the chief financial officer. While pretending to check her shoe lace, she really listened.

The CFO said, "We are a legitimate humanitarian organization. Here are backup tapes and copies of our calendar year disbursements."

The receptionist, Debbie, walked up to Hannah, looking frightened. "My mom called and said Helpers is on TV. The reporter claims we're being raided for helping terrorists!" The young woman, also an intern, choked back a sob. "Hannah, is it true? Are we going to lose our jobs?"

At least Hannah had been warned that federal agents would be snooping around. It would have been a crime for her to mention it, even to her mother. Now, the whole world knew. Still, Hannah was sorry for the shock her friend was feeling.

She held Debbie's hand, "No matter what happens, God will look out for us. Of that, I am sure."

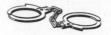

TWENTY FIVE

The doorbell rang. With the front door hanging on one hinge attached to the frame, it took all of Sari's strength to lift it up from the bottom and open it. Wordlessly, she fell into Thelma's ample arms.

"Honey, you didn't tell me they busted in your door!"

With her good hand, Sari pulled her friend into the vestibule.

"Those nosy reporters are circlin' on the sidewalk like hungry vultures. They tried to block my car and asked silly questions like 'Are the Jubayls terrorists?'"

Sari shuddered, and a sob caught in her throat. Would the reporters be bold enough to come into her house with the door broken? Her phone hadn't stopped ringing since the feds left.

Thelma squeezed her hand. "Let them hover."

Thelma ambled into the living room, took off her coat, and threw it over a chair. She eyed the magazines and newspapers strewn about the room.

Sari held up her bandaged hand, "An agent, a young woman named Hollings who looked like your daughter, put this on, but blood dripped there." She pointed to a pink stain by the couch. "She said she didn't think I needed stitches. Every room is like this, destroyed. I swept up broken glass in the kitchen."

Her knees weak under her, Sari sank into a wing-back chair. She was frightened. Those guns in her face had refreshed memories of exploding gunfire in Beirut during the civil war. Those images of terror and bloodshed, which now only visited Sari in her dreams, rushed back like a swollen river and tore her mind from its moorings. Despite her thick sweatsuit, which she had changed into after the agents left, Sari shivered.

Thelma lifted up a canvas bag. "Honey, I thought you might be hungry. I brought you some sandwiches and fruit."

Sari shook her head, her hands to her temples. She whispered, "Before my parents got us out, I thought I would be killed. I almost—" Her hands slumped to her sides.

Thelma lightly touched her shoulder. "Don't let this take you back there. You're over it. Come with me to the kitchen."

Thelma was right. If she was frozen by past fears, those wrongly accusing them would win. Sari got a jacket from the closet and put it on. Thelma closed the door as best she could. The reporters by the curb shouted when they saw her.

"That door needs fixin', with due speed," she said. "You make tea. I'll call Ben Atlee and see if he can fix this door so it will lock, or you'll stay at my house tonight."

The two women threaded their way to the spacious kitchen, where Sari often cooked casseroles for those in need. Today, she was glad her friend was there. Otherwise, she'd be lying on her bed, crying her eyes out.

Sari turned on the electric kettle. "Mrs. Palmer offered to let me stay with them, too."

"Good neighbors are like a pocketful of gold, I always say." Thelma thumbed through the directory for Ben's number. Finding it, she asked, "Sari, did the police say what they were lookin' for? Is it because your son was in that protest when the bomb went off?"

Sari dissolved into fresh tears.

Thelma walked her over to a cushioned stool and made her sit. "I'll make tea and call Ben. I brought the church directory to call Eva Montanna. She'll know what to do."

An hour later, the ladies had finished their tea, cried together and were upstairs, putting the Jubayl house back together, when they were interrupted by the doorbell.

Thelma inserted a drawer into the nightstand. "If it's a reporter, I'll send 'em away."

Sari rolled up the sheets from her bed. Agents had torn them off, along with the mattress cover, and tipped the mattress upside down. All the stripped bedding needed washing. Even her clean sheets had been tossed from the linen closet. It was going to be a late night.

Sari met Thelma at the top of the stairs and Thelma told her, "Ben will secure the door tonight. Tomorrow, he'll put in a new door jam. Meantime, use the garage door. Do you want to see him?"

Sari shrank back into the bedroom and held out the linens. "I don't think I'll go down. Could you wash these? They've been trampled on."

Thelma took the bundle from Sari and went back downstairs.

A photo of her family, in a silver frame, lay on the floor. Sari picked it up and examined it. Their eyes had vacant stares. They all looked sad. Sari put the photo on her dresser. It was good Emile was not home. Once the door was fixed and the house back in order, it would be easier for him to handle it all.

"Sari! What on earth is going on here?"

That sounded like a man, not Thelma. As if waking from a deep dream, Sari turned to look at the figure in the doorway and thought it was her husband. He was supposed to be in Lebanon. Was he for real?

"Emile?"

"Of course it's me," he snapped. "What are you doing? A man pounding nails in the door frame told me nothing. The house looks like a tornado hit it. Did someone break in?"

Speechless, Sari wanted to ask what he was doing home. In her state of mind, she was no match for his questions. She heard Thelma singing, coming up the stairs.

"Mr. Jubayl, did they cancel your flight to Lebanon?" Thelma asked.

"My flight wasn't canceled! Federal agents pulled us off the plane. They questioned me and George for hours. When he was arrested, George signed papers for his bond that made it clear he was not to leave the country. But, he says he didn't read them. George never showed them to me. Did he show them to you?"

His wife shook her head. Could their lives get more complicated? Why did George ever go to that silly protest?

"They claim that because the airplane door was closed, it proves he was fleeing the country."

Thelma asked, "Emile, did you tell them your Mama died and you were going to her funeral?"

"I spent five hours telling them. They finally released me. George is being held. His bond is revoked. Tell me what happened here!"

Sari's heart pounded as she blurted, "Agents searched the house. It was terrible." Sobs overpowered her.

Thelma intervened. "I got here 'bout two hours ago. I called Mr. Atlee from church to give the door a bandaid until tomorrow.

Sari's hand is cut. She may need a doctor." Thelma placed both hands on her wide hips. "They showed Sari a search warrant. There may be a copy around here someplace. If you don't mind my sayin' so, if I were you, I'd get a lawyer right away."

"What has George gotten us into?" Sari sagged onto the bed.

Thelma walked to the bathroom, brought Sari a box of tissues, and said, "I'll leave you two alone. The livin' room needs help. Have you talked to anyone at Helpers? I just turned on the TV and the news showed the feds cartin' out computers and boxes."

Emile turned on his heel and said, "I'm calling my lawyer."

The visitor's room had no windows, was sparsely furnished and cold. Eva was glad she wore a wool jacket over a black turtleneck sweater. She could not see the falling rain, but her aching bones felt the constant dampness. In this strange environment, as she waited for Camille, her mind jumped to another thought. Was thirty-eight too old to have another baby?

Her doctor said it wasn't. Eva forced her mind to obey. It felt funny even to think of personal matters at a time like this. She intended for Camille to meet a committed agent doing her job. Brewster's foray to Camille's apartment gleaned further links in the case, and a new plan. Eva thought it was a good one, if Camille cooperated.

The metal door scraped open. Brewster's coworker shoved a small woman through the door. She had black hair that had seen neither shampoo nor brush in days. She practically fell into a metal chair near the cement block wall.

"I'll be outside the door." He glowered at Camille and warned, "This is your last chance to get out of here." Then he was gone.

Eva pulled up the other chair to face Camille. She introduced herself without holding out her hand.

As she had practiced, Eva said gently, "My government has a vital interest in you, but I cannot make you talk to me." Eva paused to study Camille's aloof demeanor. "I flew a long way to speak with you."

Camille cast her eyes to the tiled floor. Eva leaned forward and said, "Please look at me, Camille. I don't bite."

The prisoner's eyes flickered to Eva's face, then went right back down. This was not going to be easy. A supervisory job had advantages, including a hefty raise, but Eva hadn't been promoted for her interviewing techniques.

"Your friend, Farouk Hamdi, told us of your part in the diamond smuggling. Let me say, his passion for the cause does not run as deep as yours. He values his life outside prison walls."

Camille's cheek muscle twitched, but she kept silent.

"Farouk's main reason for helping us is to get you free. Do you share his interest?"

If Camille did, she refused to say. She simply stared at the floor.

Eva tried a different tack. "Because he does not know all your connections, his freedom and yours depend on what you tell us about ARC and El Samoud."

Camille folded her hands. Her coal-black eyes bored into Eva's blue ones. "You should know I have no interest in my freedom. I would rather be martyred." Her affect was flat, her voice stripped of emotion. There was something about Camille that reminded Eva of a woman who had been physically abused.

"What about your brother? Does he interest you?"

Camille's eyes blazed. "What do you mean?"

"Jacques left a message on your answering machine that he was coming to visit you."

Camille said softly, "My brother will have nothing to do with you."

"That's where you are wrong. British and American agents were at your flat to receive him. It seems he knew nothing of your arrest and got quite a welcoming committee."

Camille began to pace in the tiny room. " I don't believe you!" She shoved a chair against the wall, which brought the MI-5 agent into the room.

Eva held up her hand. "It's all right. Give us five more minutes." Eva purposely said "us" to impress upon Camille that they were in this together.

The agent glared at Camille as if to say that more time was useless, then closed the door behind him.

Eva returned her attention to the surprised prisoner. "It is true. He called your apartment last week to say he was coming to see you. We know he pilots a ship for El Samoud. We want to know where his boss is, where he is going, and what he is planning."

Camille said through clenched teeth, "He will never talk."

Eva smiled for the first time. "No? Not even to save you? Britain is going to extradite you and your brother to America. You may not value your life, but your brother does. We have a saying, blood is thicker than water."

Camille spat on the floor. "I hate Americans."

Eva had dealt with many criminals, but most of them, except for a few tax protestors, usually knew what was in their best interest. Camille de Berg was a different breed of militant. The cause meant more to her than the people, who were tools to an end.

Eva stood and looked into the hardened face. "Why hate Americans? We want people around the world to have the freedoms we have, to marry, earn a living, and elect a government. We don't invade other countries to control them, but to set the people free." Her speech finished, Eva reached for the door handle.

Camille's hand gripped the back of the metal chair. "Why, you ask? Because you killed my Papa." There were no tears, just vials of venom in her voice. "He died helping to arm the brothers in our struggle. I will never, never help you or your country. I hope you die."

Eva felt a blast of hate, such as she had never experienced in all her years arresting money launderers, low level mobsters, and corrupt corporate executives. Whatever Camille had been as a child, Eva saw before her a terrorist driven to destroy those in her way. Camille de Berg needed to stay where she was, in prison. Eva would never agree to Farouk's request that they help her.

Eva responded carefully, with words she had not used before in any of her cases. "I pray to God that one day you will see the bleak condition of your twisted soul."

Camille's face filled with rage.

This was a battle of good and evil that went far beyond agent and terrorist. Eva knocked on the door to signal MI-5.

To Camille, she said, "To prove I am not lying, I will permit you to talk with your brother. He is here, now."

The MI-5 agent pulled open the door. "They can have ten minutes."

Eva added to her French detainee, "Jacques is willing to save his life and yours."

While Camille stood defiantly in the grim room, Eva watched her eyes travel outside the doorway to see if her brother was really there.

"If you and Jacques do not help us, you will be extradited to the U.S. for trial, and probably execution."

Eva stepped aside, and the MI-5 officer pushed Jacques into the room. From the corner of her eye, Eva saw Jacques bend down and wrap huge arms around his sister. Her face peered over his shoulder. Eva thought she saw tears in Camille's eyes.

As Eva put the key in the door to her room, she heard the phone ringing. In her haste, she turned it in the wrong direction. The phone continued to ring. Finally, the door lock opened. She pushed open the door and ran to the phone. Out of breath, she answered, "Hello."

"Hi, love."

Eva sat on the bed to relish her first trans-Atlantic conversation with Scott.

"The phone rang twenty times. When no voicemail came on, I let her rip." Scott laughed.

"How are you and the kids?"

"Glad my trip to Central Asia was postponed. And we're all sick of pizza."

Eva kicked off her pumps. "I can't say much, but I'm making progress. Pray for me?"

"I do. Your empty pillow makes me sad."

Eva rubbed her feet. "What's new back home?"

"Zak is litter trained, to Kaley's credit. For almost ten years old, she is so focused. You must have been like her growing up."

Eva pictured how at ten she had entered a dressage competition and Jillie cheered her when she won. Tonight, Eva thought of her sister with love, not tears. "And Andy has your energy and big heart. Did the kids go to the club program at church tonight?"

"I nearly forgot. Remember the African director who spoke at the mission's dinner?"

"What about it?" Eva's body tensed.

"Helpers International was on TV tonight. I just caught the news."

"So?"

"You sound testy. Are you tired?"

Eva closed her eyes. "Sorry, but I am interested." More than she could admit.

"Federal agents raided their headquarters and Jubayl's home for giving aid to Middle East terrorists. I wonder if Pastor Greene or anyone at church knows. "

A dozen questions she couldn't ask Scott flooded Eva's mind, like which agency did the raid, and was Trenton still investigating Emile? What happened in Virginia could impact upon what she was doing in London.

Eva changed the subject. "Is your trip rescheduled?"

Scott would fly to Kazakhstan next week. Due to security, he'd only learn his exact itinerary the day before. "When will you be home? Should I ask Grandpa to come, since he didn't have to this week?"

"Honey, my feet ache. Call me tomorrow? I should know more by then." It was too late to call Dan Simmons tonight. Then she remembered that Virginia was five hours behind London.

Scott blew a kiss into the phone. "Be careful, and sleep tight."

"Have a good night, Scott, and hug the kids for me."

Eva found her PDA in her briefcase, looked up Dan's home number, and dialed. The phone rang and rang.

At least, she could soak in the tub. When she checked the bathroom, there was no bath tub. A hot shower then. Eva placed her hand under the running water. Barely warm. She'd find solace another way. In the kitchenette, as Brewster promised, the small refrigerator was stacked with scones, cream, and jam. Eva ate one, piled high with jam. It tasted so good, she ate another, washing it down with a cup of tea. Morning would come soon enough and, with it, fresh problems.

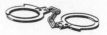

TWENTY SIX

Kaley and Andy ran to their rooms, and Scott eased a bag of Chinese takeout onto the kitchen counter. He could already taste the moo shoo pork with plum sauce, which would be a nice change from the pizza they'd eaten nearly every night since Eva went to England. He set the table with paper plates and cups, grabbed forks for the kids and chopsticks for himself, and they were ready to eat dinner.

Scott walked to the foyer and yelled up the stairs, "Wash your hands and come eat."

The doorbell clamored in his ear. A dish towel slung over his shoulder, Scott flipped on the outdoor light and opened wide the front door. It was not his neighbor as he expected, but a woman in a black trenchcoat. She looked familiar.

"May I help you?" he asked.

"Is Eva home?" Her face was blotchy, like she'd been crying. She held a crumpled tissue in a bandaged hand.

Kaley chased Andy down the stairs. "Gotcha. You have to clear the table," she said.

"Daddy, no I don't," Andy whined.

Scott turned to his children. "Go upstairs and play till I call you."

Andy chased his sister back up the stairs, laughing.

Facing his guest, Scott asked, "I'm sorry, what was your name?"

Her red face deepened a shade. "Sari Jubayl. I met you at church with Thelma."

Scott knew instantly this was the woman whose house was raided. He had seen a TV news report about it. He drew her inside. "Eva is out of town on business. Can I help?" Thoughts of eating the delectable Chinese dinner evaporated.

Sari wiped her nose with the tissue. "It is her business I came to see her about."

Scott shut the door. "I saw the news about the search of your home. Eva is not involved. If you want to talk about it, we can sit in the living room."

Sari looked dazed. "If you don't mind, I will sit a moment."

Still wearing her trenchcoat, Sari perched on the edge of the sofa. Scott had said he was going to get her some tissues. The sofa was the same red-flowered fabric as hers! Vivid scenes of being handcuffed and cowering on her couch rushed to her mind, and dark memories evoked a flood of bitter tears.

Scott returned and handed her the whole box of tissues.

Sari burst, "I am no terrorist! We are innocent, yet they treat us like criminals. At first, I thought the police were after us because my son did a foolish thing."

"Tell me about your son."

Her head slumped back against the sofa. How to find the energy and the words to tell the story? Soon, Scott's kind look and caring manner coaxed her to tell everything. The bomb, garbage searches, subpoenas, and the raid. She could not bring herself to admit she wrote the letter and placed it in the garbage with spoiled salmon.

"With Eva's job, I have only seen her side of a federal investigation. Is it possible your son is involved in things of which you are not aware?"

Sari wiped fresh tears from her face. "George is a typical college kid, doing goofy things, but he's no criminal."

Scott said, "Sari, you hinted this may involve more than your son."

She crumpled the used tissue into her coat pocket and said softly, "I am not sure. Emile's organization was raided, too."

"What do you make of that?"

Sari looked at her nails; they were chewed to the quick. "Things have bothered me, which I have prayed over. " She glanced around. It was so quiet. She would tell him now.

"Emile is weighed down by some great burden. Dark circles appeared under his eyes, and he travels to the Middle East all the time." She stopped, closed her eyes.

"Please go on. I'm listening."

Warmer now, she unbuttoned her overcoat. After she told Scott how she and Emile fled with their parents during the Civil War, she said, "We met in Baltimore in our late teens. Emile's brother refused to leave Lebanon. He stayed with his cousin and uncle. The fighting got worse. Beirut was demolished."

"The Civil War began in the 1970s. Is that when you left?" Scott asked.

Sari nodded. "In 1978. Then the kidnapping started. Some made news, like Terry Anderson's, but many did not. The militia knew Emile's uncle was a banker with ties to the West. Emile's brother, Claude, was snatched off the street on his way to American University. Their uncle got one ransom note, which he ignored at first, thinking it was a prank. They got no more letters. Claude's body was found a week later, in a ditch. He was shot in the head."

She shut her eyes at the memory of that awful death. When she opened them, Scott urged her to continue.

Thump, thump, sounded above their heads.

"Your children. Are they all right?" Sari asked.

"I'll check in a few minutes."

Sari blew her nose on a clean tissue. "Emile's heart was broken. He has never forgiven himself for leaving Lebanon. He believes if he had been there he could have saved his brother."

Scott said, "He was still a kid himself."

"He wants to save the Middle East from violence and poverty, all in his own strength." Sari blew her nose again. "Because of the pressure, he was diagnosed with prostate cancer. We went to the Mayo Clinic in Minnesota for surgery. With these raids, he might relapse. I think the government pursues Emile because he loves Lebanon."

Scott replied, "Eva would never do that. There must be more."

Sari looked up from her chewed nails. "When agents took them off the plane, Emile and George were on the way to bury his mother."

"I am sorry. Let me get you something cold to drink."

He returned with orange juice. As she drank it, Scott asked her to stay for dinner.

She shook her head and handed him the glass. "I should go. Emile will want his supper, if he is home. I never know any more."

Scott lightly touched her arm. "Have you spoken with a lawyer?"

"Emile spent the afternoon with one. That's another reason I am worried. George has a court appointed lawyer. Why does my husband need one of his own?"

Eva tossed and turned, wrestling with the overstuffed pillow. Snippets of details from the agreement she hammered out with Jacques and his sister floated into her mind. It was no use. She could not sleep. Throwing the monster to the floor, Eva recalled Camille's surprise when Brewster explained that she had to stay in solitary confinement until El Samoud's capture.

Jacques insisted that Camille spill what she knew about the Paris terrorist cell. She must have told everything because, afterward, she passed a rigorous polygraph exam. Eva shook her head at the image of the giant man hugging his hardboiled sister. Leaving them alone had been a stroke of genius, but it wasn't her idea. Griff had suggested it. Eva turned on a table lamp by her bed. It was seven in the evening at home. Scott and the kids might be playing hide-and-seek. She really missed them. Being an ICE supervisor, responsible for a whole team, was tough. But, if she and Griff pulled off their plan, it would be worth every lost night's sleep and the distance from her family. It was one giant "if."

The room was chilly. Eva put on her robe and stuffed her feet into suede moccasins that Scott had bought for her on a trip out West. She roamed to the refrigerator where she selected cheese and tomato juice. In the cupboard, she found a tin of biscuits. Eating her late-night snack, the enormity of what was before her startled her like a door closing in the middle of the night. Even if the intelligence she and Griff gathered was credible, was it possible to capture El Samoud?

Eva bit into a buttery biscuit. She and Scott had been allowed to see the burned out Pentagon when the fires were finally put out. These years later, Al Qaeda was on the run, but ARC was strong. Her thoughts ranged over the meetings of the past few days. It was ironic that she and Griff, financial crime experts, had found Jacques when terrorist specialists at CIA and NSA did not.

Even if Jacques returned to the ship, which made the most sense because he could lead them to El Samoud, the arrest of the world's most wanted terrorist was not assured. On a legal pad, Eva wrote down all the circumstances that had come together under her watch. When done, she marveled. It was more than good planning that had produced these results.

FIG worked on Operation Stitch for nine months and, the day they hit, Farouk was home, not in London or New York. Farouk meant to deceive Trenton in London, but revealed his ties to Camille. Eva and Griff "chanced" to meet Brewster at a financial briefing. Griff had British ancestry. Brewster took to him as a brother.

Farouk called Griff to meet and gave them startling information—Jacques and Camille were siblings. He told them about the hidden key, names, and account numbers. Jacques' radio needed fixing. He left a message saying he was coming to see Camille at the same time Eva and Griff were in London. All they had to do was wait for Jacques to show up. When he did, he was willing to deal to save his sister and claim a share in the 50-million-dollar reward.

Some of Eva's other cases had gone well, some had not. Were the breaks in this one mere happenstance, or was God answering Scott's prayers? Sipping the spicy juice, Eva considered that, while Jacques was acquainted with El Samoud's ship, Zayed had pieces of the puzzle Jacques did not. In their debrief earlier today, Zayed confided that Farouk had a highly placed source at the Department of Homeland Security. While Zayed's understanding of the level was incorrect, he told what he knew.

Eva tended to believe Zayed, who had everything to lose by co-operating. An architect by profession, at Brewster's urging he drew an exact likeness of El Samoud's villa from memory. He provided the code words to begin ARC's massive attack. Not only that, he had glimpsed El Samoud's face. If that became known, his life was in danger.

Where did Emile fit into the scheme? Zayed and Camille claimed they had never heard of Emile or George. That was not surprising, because ARC kept its cells separate; each functioned without knowledge of the others.

Eva had not yet reached Dan about the raid at Helpers. In a few hours, she'd contact the Justice Department about the 50-million-dollar reward. How to split it among the three was someone else's decision. If asked, she would recommend an equal split, even though Zayed demanded the lion's share. It all hinged on getting El Samoud.

They could storm Socotra. Yet that plan was filled with danger. While Zayed had seen only a few guards with weapons, sending in the U.S. military to capture a terrorist in a sovereign nation was an unlikely option. There had to be another way.

El Samoud expected Jacques back at Socotra in a few days. He was bringing with him new radios and a secret satellite phone from Griff. There was no way they could place an agent on the inside, but was there a way to track the terrorist's movements? Eva finished her juice. Hmm. Track his movements. She had done that before.

Her mind scanned memories of old cases, then stopped at one involving a violent and elusive mob boss, who transferred to offshore accounts all proceeds in his waste-hauling business. It was Griff's informant who told how his boss flew into a small airport outside of Manassas. Eva had it! They could get El Samoud the same way they arrested that mobster.

Excited with her theory, Eva called Griff's room. No answer. He often ran at odd hours. Helped to clear his mind, he said. Eva wrote out her plan with as much detail as her mind could muster at this late hour.

Twenty minutes later, Eva dialed a different number. Kaley answered.

"Mommy! Daddy said you'd call. My teacher gave me a gold star for my solar system in a blue box. Daddy got me glow stars. I wish you could see it."

She was homesick! Eva tried to sound happy. "You are a smart girl and I am so proud of you. How is Andy?"

"Playing with a racetrack that great grandpa got him. My car goes faster."

Eva chuckled at her high achieving daughter, then said, "He's still a little boy. Give him a chance to catch up. Is Daddy there?"

"He's in the kitchen. Andy spilled cereal on the floor. I'll get him. Love you, Mommy."

"I love you, too, honey."

The next voice she heard was Scott's strained one. He said, "Are you flying home tomorrow? I leave in two days."

Eva held the phone away from her ear, her high hopes for her case dashed by Scott's curt words. "Hello to you, too. I need to stay one more day. Maybe I can fly out tomorrow night."

"Let me start over," Scott said. "I wanted to have some time together before I leave. The last twenty-four hours have been so crazy, I can't keep up. That's why your grandfather is here." He tried to laugh.

"Kaley told me about the cereal."

A small moan escaped his throat. "That's not the half of it. Besides the trip getting sprung on me at the last minute, the van's transmission went. We're driving your bug. Last night, Sari Jubayl came over. Maybe I should not have spoken with her. What if I'm called to testify at trial?"

Eva was stunned. Sari came to their house? "You let her in? What did she say?"

Scott defended himself. "She came for you. Eva, did you know Emile had prostate cancer and that he was flying to Beirut for his mother's funeral when agents grabbed him and his son from the plane?"

Eva felt sympathy for Sari, but Emile and George were another matter. "George is out on bond. He can't leave the country."

"I knew you'd know more about it. Sari is convinced Emile is in trouble, too. He hired a lawyer and spent all day with him. His brother was kidnapped by rebels years ago in Lebanon and was killed because his family wouldn't pay the ransom."

"Scott, you lost me," Eva interrupted. "Whose brother?"

Scott told Eva about Claude's kidnapping and death.

"What does that have to do with the searches?" she asked.

"Maybe nothing," Scott said. "Sari says because of guilt over his brother's death, he is fanatical about helping the Middle East. She insists he is no terrorist and I believe her. Enough about them. I love you. Come home to me?"

"I'll arrange for the flight and let you know. Love you back."

Eva hung up, alone with the questions that plagued her. Was the plan she conceived earlier really possible? She turned off the lights and got into the small bed to try to get some sleep. It never came. By morning, she was convinced her idea could work if all the pieces came together as they had so far.

In a hastily scheduled Saturday meeting, Trenton sat at Nathan Barlow's large conference table with Ari and AUSA Midge Hopper. Trenton believed the searches proved, just as his source predicted, that Emile and his son were leaving the country. Nathan Barlow, Assistant Director of the FBI for Terrorism, had the floor. Trenton had to at least pretend he was listening.

Barlow tapped the table with his pen. In a grave voice, he asked, "Need I remind you, searches of Emile and George Jubayl and their luggage revealed no evidence of support for terrorism?"

When no one replied, he added, "Their home computers and papers produced no links to terrorists. Computers from Helpers contain a wealth of financial data that still needs review. So far, however, it all looks legitimate."

Irritated by more than the *tap* sounds, Trenton followed the Assistant FBI Director's eyes as he cast them around the group. With

no clue what he'd say next, Trenton could do without Midge's sullen
face. She looked like she'd lost her favorite dog. Ari's eyes were on
his notes. And Barlow wore a huge watch that banged the table every
time he moved his left hand.

The tapping stopped. Barlow was talking again. "Helpers' financial officer gave our agents their donor support records and CPA's
audit. The raid appears to be a washout. I want to know how we are
going to put a positive slant on this for the public."

Barlow narrowed his deepset eyes at Trenton, who refused to reveal any worry.

Unsatisfied, Barlow said, "It looks bad when we rummage around
in a citizen's home and the media identify them as terrorists."

Ari rapped his pen on a notepad. When the assistant director
looked at him, Ari said, "Trenton has an informant. Perhaps it is time
to bring him, or her, in for questioning."

His arms folded, Trenton failed to see Barlow's problem. Steadfast
in his belief that Emile supplied terrorists with money and even medical supplies, Trenton was not going to divulge his informant's identity.

"My source knew all about George's anti-American feelings. He
was at the State Department bombing, remember? My source told me
when Emile gets certain phone calls he speaks in Arabic. What about
that letter and his huge deposit? It's not a coincidence."

Barlow cut him off. "I want your informant's name and address."

Trenton's pulse raced. "I cannot identify my informant. He or she
is too sensitive. Besides, I gave my assurance the informant's identity
would never be revealed."

Then to keep the focus off his newest source, Trenton added, "My
affidavit was accurate. Emile and George were on a plane headed for
Lebanon. When you analyze the seized computers and bank records,
you'll see that the Jubayls are aiding terrorists."

Barlow shot out of his chair. "The FBI does not like to be embarrassed. Any ideas how the media got their hooks in this?" His gaze
around the table was met by blank stares. "What's worse, it involves an
American religious humanitarian organization. The President will not
be pleased if this becomes a public relations fiasco. Heads could roll."

He must have liked the sound of that, because he repeated, "Heads
could roll."

Trenton noticed the somber look on Ari's face. Was this a serious
problem?

Barlow opened his office door and warned, "If this doesn't turn around in thirty-six hours, I assure you, it won't be my head. Internal Affairs will investigate the media involvement and anything else that smells. You better hope Trenton's claims are true and that analysis produces the punch we need. If not, some—or all—of you, could be fired—or at new lows in your careers."

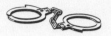

TWENTY SEVEN

Only days before Christmas, in the second meeting that week with Emile Jubayl, Attorney Harlan Scribbs quit writing. After filling ten pages of background and concerns from Emile, including one that every lawyer heard, his fingers ached. His newest client insisted his phone was tapped. A former federal prosecutor, Harlan knew that less than two percent of federal cases had a phone tap. Yet, almost every target believed his phone had one. If Emile's was tapped, there would be incriminating tapes in his client's own voice. Such tapes were virtually impossible to beat in court.

With a full head of white hair, Harlan looked every bit the top criminal defense lawyer that he was. Gold cufflinks sparkled on his white shirt as he picked up the fountain pen and made a note to check out the claim. Emile thought he was a target because of his Middle East connections. The evidence seemed tenuous, yet it was Harlan's duty to his client not to jump to conclusions.

Prepared to probe more deeply with his eyes and specially chosen words, he took off his reading glasses. "I combed through the search warrant affidavit. What do you know about a handwritten letter that refers to helping terrorists?"

Emile undid the top button of his blue starched shirt. "I have no idea."

"I see." Harlan wrote on his yellow legal pad, *Find out who wrote the letter.*

Emile crossed his legs and adjusted the crease on his wool slacks. "Harlan, help me understand what is happening. Growing up, I remember how my parents could not wait to emigrate. All I heard was the beauty of the American system, that you are innocent until proven guilty. In Lebanon, persons on the wrong side of political power were killed. There were no judges, juries, or trials."

"At this point, you are innocent in the eyes of the law. Remember, you have not been charged with any wrongdoing."

Emile pushed himself back from the massive conference room table and walked over to the large window that overlooked Pennsylvania Avenue. "That's my problem. How do I prove I am not guilty when the government piles on evidence to make it look that way, then leaks it to the media?"

Harlan did not want to get distracted—he had to find out the extent of Emile's involvement. When a client waxed eloquent about philosophy of justice, it meant one thing: He was guilty and didn't want to spend money to prove his innocence. Yet Emile had brought in a 20-thousand-dollar retainer and signed an agreement to pay another twenty thousand if he was indicted.

"Emile, sit and listen." Harlan paused. "Thank you. Your situation is tough right now. But you need to help me analyze the government's evidence. They say an incriminating letter was found in the trash from your home."

Emile shook his head and picked lint from his slacks. "Sari warned me someone was scouring our trash. What will they stoop to next? They leaked the raids to the press. The front pages of the local papers splashed color photos of agents carting boxes out of Helpers."

The renowned lawyer studied his client. Was Emile innocent as he claimed? Harlan pursed his lips. There was a way to test him. He would push the well-dressed, soft-spoken humanitarian out of his comfort zone.

"Well, your conduct looks suspicious. Allowing George to fly out of the country while on bail was a reckless thing to do, even if he was going to Grandma's funeral. Why didn't you call Court Services or ask his attorney to file a motion so he could legally attend?"

Emile looked at his attorney. "Sari mentioned he had a lawyer, but this is all new to me. George is an adult. His lawyer never called me. My son is," Emile paused as if reluctant to reveal much, "unlike me at that age. I knew what I wanted and set about finding a way to get it. George has no vision and thinks only of himself. I was taking him to Lebanon for his grandmother's funeral to please my wife."

Harlan used his authority to impress on Emile that his lack of attention to his son was part of the problem. "If you want my opinion, you should wise up. After the subpoenas and the feds searching your garbage, you could have called me to see what I thought about a trip to Lebanon, especially with you carrying jewelry and cash. How do you expect me to help you now?"

Emile leapt to his feet. "Because I am paying you good money to protect my reputation, Harlan! Do you think I am guilty? Because if you do, perhaps I should go elsewhere."

Harlan did not flinch. He stayed seated. "If you feel you cannot work with me, say the word. That is your business. Mine is to represent you to the fullest extent of the law, and I will. I told you I thought the evidence was weak. But I am still evaluating it." The former United States Attorney put on his glasses. "And, it helps when my clients are honest with me."

Emile blinked rapidly, then sat. "I like directness. You are the best, and I want you to be my attorney."

"All right," Harlan responded. Maybe now they could get down to business.

Emile took a deep breath. "I was approached twice by people I suspected were terrorists trying to use my organization to funnel money to forbidden groups. I was smart enough not to go along with them."

"When and where did these contacts occur?"

"The first time, a man phoned my office and left a message. I am known throughout the Middle East for the work I do there for the poor."

Harlan nodded. "I know of your reputation, which is why I agreed to handle this case. What did you do with the message? Do you still have the number?"

"I called back and the man told me he wanted to establish a relationship with us. He is a friend of my cousin, Duma, who is the director of a large bank in Beirut. Thinking he was legit, I promised to get back in touch."

Emile cleared his throat. "I found out his group was on the State Department list of restricted organizations that cannot receive American funds. When I called him the second time, I told him we could not work together."

As Harlan furiously took notes, he wondered if there was more to that call. "Emile, I am sure the agents who searched your home and office know about those calls. This could be damaging. It's too soon to know if there are tapes verifying what you said."

Emile interrupted. "What do you mean, tapes?"

Harlan answered indirectly. "If there are tapes, a Title III wiretap warrant was issued, which means there is more than probable cause against you. I assume you asked Duma about the man who called."

Emile did not answer that question. Instead, he replied, "The second time was more subtle. Helpers received a ten-thousand-dollar contribution from Mr. Ashur Wadi, who claimed to live near Detroit. I flew to meet him, and he offered me two million." Emile stared at his lawyer. "Can you imagine what I could do with that kind of money? It took all my strength to shut him down."

Harlan looked into Emile's dark eyes. "Why did you turn it down?"

"He wanted me to designate part of the donation to a group tied to Hezbollah."

Harlan nodded. "Hezbollah is also on the State Department's list of prohibited organizations. But I see you knew that." The attorney scanned his list, then asked, "What did Mr. Wadi look like?"

Emile took a circuitous route, of which Harlan was growing wary. "I learned long ago some in my business have less than pure motives. In the Middle East, it is crucial to know with whom one is dealing. I checked on Mr. Wadi before I met with him. None of my Arab friends in Dearborn or Detroit ever heard of him."

"What does Mr. Wadi look like?" Harlan asked.

Emile replied, "Contributions have fallen in the last year. It was hard to turn it down."

"I asked what he looks like."

It took a moment for Emile's eyes to shift from his hands to Harlan's intense face.

"The more we talked, the more I suspected he was not Arab. Besides not knowing my contacts in the area, his hair had a slight curl that gave him a Hispanic appearance. He was about six foot one, which some say is tall for an Arab."

Harlan twirled the cap on his fountain pen. "You are more observant than I guessed."

Emile broached a new subject. "These reporters nosing around, Harlan, what can I do? They show up unannounced at the office and bother the staff. They camped on our street for two days. I am glad George is in jail. Who knows what crazy stuff he would say."

Harlan stood. "I'll draft a statement for the media, but I have no news conference planned."

Not yet, anyway. Harlan first had to be sure his client was not a terrorist before vouching for him on live television. "But," he added, "I have an idea how to find Mr. Wadi."

On the way home, Harlan stopped at Eva's office. She was expecting him, and he was punctual, as always. Eva thought he looked older and more tired than she remembered, but it had been almost five years. His hair was elegantly white now.

Unsure of his reason for asking for the meeting, Eva showed him into her private office. Their years of being on the same side gave him priority over other defense attorneys. "I only have a few minutes. Scott's leaving tomorrow, and I promised to be home by five."

Harlan had not brought in a file or legal pad. "You mean, you don't have time to reminisce about our stolen airplane case? Too bad. We had Judge Pendergast on the edge of his bench on that one."

The memory of the crusty Korean war pilot who testified as an expert defense witness, wearing a white scarf around his neck, evoked laughter from Eva. "Do you miss being a federal prosecutor?"

Harlan pointed to his head. "See this white hair? My wife is glad I can now pick and choose cases, which gives us time every winter to get away for a few weeks. Logging in ten hours a day is what associates are for."

"You didn't send one of your associates to see me today. What can I help you with?" Eva checked her watch to gauge her time.

Harlan dropped his casual demeanor. "I checked. FIG was initially on Emile Jubayl's case. I'll try not to ask questions to put you in a compromising position."

"Good." Even though he was an old friend, there were limits to her hospitality. The need for secrecy was one of them. Despite her reticence, she smiled. Harlan was not only the brightest lawyer she had worked with, he was the most ethical.

"Because the affidavit for the search warrants was not sealed, I reviewed it. Emile said he attends your church and met you once."

Eva nodded. She could have kept what she said next to herself, but she had too much respect for Harlan not to tell him. "I know his wife slightly. She also came to my home a couple of days ago when I was not there. Scott talked with her and told me what she said." Crossing her arms, Eva waited for Harlan to speak.

"Can I ask you one question?"

"That depends on what it is." Her arms remained crossed.

"Is there a sealed warrant for a wiretap of the Jubayl home?"

After an instant mental calculation, Eva replied, "I cannot answer that."

Harlan laid out what he thought, with a caveat. "This is, of course, off the record. Emile is certain there is a tap on his phone because the FBI grabbed him off a flight to Lebanon. Except for a single phone call, no one besides his wife knew he was leaving for Lebanon. The affidavit for a search warrant mentioned a 'very reliable' source. Eva, you and I both know such language is often used to disguise a wire tap."

She did not want to be rude, but it was time to leave. "George was on that plane, too. Maybe he or their travel agent has a big mouth." Eva stood. "Harlan, this has been interesting, but I am in the dark on this case. Call me again and we'll have lunch."

Harlan wrinkled his brow. "One more question. Does Griff Topping work for the FBI Task force that raided the Jubayl home?"

"No. Why?" Eva edged around her desk toward the door and Harlan followed.

"That blows my theory."

"Which is?" She almost did not want to ask.

Harlan chuckled. "I recall Griff was undercover in his New York City days. Emile described meeting in Detroit with a man claiming to be a donor, but whom Emile suspected was a terrorist. He fits the description of Griff perfectly. Is Griff still working undercover?"

"One question too many," Eva said. "Sorry. Got to run."

"I can't get Sari's devastated face from my mind," Scott lowered his large frame onto a stool at the breakfast counter. Eva threaded thin spaghetti into a boiling pot, then wiped her hands on her blue and white apron printed with Dutch windmills.

Her earlier dream of Sari in the hospital flashed in her mind, but she said, "In answer to the question you want to ask, I haven't found out anything about Emile's case. We have one night home together as a family." Eva blew him a kiss, "I prefer to think about you."

She covered the spaghetti and walked around the counter. Scott stood and put his arms around her. "And I will enjoy seeing your beautiful face eat a proper meal for a change." He squeezed her against him. "You feel like you're losing weight."

She snuggled against him. "All that travel and no time to eat. Why do you think I'm cooking eight pounds of pasta tonight?"

They both laughed. Eva liked feeling Scott's solid arms around her. She was home, and his love for her was real, no matter if she was too thin or whether they had another baby. "Glad you arranged to meet Secretary Cabrini tomorrow, rather than fly out tonight," she murmured.

"Sshh. I just want to hold you like this. When your current cases wrap up, promise me we'll take a vacation, since we had to cancel going to Disney World for Christmas." Scott kissed the top of her head.

Eva liked the sound of planning a trip, even if it did not happen until summer. She pulled back to look up into his eyes and asked, "Where to?"

"Andy wants to meet Shamu, and Kaley is determined to visit Africa to see her friend from the mission's dinner. I want to go to the Smokey Mountains. Sit by a campfire, roast hot dogs—"

The sound of water spitting on the stove spoiled their dreams.

"The spaghetti is boiling over!" Eva tore herself from his arms, turned off the burner, and lifted the pot onto a hot pad. Sticky pasta water lay in pools on the counter and trickled down the cupboards to the floor.

"What a mess," she sighed.

"I'll get paper towels. Not to worry, I found a great Chinese place while you were gone."

Scott went to the pantry while Eva opened the pot. All the water had boiled out. Most of the noodles were stuck to the bottom. She heaved the gooey mass into the garbage disposal. Cheered by the thought of going out, she refused to get upset over a damaged dinner.

Scott helped her wipe up the liquid. Eva asked, "Do I need to get back with Sari?"

Scott shrugged. "I said we'd pray for her."

Eva turned off the faucet. "I have prayed for her. Get the keys, I'll round up our two sweeties and we'll see what delights await us."

"And I told her if you could tell her anything, you would. Can you?"

Eva turned around in the doorway. "Emile's lawyer came to see me, off the record. Remember Harlan Scribbs, the U.S. Attorney who tried my airplane conspiracy case? I respect him. He posed a perplexing question. The problem is, I am no longer working that case and have no authority to find the answer."

"You'll figure out what to do. Ready?"

Something in the back of her mind goaded her. Once she had authority over Emile's case. Was there a way to exercise it now? Even if there was, wouldn't Emile's case sidetrack her? In London, Griff and Brewster thought her idea to capture El Samoud had merit. She should forget Emile and focus all of her energies on getting the known terrorist.

Eva walked up the stairs, tempted to see Gus in the Tech Op Group tomorrow. And say what? Then, like getting an answer to a prayer she never prayed, she remembered—she never made sure Trenton disconnected the pen registers! Eva could ask Gus tomorrow and sneak in a question or two about a wiretap of Emile's home. She would not tell anyone what she learned. She needed to know for herself.

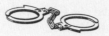

TWENTY EIGHT

S ari stared at the small television set on her bedroom dresser. The camera shot of their street narrowed down to the front of their house. There was George, looking like a street thug with torn jeans and black leather jacket, his hand on the doorknob. This time, the reporter used his upcoming trial as an excuse for reminding the world that their home was searched and evidence taken because they were suspected of helping terrorists.

George gestured at the camera, and shouted angry words. She felt helpless watching him stick out his tongue, show off his stud, and ring the door bell. The camera zoomed in. Sari opened the door for George. Her eyes looked frightened. George brushed past his mother and slammed the door in the reporter's face.

Sari flipped off the TV. She looked awful on that clip. Her hair was a mess, and dark circles ringed her eyes. Emile's attorney, Harlan Scribbs, arranged with George's attorney to get him out on a higher bond, so at least George had been home for Christmas, such as it was. Sari forced herself from the bed.

Sari changed into a pair of black slacks and slipped on a wool sweater. Her purse under her arm, she left the master bedroom and forced herself to go past George's room without knocking. Since he got home yesterday, he came downstairs long enough to load up on pizza and cookies. She tried not to mentally count the dirty dishes in his room.

Sari skipped breakfast and went straight to the back door. Yesterday, when she weighed herself, she was surprised to see she had lost seven pounds since George's arrest. Who cared for food when your life was turned inside out?

As she opened the garage door, the phone rang. It was probably an annoying reporter who refused to take no for an answer. Thelma was the only person she wanted to talk with. Everyone else had an ulterior motive for calling. But what if it was Eva Montanna? Sari decided to answer. She picked up the phone but the caller had already hung up. If it was Eva, maybe she would call again.

Sari slid onto the leather seat of their SUV. When she got back home, she would change their number and make it unlisted. The expense was worth the peace of mind. As she backed out of the garage, she waved at Mr. Palmer taking Christmas lights off his house. He looked over but didn't wave. Maybe he didn't see her.

Ten minutes later, Sari pulled into her favorite market where she shopped for fresh meat and vegetables. While she didn't feel like eating, Emile's appetite had doubled. In the lively shop, smells of garlic and spices overwhelmed her, turning her empty stomach upside down. Well, she was here now. She'd buy her supplies and leave.

Sari greeted the owner, whom she had known for years. "Hi Joe."

"Mrs. Jubayl," he said loudly in a thick Bulgarian accent. "Vhat vill it be today?"

A woman in a camel-colored coat, whom Sari often saw at Joe's Market, looked at her and walked away. What did that shake of her head mean?

"Two lamb chops, six chicken breasts, and a pound of homemade summer sausage."

"Just made a new batch. Vant to taste?" Joe held out a slice of the peppery sausage.

But Sari was more interested in watching the woman whisper to a young woman, who, in turn, eyed Sari and shook her head.

The smell of the sausage made Sari's stomach reel. "No thanks, Joe, just wrap my order, please."

Joe completed her order while Sari tried to ignore their glances. Those women must have seen the news and recognized her. Sari's face burned with shame. How could she, a Christian woman, ever live this down? Even Thelma did not understand. No one did!

She grabbed her packages from Joe, muttered a kind word to him, and hurried to the cashier, not bothering with the other items. Barely able to breathe, she had to leave the store this instant or she would faint!

By the glass doors, she heard the older woman say, "Don't come back. Terrorists are not welcome here."

Sari found refuge in her car. Until a man in the next car pointed at her. She accelerated out of the parking lot. She'd shop at another store, in another neighborhood. That comfort was short-lived. As she fled for home, it slowly dawned on her. Wherever she went, people would recognize her. Her face and name had been plastered all over the news. Maybe Joe would deliver her groceries. He was a dear man, and she had been a loyal customer for years. Surely he would not snub her.

As Sari eased the SUV into the driveway, she saw the Palmers. Sari stopped the car and waved. They just stared at something in their yard. Sari straightened to see. It was a sign that read, "For Sale by Owner." The Palmers were moving out of the neighborhood. Moving to get away from them!

Her meat put away in the freezer, Sari knocked on George's door. There was no answer. She tried the knob. It was unlocked. Unsure what she'd find in there, she swung the door slowly. It was worse than she imagined. CDs littered the floor. His bed was unmade. A blanket was thrown on the bathroom floor. Dishes and glasses cluttered his dresser.

"George?"

Her call was met by silence. For a moment, Sari considered cleaning his room, when an idea stopped her. It was time George took care of himself. Sari shut his door with a snap.

She hurried to her own bathroom. Inside the cabinet, the aspirin bottle stared at her. Opposed to medicine of any kind, this time she took two with a glass of water. Sari put on an old robe and lay on top of her bed. Her sleep was not restful. She dreamed she was lost, first in a broken-down building, then on an unknown highway. She wanted to cry out, but words were stuck in her throat.

A car door slammed. She woke suddenly. Disoriented, Sari tried to stand. Her trembling legs refused to hold her. She fell next to the bed. Thankfully, the floor was carpeted and she was not hurt. But her mind, now that was a different matter. Sari pushed herself to her feet. Of course she was weak. She'd eaten nothing all day. Still, she wasn't hungry. Food held no solace for a heart that was broken.

The cut in her finger throbbed. She removed the bandage and saw it was red and puffy. Should she go to the Care Center and get it looked at? An ugly voice taunted her mind. "Don't come back. Terrorists are not welcome." No, she'd treat the wound herself.

Sari drizzled hydrogen peroxide over the cut. Tiny bubbles formed. She longed to pour tonic over her life. A few words at a time, verses she had memorized from the Bible trickled through her mind. "If God is for us, who can be against us?"

How did the rest go? Sari's mind went blank. She fiddled with a tube of antibiotic cream, spread it over her finger, then wrapped a bandage over it. She flexed her finger; it was not on too tight.

Sari went to the kitchen, and turned on the kettle for tea. Her Bible lay closed on the counter. In it, she looked for the verse in the Concordance, but couldn't find the right one. Sari drank her tea and ate a slice of toast with blackberry jam.

Suddenly, she remembered. She leafed to the back of her Bible and found a slip of paper where she had written *Romans 8:31.* The words of God flowed like a river of comfort. Words that came from him to heal her at this moment. She read them aloud, "If God is for us, who can be against us? He who did not spare his own Son, but gave him up for us all—how could he not also, along with Jesus, graciously give us all things?"

Sari stretched her hands over the parchment, as if she could absorb the truth through her fingertips. She felt a measure of peace for the first time since she found out about the garbage raider. With that peace came a kernel of hope for this new year. All was not lost. She repeated the verse.

"Sari, what are you doing sitting alone, talking to yourself? Have you lost your mind?"

Emile looked at her as if had he caught her doing something wrong.

She held onto the power of God's word in her heart and refused to feel guilty at his reprimand. He was stressed, with no clear way out. "Emile, we need to talk."

To her surprise, he sat without protest. Sari found a ceramic mug and reheated the water. While she made him tea, she saw him look curiously at her Bible, which was open to the passage she had marked in Romans. Sari hoped he was reading it. That hope came to nothing. When she sat at the table, he pushed away her Bible.

She said, "We need to pull our family together. You have left George to me these last few years. Can't you see he needs your attention?"

Her husband looked at the tea inside the cup.

"You think George is nothing like you were at his age. You wanted to accomplish something for your brother. We met and got married. You are right. George *is* at loose ends." Sari touched Emile's arm. "But he is more like you than you know. He wants to make a difference in the world. If you would talk with him or show interest in his ideas, you could influence him for the better."

Emile remained still, Sari's hand on his arm. When he finally spoke, his words were forced. "I tried to take him to Lebanon. Look where that got us." He blew air out his lips like steam from an engine. "I hate to say my own son is trouble, but he is. He thinks only of himself. I see too much suffering in the world to be moved by a kid who has everything and is unable to figure out what to do with it."

Sari tried again. This was too important to her. "Please try, Emile. If we do not reach him now, he will be lost to us forever."

Emile rose from the table and said, "I'll think about it."

He waited in his den for Sari to call him for dinner. It was after seven and she had not shown her face. Was this some kind of message? No food unless he went with George to a movie or some other father-son outing?

For all his bluster, something about Sari's plea touched his heart. He flashed back to her white smile when he met her at the Lebanese Community Center all those years ago. He handed her a glass of lemonade, and she replied in perfect French, "Merci." Her almond-shaped brown eyes danced. He was smitten by her beautiful face.

The more they talked that day, the more he liked her spirit. She was eighteen, had been in America a little over a year, and was studying to be a legal secretary. Her English was very good. What was it she had said to him? Emile had difficulty retrieving the rest of the memory; he blocked those years from his mind. But he recalled telling her about his dream to rebuild Beirut.

Tonight, he painted a mental picture of her face. For the first time in months, he saw her. Truly saw her. Sari's skin had lost its luster. Her face was drawn. Purple streaks lurked under her eyes. The pain of a wayward son and all their present troubles were hurting her.

Her words from so many years ago streamed in his conscience. "Emile, we are free here. You can do anything you want in America! I believe in you."

She was the one who urged him to finish high school at night, then go on to community college before transferring to the university. He proposed to her before graduation, and she did not hesitate. Her parents were dead; she was anxious to start a family. Their only living child was George, and he came only after three miscarriages.

Sari saw their baby boy as a gift. Emile swallowed. Where had they gone wrong? Had he been too distant as she claimed? To compensate, didn't she spoil him endlessly? And now, after he survived surgery for prostate cancer, their family was the target of a federal investigation. Sari was right, they had to do things differently.

Emile sighed and went to find his wife. She was mashing potatoes. Apparently, Sari was not withholding food as a weapon. How could he think that of her? He rubbed her shoulders with his hands. She stopped mashing.

He said, "Sari, I agree with you. I am not sure what we can do about George. We may insist he move. I will talk with him. Where is he?"

Sari faced Emile. "I don't know. His room is a mess. Today, I decided I would no longer clean it. He is old enough to do it himself."

That was progress! Sensing Sari was willing to change, Emile offered, "I will attend church with you tomorrow and insist that George come along."

Sari cast a sideways glance at Emile, who sat stiffly at the end of the pew. She wished he would quit doodling on the church bulletin and listen to the choir and orchestra. Their rendition of "Behold the Lamb" was beautiful. Rather than dwell on the negative, she recalled her joy when Emile told her last night he would worship with her today. He had refused to come on Christmas Eve, something they had done as a family for years. Sari squeezed from her mind their dark house on Christmas morning, when Emile would not string lights or allow them to exchange gifts. The holiday was over, a new year was here.

As the one-hundred-voice choir reached its crescendo and sang Amen in harmony, Sari tried to see what Emile was writing. He didn't seem to be joining in the spirit of things. His mind was always churning. She read on his bulletin the words, "phone call to Armed Revolutionary Cause." Her eyes widened. She had heard that name on TV. They were a terrorist group that set off a bomb in Lebanon! Did Emile call them? Why was he writing such things in church?

Pastor Greene said, "Give a warm handshake to one another on this cold morning,"

Sari turned to the worshippers behind them, a couple from her prayer circle, which she had stopped attending after the news claimed they were terrorists. She held out her hand to them. Rather than shake it, they turned their backs on her and grabbed someone else's hand. Thelma tried to convince Sari that those in the prayer circle loved and supported her. This was proof that she was right not to believe it. Thelma now met with Sari in her home.

Sari sat with the rest of the congregation, deep in thought about George's trial being postponed until April, and Emile's silence at home. Her fists were clenched, and her fingers dug into her palms. Blood pounded in her ears. She missed hearing the solo by a young woman who was on her way to serve in Kenya.

When would she get back her old life? Her emotions spiked so high, she lamented the loss of something she did not have. Sari's head felt on the verge of bursting. Emile squirmed next to her, loosened his tie. A rush of heat cascaded through her body. It may be thirty degrees outside, but it was stifling inside. Sari barely heard Pastor's final words.

"Judas betrayed our Lord for thirty pieces of silver. When we love money and material goods more than him, we also betray our love for him. I ask you, what are you willing to lay down for him?"

Emile leaned over to Sari and hissed in her ear, "Can we go now?"

The song leader announced, "All rise and sing the benediction,"

Sari stood. Sharp pains thundered in her chest. She could not breathe! Bright lights swirled around her, and she collapsed onto the padded pew. Emile had started walking up the aisle while the others sang, so it took him some moments to realize Sari was not behind him. Emile stalked back to the pew to find her.

Then, he saw her crumpled body, drool dripping from her lips. No one around them seemed to notice anything wrong. Emile's heart leapt. Groping for her pulse, he was relieved to find it was strong.

Cradling her head, he whispered, "Sari, can you hear me?"

She did not respond. Across the aisle, Emile spotted a man with a name tag.

Rushing over he asked, "Can you call an ambulance? Quickly! My wife needs help."

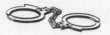

TWENTY NINE

If she could just reach the dazzling red raspberry. She lifted her arm through the branches to pluck the fruit. Ouch. Prickers stuck her fingers and arms. Sari watched drops of red blood ooze from her finger. As it flowed, the luscious berry disappeared. Her palm held nothing. A cool mist swirled about her. She heard her name. Who was calling her?

"Sari, it's me, Emile."

When she opened her eyes, they burned. She blinked to block out white light blazing above her head. Her eyes watered anyway. As she lifted her right arm to shield against it, she discovered it was held by tubes connected to a machine and IV.

"Hospital?" she asked weakly.

"Would you like ice water? That's all you can have."

He lifted to her lips a straw attached to a white foam cup. She took a sip, then her head collapsed against the pillow.

"The doctor said you are dehydrated and have not been eating. When did you lose so much weight?" Emile shook his head. "I started to see how much George has hurt you, but I didn't realize how much."

Sari closed her eyes. Worry over George was only part of her stress. Emile must also feel strain of being called a terrorist. She wished he would talk about it. He seemed so distant, like the raspberry in her dream. A tear clung to the corner of her eye, refusing to be released. He was rarely home and never talked to her.

"What happened?" Her lips didn't work right.

Emile put down the cup. "You fainted in church this morning. You need to take better care of yourself."

He cupped his hands around her free one. The warmth of his touch brought other tears to her eyes, which now dripped down her cheeks. She saw Emile's hand come up to her face and wipe away the moisture.

Emile gripped her hand. "I thought we lost you. I know I have not been attentive lately."

A small Indian doctor, wearing a blue coat and stethoscope around her neck, pulled back a curtain. "Mrs. Jubayl, it is good to see you awake. When you were admitted, your blood pressure was off the charts. I want to check it again. How do you feel?"

Sari could not feel the left side of her face. It was numb, as if she had gotten a shot of novocaine from the dentist. She tried to talk. Her lips felt huge.

Sari pointed to her face and said, "My ear hurts." Drool drizzled from her mouth.

Emile released Sari's hand. "Why is her speech slurred?" he asked the doctor.

The doctor took her blood pressure, listened to her heart, and felt her pulse. She looked into her ears using a wand with a light on the end. "The good news is, you did not have a stroke or a heart attack. Your blood pressure is sky-high. You have all the symptoms of Bell's palsy."

"What is that?" Emile asked.

Sari's eyes widened. It sounded permanent, like polio.

The doctor seemed in a hurry. "An inflammation of the nerve endings. I will have the nurse bring you some literature. You can probably go home tomorrow, once we have your blood pressure under control and get the blood test results."

As the doctor started to leave her curtained cubicle, Emile asked, "Can it be treated?" He took a square tissue from a little box and wiped Sari's chin.

"It can disappear as suddenly as it came. In the meantime, it will be hard for her to talk. The left side of her face may droop for some time. Bells palsy can be brought on by stress, lack of sleep, that kind of thing. Have you been stressed, Mrs. Jubayl?"

Sari nodded her head, her dark eyes looking even larger in her thinning, deformed face.

"Mr. Jubayl, it is your job to see that she gets de-stressed. I am going to prescribe a sedative for tonight. Her blood tests will tell us if she has anything else to worry about."

Sari did not like the sound of that.

Emile asked, "Such as?"

Fiddling with her stethoscope, the doctor explained. "Lyme disease or HIV can also trigger facial paralysis. Did she have any bites from ticks or find a red ring last fall? Ticks are common in northern Virginia."

Was that possible? Was she suffering from a terrible disease and did not know it? She muttered, "No bites."

The doctor replied, "I don't think you have either of those diseases, but we have to be sure. I will return at six in the morning. Please be here, Mr. Jubayl. I want to know what help you are going to give her."

Eva popped in a mint. Her stash had been replenished since her grandfather visited at Christmas, bearing gifts from the Netherlands.

Griff smiled. "This afternoon, I'm going to NGA," he told Eva, referring to the National Geospatial-Intelligence Agency, "to check on satellite photos over Yemen and Socotra. This morning, I met with the assistant director for the FBI's Tech Ops."

"And?" Eva interrupted.

"I explained your plan, but he was reluctant to give an opinion without more information. When I hinted it was a high-level terrorist, he became more cooperative."

"I told you not to tell him it was El Samoud. The FBI will try to steal our case."

Griff held up his hands. "Hold on. I explained that the informant is controlled by ICE and I had no influence over that. I reminded him I was trained in electronic installations by the Technical Support Group."

Eva shook her head. "Too many people are finding out, and it could compromise our strategy."

"Bottom line with FBI Tech Ops is they give us the equipment we need, and pay our expenses, if we give them part of the credit."

"That's a terrific deal," she replied. "Brewster sent me an encrypted message. The longer Camille is in solitary confinement, the more belligerent she becomes."

"Word is, Camille's the money person for The Grilled Onion as well as ARC's diamond smuggling operation. MI-5 fed a story to the London Times of a woman and man who were victims of a boating accident on the Thames. Only Brewster and a few key people know it's a cover story for Camille and Farouk."

"Is intelligence picking up chatter about their disappearance?"

Griff shook his head. "As Farouk predicted, ARC has gone underground. No talking on cell or satellite phones. No e-mails we can trace."

Eva looked at Griff. "Can Jacques be trusted not to leak our plan to El Samoud?"

Hands folded over one knee, he looked serious. "Not only is Jacques a mercenary, but he looks out for his sister's best interest. He will do exactly what he said for the thirty-three million dollars and Camille's freedom."

Eva swallowed the last of her coffee. "I hope you're right."

Wanda knocked at Eva's door jamb. Painted eyebrows drawn together, her voice quivered as she said, "My mom just called. We've been attacked."

Eva yanked the remote from her top drawer and turned on her portable TV in time to hear the reporter say, "The small plane, loaded with explosives, was shot down by the Navy after it ignored warnings to turn from its path toward the newest carrier in the Atlantic fleet. As I step aside, you can see not much is left of the plane. Authorities tell us no one survived on the plane."

Eva held her breath. Had sailors been killed?

As if anticipating that question, the reporter said, "No military personnel were killed or wounded. Authorities believe terrorists were attempting to fly the small plane into the carrier, which had just returned to port in Norfolk. They are also claiming that the shoot down demonstrates improvement to our defensive systems since 9/11. Back to you in Washington."

Eva sat in stunned silence. This attack was not in some foreign country, it was in Virginia, close to home.

Trenton zipped up his leather jacket. It was still winter, and it was cold. Hannah was late. She had agreed to meet him at the Commons before her class at 3 p.m. It was now twenty minutes after. He poured a refill into his disposable coffee cup, then called Helpers International on his cell phone. The receptionist said Hannah was not in.

"Is she sick?"

The receptionist asked, "Who is calling?"

"A friend from school. She called me this morning and said she would meet me here."

The receptionist chuckled. "I see. Well, she must not have known at that time that Mr. Jubayl would send her on a special errand."

What did Emile have her doing? Trenton should have insisted she quit! Of course, he had no right to tell her anything.

"Want to leave a message?" the lady repeated.

Trenton was all business now. "Will you tell me what her errand was? Maybe I could catch up to her there. I forgot to turn on my cell phone, so if she tried to call me, she would have gotten no answer," Trenton fibbed.

"Mr. Jubayl asked her to go to the bank and travel agency. What is your name?"

"My friends call me "T." Please let her know I called."

Trenton hung up. Hannah probably went straight to class. It was odd she didn't call him on his cell, which was turned on. She usually did exactly what she said she would. He called her at home, left a message for her to call him. Then he phoned his dad.

"You busy? Thought I would drive out this evening." Trenton wanted to get an idea of what he should do while the analysts combed through Emile's financial and personal data, which was taking longer than he or Ari thought it would.

"Great. Your mom's making burritos. Did you hear the terrible news?"

His dad was not one to exaggerate problems. "I'm in the field. What happened?"

Duke took a deep breath and let it out all at once. "ARC tried to crash a Cessna into our newest carrier. The Navy blasted it out of the air. The terrorist died on impact."

Trenton replied, "Catching those terrorists is what I wanted to talk with you about." He added, "But without Mom."

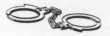

THIRTY

Eva was a few minutes late. The Channel 14 reporter had called wanting Eva's reaction to the shoot-down of the ARC terrorist. After telling Kat she had no comment, Eva rushed to her meeting with Gus Grant, Supervisor of the FBI Technical Operations Group. The agent who let her in pointed to Gus's cubicle.

Eva walked over and said, "Glad you're back. When I last stopped by, your secretary said you'd be out several weeks."

Gus pushed himself up from his chair then leaned against a cane to remain standing. "I wanted to stay home a few more days, but duty calls." He winced as though in pain. "I was telling Trenton when we installed the pen register that I blew my knee out playing soccer. It will heal. You know how busy it is around here."

Eva understood the pull of duty. Last week, she postponed her follow-up visit to the fertility specialist until next month. Scott had not been thrilled, but he didn't seem surprised either.

"Speaking of pen registers and Emile Jubayl, we closed it and shut down the pen registers."

From Gus's expression, Eva sensed he did not comprehend what she was saying. "Maybe you missed that because of your surgery. With Trenton's help, Ari's Terrorism Task Force searched Emile Jubayl's home and business, Helpers International. Is there is a wiretap on his home phone?"

Just watching Gus shift his weight from one leg to the other, Eva's knee felt sore.

After a moment, he nodded fiercely. "Trenton's stinker case? I would know if there was a wiretap on that, it's the talk of the office. We smelled it in here for days." Gus shifted the cane to his other hand, then sat on the corner of his desk. "Nope. No wiretaps. You should have told me you closed the case. The pen registers are still working."

"Still working? Trenton was supposed to tell you to shut down *all* registers on the Jubayls' phones."

"I haven't seen Trenton in awhile. But, I *was* on a lot of pain medication before the surgery. Let's take a look."

Gus stood and hobbled toward the wire room. Eva followed, trying to deal with the news that the registers were still active. She should have checked sooner. He took her to the three pen registers assigned to Emile Jubayl. The register lights were lit. Paper tapes containing called numbers hung from the machines like grocery store receipts.

"Trenton or someone must be servicing the machines, or the tapes would be winding all over the floor. He's a good kid. Ari probably extended the court order and transferred the registers to his group while I was on sick leave."

Gus leaned over and squinted at the court order, taped on the wall above the machines, as did Eva. It was the old one. Nothing new was added.

Gus looked at Eva. "Is it possible that Trenton forgot?"

"Are you sure no wire taps were added to the pen registers while you were out?"

"Positive," Gus said. "If they were, these machines would have been moved next door for monitoring 24/7."

Trouble, like an alarm, rang in her head. Gus was the expert, he should know.

Eva asked, "Could I listen to a call as it comes in through the register?" She hoped Gus said no.

Gus needed a chair to sit on, but the only one in the room was too far away. "Mind if we head back to my office? My knee hurts."

Back in his office, his leg propped on the corner of his desk, Gus said, "I assume you have a good reason for that question and are not trying to see if I'd break the law."

Eva stepped back. "My goodness, Gus. I should have explained. I don't want to listen in, I only need to know if it's possible. Recently, I was told that a piece of evidence used to get the Jubayl search warrant could have come only from someone listening to a telephone conversation. If it is possible, I have an obligation to find out who did it."

Gus thrust back his head so far behind his chair, Eva was afraid he might tip over. When he looked back at Eva, he wore a strange expression. "Remember, I was gone for my operation and not here to monitor everything." His voice ebbed away.

Eva had not meant to put him on the defensive. "Let's get past the fact that the registers are still operating. The question remains, what do we do about an illegal overhear?"

Gus lowered his voice, even though there was no one else in his office, "If a technician or agent had a telephone repairer's handset, he or she could intercept what was being said on the phone call. The caller would not know. I trust you won't broadcast this."

The rubber band holding her hair tightened against her head. Eva ripped it off and ran her fingers through her hair. Harlan might be wrong. Maybe the agents found out about Emile's trip from his travel agent or from George. Yet she had to admit, Harlan had a reputation for scrupulous ethics both before and after leaving the U.S. Attorney's office. Eva had to pursue this, even if it meant finding out things she'd rather not know.

She asked Gus, "Do you keep handsets in the wire room?"

"I'll call you once I find out. Have you told anyone else of your suspicions?"

"Not yet. If a handset was used to listen into a phone call, can we find out who did it?"

As he moved his leg from his desk, Gus stifled a cry. "I have to think about that."

Wednesday morning, Thelma drove Sari home from the hospital. Emile was meeting with his Board of Directors for damage control. While Helpers International issued a statement declaring its innocence, only a few local newspapers carried it. None of the television stations thought it worthy of mentioning.

Sari invited her friend in for tea. "I doubt there is much food. Emile's not a shopper," she said through lips still twisted from the effects of her illness.

"I made him a chicken casserole and brought it over yesterday. Set it on the step over there. I don't see the pan, do you? Let me get your door."

Thelma's help warmed Sari's torn heart. Wintry weather had given way to balmier temperatures. Still, both women were bundled in coats to guard against a howling wind. Sari spied the Palmer's "For Sale" sign and was glad they weren't outside. She had no desire to talk to them. Thelma carried the pink carnations Emile bought, while Sari used her key to open the new solid wood door.

Inside, Sari felt a rush of cold air. Had Emile turned off the heat? Sari closed the front door, but a cold draft blew through the hall.

"My land, what have your two men been doin'? It feels like a window is open," Thelma cried. She set the vase on a hall table and hustled to the living room.

"Sari, come see this!" Thelma called.

Sari drew her jacket around her. She joined her friend, and the two of them faced a broken window. Celery-colored sheer curtains blew in the stiff breeze. Bits of glass glistened on the carpet.

"Look at that!" Thelma pointed to a dark object.

It was a brick with paper tied around it. Icicles of fear lodged in Sari's heart. The doorbell rang.

"Let me answer it," Thelma said efficiently. "Don't touch that brick."

She opened the door a crack, and saw a young woman in a hooded jacket, carrying a pad of paper. Correctly assuming she was a reporter, Thelma put her hands on her hips and declared, "No one's here for you to talk to."

Channel 14's Mary Katherine Kowicki protested. "I was in the car across the street and saw you with another woman. I recognized her face. It was Mrs. Jubayl. It is better for her if she talks."

Instead of saying, 'Or you will make up what you want,' Thelma stuck to her mother's wise words, 'you catch more flies with honey than vinegar,' and said, "She is not able to talk just now. Leave your card. Then she can set up a convenient time. Is that all right?"

With pursed lips, the reporter handed a card to Thelma. "Everyone calls me Kat. If she calls by four, I'll get it on the five o'clock news."

A pinched smile on her face, Thelma closed the door with a click and shoved the card in her pocket. She found Sari staring at the brick.

"I should call the police. Better come with me. There might be someone in the house or maybe somethin's been stolen." Thelma took Sari by the arm to the kitchen, where she dialed 911.

At the kitchen table, Sari held her head in her hands. Her faith had shriveled to a size smaller than a mustard seed. Would their torment never end?

"Officer, what took so long? I called hours ago. Fortunately, there were no bad'uns in the house!" Thelma steamed.

"I had other calls, but I'm here now. What's the problem?" A Jefferson County Sheriff's Deputy, wearing a gray and blue uniform and Stetson hat, removed a notebook and pen from his back pocket.

From the front hall, Sari watched Thelma take the deputy to the living room. He nudged the brick with his boot. She imagined he was thinking he had more important things to do than protect suspected terrorists.

The well scrubbed Deputy turned to Sari and asked, "Do you have any enemies?" Unsmiling, he prepared to write.

"Sir," her mouth drooped, "I've been in the hospital."

As she swayed in the hall, Thelma took over.

"You lie down, honey. I'll take care of this. Go on now."

Sari sighed. With great determination she climbed the stairs. She knew not what Thelma would say. Finding out who threw the brick was impossible. It might have been any one of the millions who saw their faces splashed on television. From habit, she stopped at George's door and put her ear to the wood. He had not come in since she returned from the hospital. She knocked lightly.

No response. Sari opened the door to the worst disaster area she'd ever seen in his room since the agents searched it. The curtains were ripped from the window, which stood open. Clothes spilled from his drawers to the floor. Potato chip wrappers littered the floor. Did George do this or had someone entered the house? Maybe she should get the Sheriff's Deputy to come upstairs.

Even the heat register popped up from the carpet. She walked over to it, stooped to press it down, and saw an object underneath the metal. Sari poked her fingers through the thin metal slats, but her fingers were too large to fit between them. When she pulled back her fingers, they got stuck, which raised the register completely from its position. The register was not attached, but it rested inside the rectangular heat duct. Sari lifted it out and saw duct tape sticking out.

She examined it, and became dizzy. The room spun around her like some carnival ride. Knowing someone hated them enough to throw a brick in their window prevented her from eating any of the chicken casserole Thelma heated earlier. Sari focused her eyes on the dresser. Looking straight ahead helped. Sari tilted her head to the side and pulled on the tape. Like a snake being dragged from its hole, the foot long tape revealed its catch—a small brass box. Sari had never seen it before. She removed the ornate box from the sticky tape.

Inside was a small leather pouch. Curious Sari pulled open the top, but couldn't see the bottom. Over her hand, she held it upside down and shook it. Several stones rolled out. They looked like diamonds, sparkling on her palm. She picked up the largest one, a soft pink gem.

It looked too valuable to be taped under the floor. She put the jewels, if that's what they were, back into the pouch. There was something else in the box. It was a metal key on a gold ring, adorned with a carved cedar tree of Lebanon. As a child, she made drawings of the same tree. The cedar trees of Lebanon were legendary, a national treasure. Sari held the key in her hand. It was too small to fit a car or a door lock.

Sari raised herself from the floor, the box in one hand. After closing the window, she decided not to bother the police officer. No doubt, George was on a tear looking for something and had opened the window. Their son was selfish. Yes, she dared to think that word; he had rushed out and let the cold air stream in.

She rolled the pouch with the gems and the key in her hand. Did Emile give George this key? If so, why was it hidden? Did Emile even know of it? Maybe the gems belonged to one of George's weird friends. But it was all so strange. As she tried to sort it out, an idea formed in her mind. Without replacing the key and pouch, she slid the box back inside the heat duct, re-attached the tape and pressed the metal grate back into the carpet. Sari closed George's door and went to her master bedroom sitting area.

It took her a few moments to decide what to do. Then she pushed the secret find to the back of the bookshelf, her Matthew Henry Commentary as a solid guardian. Neither Emile nor George ever touched her Christian books. But they might. She needed a better hiding place.

It came to her in a flash. Sari emptied the contents of a cold cream jar into a plastic bag. She rinsed the jar out in the sink. The key and pouch went into the jar, covered by a few cotton balls. Sari closed the lid.

Sounds of pounding drew her attention downstairs. Sari changed into her good slacks and turtleneck and packed an overnight bag, including the cold cream jar. She met Thelma at the bottom of the stairs.

"Sorry if Ben woke you. He's boardin' up the window for now. The deputy promised to get right on this." Thelma was all words, as usual, until she saw the overnight bag in her friend's hand.

Sari lifted it slightly and worked her mouth the best she could. "Your house."

"That's more like it, honey. Want to call Emile?"

Sari shook her head.

"Write him a note?"

Sari handed her bag to Thelma. At the hallway table, which was supplied with paper and pens, she dashed off a note that she was staying the night at Thelma's. She folded it in half and wrote his name on the front. Emile could have brought her home. Instead, he came before the doctor arrived, stayed a mere ten minutes, then disappeared again. She knew he had a lot on his mind, but so did she. And he was supposed to be helping her experience less stress. So far, he was failing.

Thelma loaded Sari's bag into the trunk and told Ben they were leaving. He nailed a slab of plywood outside the broken window, then gathered up his tools. Sari locked the front door and walked over to Thelma's car. Ben tipped his ball cap, fired up his diesel truck, and drove away.

Once in Thelma's sedan, Sari began to relax. She needed a full night's sleep and time away to plan what to do. The key and gems disturbed her more than the broken window. They signified something important, hidden like that.

Thelma drove out the driveway, but Sari did not look at her house.

"Your neighbors, the Palmers, are nice people. When the deputy left, they stopped by to see if you were all right. Too bad about their daughter." Thelma sounded worried.

Sari looked at her friend. "What?"

"She had twins, then that terrible car accident. Broke both legs. Her husband is on a Navy carrier. He's on three weeks' leave. The Palmers are sellin' their house to care for their daughter and grand babies."

Sari felt terrible. She was so absorbed with her own misery, she failed to know a tragedy had visited her neighbors. Tomorrow, calling them would be the second thing she would do. The first thing, she would tell to no one, except Thelma. She had to find the answer to the secret key and diamonds.

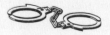

THIRTY ONE

Eva penned approval for Earl to begin a new case. Between him and Griff, her year-end numbers for asset seizures and arrests exceeded last year's. Her mind drifted to the fiftieth anniversary party she was planning for her parents in six weeks. It was to be a surprise. From the guest list, she crossed off the names of those she'd already invited. Marty promised to come to the party on March 14, even though he was flying back from the Netherlands the day before.

Eva missed spending time with her father's father. As a girl, she loved to hear his stories about how his family hid Jews during World War II. She tried to imagine what Marty experienced, losing both parents in less than a month. Alone in the world, except for an aunt in the Netherlands, he sailed there only to be caught in the war when Germany invaded. Eva tried to convince him to write down his experiences. Maybe she should help him.

Her phone rang. Eva flipped shut her personal notebook and answered it.

"Can you come to my office, now?" Gus was all business.

"In two minutes," was her quick reply.

As usual, Wanda was not at her desk. Eva continued down the hall to Griff's office, where he was on the phone. She drew her hands into the shape of a T, signaling time out.

Griff placed his hand over the receiver and mouthed, "What's up?"

She whispered, "I'm going down to the Tech Room. If Brewster calls, we'll call him back at four-thirty his time. Wanda's out for a smoke."

"She needs to quit," Griff mouthed and returned to his call.

A few minutes later, Eva was in Gus's office with the door shut.

He ran a hand along his pant leg, and cleared his throat. "Uh, how do I say this? I guess, I'll just tell you. Sitting in my outbox, was a written request from Trenton to close the pen register. How it got in there without my seeing or signing it remains a mystery."

Eva held up her hand. "No need to explain. You were out with surgery. I'm relieved Trenton gave you the paperwork."

"Me, too," said Gus. "What I'm about to say, keep confidential. I don't want it known to the agents within either of our groups."

Puzzled, Eva said, "All right."

His face red, Gus seemed uncomfortable. "When I worked at the Los Angeles office, someone used monitoring equipment without authorization. We never found out who. Ever since, I install hidden pinhole cameras in the ceiling over the wire and monitoring rooms to film the activities in there."

"Legally, can you do that?"

"It's never been challenged. Persons working in these areas have no expectation of privacy. I don't need a court order, and because they are like public areas, a search warrant is not required. Anyway, in this case, my system worked. It's a time lapse camera that operates at slow motion, with the time and the date recorded in the memory."

Gus turned on a TV monitor and fast forwarded the frame meter on the black-and-white screen. "I went through the wire room pictures for the week before the search warrant was obtained. The night before the search warrant, I found an anomaly. Watch."

He stopped at his intended frame. On the dark screen, the wire room suddenly grew bright. The pen registers were visible with a bird's eye view from the ceiling.

Gus narrated, "Someone just entered the room and turned on the light."

A well built man of medium height, wearing a ball cap, examined the tape protruding from the pen register. Several frames lapsed, and he disappeared from the picture.

"There is a supply cabinet in the corner of the room, which according to my log of equipment, contained a phone repair handset. See what he does," said Gus.

The man returned to the pen register machine and moved it away from the wall. In the jerky movements of the picture, Eva saw that he attached wires at the rear and placed a device similar to a telephone receiver to his ear, resting it on his shoulder.

She drew in her breath. Was he listening to a call?

Gus slapped his thigh with the palm of his hand. "He's violating the Fourth Amendment and the federal eavesdropping law! Who is it?"

Squinting, Eva said, "Zoom in on the ball cap. Are those initials on the front of it?"

"I can't zoom, but I can freeze the frame. Wait a minute. He moves to a better view."

The man stood by the pen register for several minutes, the receiver pressed against his ear. Then he wrote something down. It was too far away for Eva to read anything. He disconnected the handset and shoved the pen register against the wall. When he turned, the front of the baseball cap came into clear view.

"Stop there!" In a circular logo, she saw "Cubs." Eva whispered, "Who could that be? I don't recognize that cap."

Gus unfroze the frame. The picture showed the man walk out of the camera's view. Gus turned off the tape. There was nothing more to see.

"Where did he go when he left the register?" Eva asked.

She still could not believe she witnessed an official violate the law. Maybe he had a court order and that was in Gus's outbox, too. She asked Gus if this was possible.

He shook his head. "No court orders here. Maybe you should ask Ari. I assume whoever listened returned the handset to the cabinet. There are none, now. Maybe it's been discarded. It would have fingerprints."

Eva started to cough. She found a peppermint in her pocket. Savoring it for a moment, she wondered aloud, "I worried it might be Trenton, but I've never seen him in a Chicago Cubs cap. It must be someone else." Eva paused. "Trenton may have lived in Chicago when his dad was an FBI agent there."

Gus replied, "We need to know who was wearing that cap, but the visor shields the face. We need more than that to make a case of eavesdropping,"

"Lock the memory card in your safe, Gus. The Jubayl case was in my group when the pen register warrants were obtained, and I'm Homeland Security. But the listening offense occurred in your group and you are the FBI. I need to decide which agency has jurisdiction."

Eva returned to her office with more questions than answers. She would not investigate it herself. Before she dealt with this new crime, she'd find out if Brewster called. She needed good news, first.

It was 8:42 the next morning. Eva had tossed all night, thinking of the man listening to a phone call without a court order. The ethics officer at the Department of Justice should be in by now. She was wrong. The secretary said he was on vacation in the Bahamas, a good place to be at the end of January. Eva hung up. So much for that idea. Maybe she should let Gus handle this. It was his wire room. Or Ari. The case was assigned to him now. Maybe the man was Ari. She had seen him in a ball cap. Was it a Cubs cap?

Eva swiveled her chair to face the window. On her credenza were snapshots of her family. It was for them that she was trying so hard to shut down the terrorist's money flow, before they hurt more innocent people. Despite her efforts, ARC continued to bomb Americans. Whoever listened to that call was probably driven to catch extremists, too.

What if she and Gus did nothing, for a little while? Their current cases could be compromised if an agent or task force officer was investigated and charged. Defense attorneys would file zillions of suppression motions and argue that evidence in other cases was tainted. Eva knew it wasn't, but it might be hard to convince a judge or jury of that.

Eva touched her family's faces. Scott in shorts and tee shirt hiking in the Blue Ridge last spring. The kids swinging on a tire in her parents' backyard. Kalcy dressed up as Queen Esther, holding Zak. Eva recalled the story of Esther.

Haman wanted to kill the Jews, but Esther was afraid to visit the King and beg him to save her people. If the King refused to hold out a golden scepter when Esther approached him, she would be killed. A message from Esther's uncle, Mordecai, changed her mind. He said that if she remained silent the Jews would be saved by other means, but her family would perish.

Mordecai's next words came to Eva's mind as if they had been there all the time. "And who knows but that you have come to royal position for such a time as this." Eva folded her hands, brought them under her chin, and rested her elbows on her desk.

She remembered her dream of the woman in the yellow silk robe who was the image of Queen Esther and who whispered, "Save my people." Who was she supposed to save? Sari and Emile from Trenton? Or someone else?

Like connecting underground tunnels, one question led to another. She even questioned Trenton's version of the valise. He claimed

Farouk dropped the valise on his foot, but did he really? If law enforcement used illegal evidence, the public would lose faith in the whole American justice system.

For such a time as this. If you do not act, relief will come from another. There was no question really. It was her sworn oath. A crime may have been committed. Maybe God had a special mission for her, to uphold justice in the face of ever-increasing pressure to capture America's enemies.

When her phone rang she was so deep in thought she almost didn't pick it up. Her hand finally put a stop to the persistent ring by lifting the receiver. It was Alexia Kyros, the U.S. Attorney.

Amazed by the timing of the call, Eva said, "I thought of calling you."

"It's funny when that happens. What about?" she asked.

"You first."

"You're on the cutting edge of thorny issues posed by the war on terror. At the next Agency Head meeting, I would like you to update us on the ethical questions, such as, using religious leaders or elected officials as informants."

Alexia had to be kidding. Did she know about the video? Eva gripped the receiver and admitted, "I've just been stuck by one of those thorns."

"Can I help?"

Eva told her about the guy in the wire room. "Which agency has jurisdiction?"

Alexia was quiet a moment, then said, "We must confirm the identity of the listener. How about fingerprints?"

"The handset is missing. The most likely suspects had keys and a right to be in the room so their prints would be there anyway."

"Eva!" Alexia yelled in the phone. "You weren't in management then and you may not know this, but when I leased that building for the Task Force groups, I had a card security system installed."

"We swipe cards when we enter. So what?"

Alexia explained, "The system does more than unlock doors. Our cards are coded. Because each employee's card is distinct, the system can tell which card enters the building as well as the time of entry. It's on a retrievable memory. Do you have a date and time of the illegal overhear?"

"They're on the memory card," Eva breathed.

"My administrator will retrieve the entry data. Can you come over at eleven o'clock?"

Ready to pursue the new lead, Eva remembered something else she wanted to ask Alexia. "Do you have time for another hypothetical?"

"Sure."

"FIG indicted several people for funneling funds to ARC and El Samoud. Hypothetically, if El Samoud can be arrested and delivered to the U.S., can we indict him here in the Eastern District of Virginia?"

"Does it snow in Alaska? What are you saying?"

"We may be in a position to arrest him." She didn't mention she was concerned the ARC leader would disappear like a vapor before her eyes. "I don't want the FBI or military trying to steal away our case."

Alexia said, "As a political appointee, I will go right to the President. El Samoud can be indicted as a continuation of your existing terrorist case. What do you need me to do?"

"The plan is risky. We have an informant who claims he can deliver El Samoud. The Brits are involved but keeping a low profile." Eva forced her mind one step ahead. "I'm going to a strategy meeting tomorrow at three o'clock. If you came with some heavyweights from FBI and Justice that would be a show of force."

Alexia laughed. "The Attorney General and I went to law school together. And Eva, I want to try this case."

A smile appeared on Eva's face. It felt good to have such a respected ally. "Alexia, I am glad you called."

Eva hung up and penciled eleven o'clock on her calendar. Griff walked in.

He said, "NGA has new satellite photos of Socotra in the Indian Ocean. I'm going over, now."

"I want to eyeball those photos myself. It's after nine. Can we make it back by eleven o'clock? I have another meeting."

Griff treated her to a grin. "If I drive."

She followed Griff to the car, wondering if she should tell him about the secret video.

As Eva waited in Alexia's office, she used the time to review plans for the March 14 surprise party for her parents. All the invitations were now in the mail. This weekend she hoped to select a menu with the caterers and buy a dress. Alexia joined her, looking chic in a honey-colored linen suit and pearls. Eva's black slacks and gray blazer felt a bit dated.

"Sorry. I've been reassigning cases. One AUSA is on maternity leave and another just left for private practice. Know any attorneys who would enjoy working with yours truly?" Alexia settled in her chair behind her desk.

In a chair across from her, Eva pictured Jillie getting admitted to the Virginia Bar. The whole family was there. Jillie would have made a great federal prosecutor.

Alexia was pointing to a printout. Eva concentrated on the date.

The U.S. Attorney said, "After 8:30 that night, one card entered the building." She leveled a hard gaze at Eva. "This is the card number." Again she pointed. "And it belongs to Trenton Nash."

Eva asked, "Were there reports of any lost cards?"

Alexia shook her head.

Eva did not want to believe it. The evidence now focused on Trenton and appeared irrefutable.

"I want to see the surveillance pictures," Alexia said.

Eva was not surprised. That is what she told Griff about the satellite photo, and when she had seen ARC's trawler at Hadibu, no larger than a paper clip, she believed her plan could work.

"Gus Grant has secured the memory card."

Alexia replied, "In his search warrant affidavit, Trenton wrote that a confidential informant told him Emile and his son were flying the next day to Beirut."

Her throat dry, Eva needed a cup of coffee. "Harlan Scribbs insists no one knew of Emile's travel plans, except for one phone call to his cousin Duma. Trenton did not learn that from an informant, but by listening to that call, illegally."

Alexia put the printout in a file marked "Confidential" and locked that in her desk. "The evidence is circumstantial, but compelling. I've come across rogue agents who tinker with the law to fit their desired outcome. These things turn out badly for everyone."

Eva clung to a thin strand of hope. "Still, it does not prove Trenton heard anything. We can't hear any conversation he might have heard."

Alexia removed reading glasses connected to a beaded chain around her neck. "While some political appointees might not want to launch a full-scale investigation of one of their own, I must ensure that justice is applied fairly. If Trenton broke the law the trial will be

public, and Americans will see their government does not tolerate illegal searches and seizure."

Eva asked, "What now?"

"I'll refer it to FBI internal affairs. If they find evidence of wrongdoing, the federal Grand Jury will decide if Trenton should be indicted. You may need to testify about what you authorized Trenton
to do."

"The Grand Jury that heard Trenton testify has expired. He was
upset when a Juror revealed she worked at Helpers International. She
did right, while Trenton," Eva stopped. "Well, he is presumed innocent."

Testify against Trenton? If he was wrong, she'd have to, unless he
pleaded guilty.

Alexia stood, as did Eva. "The matter remains confidential. Mention it to no one." Her hand on the doorknob, she added, "Midge
Hopper's working the Jubayl case, but I will decide whether to indict
or exonerate Emile."

"And if Emile is not indicted?"

"I will issue a public apology, if necessary," Alexia replied.

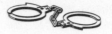

THIRTY TWO

When the sign-in sheet for the February third meeting reached Eva, she checked the titles next to the names. This was the big league. Alexia sat between Eva and Nathan Barlow, Assistant FBI Director for Counter-Terrorism. Griff sat to her right. Other high level officials sat around the long mahogany conference table. Across from Eva were the Assistant Director of Homeland Security and Assistant Attorney General for the Criminal Division. Each reported directly to cabinet officers, who reported to the President.

Eva wore a new gray pinstripe suit, a perfect match to the somber atmosphere. She signed her name and passed the sheet to Alexia, signaling Barlow to begin.

"Our greatest threat, El Samoud, continues to elude us. If we have any hope of catching him, we must find where he operates." Barlow motioned to Eva. "I understand you have a plan to do so."

Quieting her nerves, Eva provided a short overview of FIG's earlier arrests that led them to this point. "We have an idea where El Samoud was last week."

As Eva swallowed, she felt a tickle swell in her throat. She longed for a peppermint, but opted for water instead. They each had a bottle in front of them. She introduced the NGA rep sitting to Griff's right, who insisted on bringing the satellite photos rather than trusting Griff with them.

Eva cued Griff to pass the photographs around the table, then explained, "Keep them moving back to us. The first photo is a distant shot of the Island of Socotra, in the Indian Ocean, between the continents of Asia and Africa. Closer to the nation of Somalia, it belongs to Yemen. Prior to 1967, it was controlled by the British for eighty years. In 1967 it became part of Yemen."

She swallowed to moisten her throat. "It is in a remote and deso-late place, ideal for El Samoud's headquarters. Socotra is seventy-three miles long, thirty-five miles wide, and home to rare frankincense trees. This is a long-distance shot of his villa." She handed it to Griff. "Our source detailed the layout."

Several heads bobbed to see that photo. The next shot was some-what grainy, so Eva pointed to a long dark image at the harbor. "This smaller ship is a research vessel, studying the island's marine life."

She showed them another photo, with a larger object in the har-bor. "Our informant says ARC uses this 526-ton trawler, the *Crescent*, to transport their Supreme Leader and move operations around the globe."

Sounds of amazement echoed throughout the room. Eva had everyone's attention and meant to capitalize on it. She leaned forward, caught a glimmer of satisfaction in Alexia's eyes, and said, "We believe that El Samoud was on Socotra yesterday. First we want to confirm our legal basis for seizing him. Then, because he's hosted by a nation sympathetic to his cause, hammer out the logistics of seizing him."

Eva allowed her words to sink in to the minds of the leaders of the nation's security. Seconds later, she was barraged with questions. In answering them, she tried not to compromise her department's intelligence or give the FBI any room to take over their case.

"We will know El Samoud's future movements based on a highly placed source, whom we have supplied with a satellite phone. Along with British Intelligence, Agent Topping and I debriefed several sourc-es in London."

Eva smiled at Griff. Her eyes hinted it was going well.

Alexia moved her head so that she could see both Eva and Griff, then said, "El Samoud should be brought back to the Eastern District of Virginia for trial. He's linked to your earlier arrest of Farouk Ham-di and his codefendants, so we can charge him with multiple crimes."

"We have to capture him first," Barlow interjected.

Eva gave the satellite photos back to the NGA rep and said, "That's the subject of the second part of our briefing."

Barlow's watch thumped the table. He nodded.

Alexia said, "Wait."

Eva did. Besides graduating from law school with the Attorney General, Barlow's ultimate boss, Alexia was good friends with the First Lady. She was on a roll, and Eva knew enough to stay out of her way.

"I want to make it clear we have jurisdiction. Besides the con-

nection to the Hamdi case, the restaurant bombed in Beirut is head-
quartered in Virginia. Three Americans were killed. ARC took credit
for that as well as the recent attempt on the carrier in Norfolk. Agent
Topping learned that the plane that attempted to crash into the carrier departed from an airfield at Culpeper, Virginia. The U.S. Attorney
there will honor my request to have El Samoud tried in northern
Virginia before Judge Pendergast, perhaps the toughest U.S. District
Court judge in the nation."

Alexia sat back, a perfect smile on her chiseled face.

The Homeland Security official raised a new issue. "What about
the military? They might want to try him as an enemy combatant. We
should at least contact Secretary Cabrini. The Defense Department
could provide vital backup."

Wasn't that the ultimate question? But Eva knew that did not have
to be decided today.

In true diplomatic fashion, she raised a question of her own. "Is it
wise or desirable to have the American military, or law enforcement
officers for that matter, storm a sovereign nation to snatch a terrorist?"

All eyes were on hers.

She continued, "We might get cooperation, but then again we
might not. We considered having El Samoud kidnapped and delivered
to us. Our plan is more subtle."

Eva paused, looked around the table. This was the kicker. Would
they throw the ball back to her or accept it?

She said, "We seize him in international waters."

Eva first heard Barlow's watch thud, then his question, "How will
you do that without federal agents getting killed?"

She turned to the Assistant FBI Director and replied, "Our aim is
to catch him unaware. We could use the Navy's help in what we are
calling Operation Thunderbolt."

After a lively discussion of the plan's pros and cons, with Eva tal-
lying each comment in her mind, Barlow declared, "Ms. Montanna,
your plan looks solid. I will brief the FBI Director tonight."

Homeland Security agreed. The Justice Department promised
full cooperation. Since Scott worked for Defense, Eva was given the
task of securing Secretary Cabrini's help. She had no doubt he would,
but she did wonder how Scott would react to her traveling overseas
again.

In Harlan's law office, a strategy session of another kind was in play. Though his coffee had grown cold, Emile's hand cradled the cup.

He asked tentatively, "Am I going to be arrested?"

With Sari's Bell's palsy, the media attention, and recent threats, Emile doubted they could survive a rigorous trial. If the media scrutiny was this intense while he was simply a "person of interest," a full-blown trial would bring the world's attention to him in ways that might cause a lesser man to go into hiding. That Emile would never do. He intended to prove his innocence.

Harlan replied, "That's why I called the U.S. Attorney. Used to have her job."

"And?" Emile was restless. If only he could stop the imaginary video playing in his head of his being led away by uniformed officers, arms shielding his face, while TV cameras snapped his picture. He had always considered the camera a friend, a way to bring the third world to donors. Now, it was his enemy, with power to ruin their lives.

"There is no arrest warrant. I find it surprising the way they have focused on you."

Was he supposed to find that comforting? Emile had no experience with criminal lawyers. Perhaps none of them exuded empathy.

Harlan hit an intercom button and asked for fresh coffee. A gray-haired woman of about sixty appeared with a carafe. Emile's cup full, she asked if he wanted a new one. Without waiting for his reply, she set down an empty mug, took the cold one, and left.

Harlan poured his client hot coffee. "Drink it," he ordered. "Ms. Kyros said we have a small, a very small, window in which to proffer your innocence. I need you to explain a few things." Harlan's reading glasses perched on his nose. "Tell me what you know about the letter found in your garbage commending terrorists. And this time, do not lie to me."

The way Harlan scowled over the tops of his glasses, Emile thought he looked like a professor about to flunk him. He took a long drink of the hot liquid before saying, "I know nothing about it. Maybe they are lying. Have you seen it?"

"Yes. It is handwritten."

His lips pursed, Emile said nothing.

Harlan continued, "Ms. Kyros was good enough to share that your joint account had a two-hundred and fifty thousand dollar deposit. Defense attorneys usually do not get this kind of discovery until after our client is charged." A friendly smile on his face, Harlan added, "Please explain the money."

Emile jerked from his seat and stalked to the window. Through the blinds, he watched pellets of ice hit the pavement and melt. "The government is making a case against me by twisting circumstances. Do you think it's because Sari and I are Lebanese?"

"Cut the conspiracy theory, Emile. The money. Where did you get it?"

If his lawyer did not believe he was innocent, who would? He sighed. "On my last visit to my mother in London, she wanted to change her will, but there was no time. Instead of giving the five-hundred thousand dollars to Helpers, which her will provided, she wired half of that sum directly to my bank account. It was her gift to me. She did the same for Reni, my sister in London, who I am sure will give you an affidavit."

"Why did your Mother want you to have the money and not Helpers?"

Emile felt guilty enough about her gift. Now, he had to rehash her desires. Harlan probably thought he used undue pressure. Emile turned from the window.

He sat across from Harlan, and used his well formed hands to explain, "In her will—I have a copy—she gave twenty percent of her estate to Helpers International. That would have been roughly five-hundred thousand dollars. By gifting that sum to me and my sister before she died, she reduced the size of her estate. So Helpers got less."

Harlan did some quick math. "Your mother's estate was worth two and a half million? I would like to see that will." His eyes peering over his spectacles, Harlan lectured, "You did not answer my original question."

Emile threw up his hands. "Why she changed her mind? I don't know! She was sick for a while, which gave her time to think. All I know is that out of my gift, I was to wire fifty-thousand dollars to my cousin in Beirut."

"Have you?"

Emile shook his groomed head. "Not once the feds pulled me off the airplane! I was taking Duma an heirloom gold watch from my mother, which they've never returned."

"I'll find out." Harlan made a written note.

Emile leaned over the table, as close to Harlan's face as the wide table allowed. "Get this thing over with! Someone smashed our window with a brick. The police are not banging down any doors to find out who did it. My wife is ill and afraid to stay in the house. I'll do anything to show the government I have not done what they claim!"

Harlan worked up a benign smile. "I hoped you would feel that way. The U.S. Attorney wants you to take an FBI polygraph next week. To prepare, you take a private one first. Be here tomorrow morning at nine o'clock."

"I can't. I have an appointment."

Harlan was out of his seat. "Excuse me. You said you would do *anything* to show the government you are not guilty of what they allege. I suggest you cancel your appointment and get here by eight-thirty to go over the questions."

Thelma ushered Emile into her living room, where soft piano music played on the stereo. She rested her hand on his arm.

"Please sit. Sari is fixin' her hair. Will you stay for dinner? I made two meat loaves."

Emile stayed standing. "Thank you, no. A pile of work awaits me at home."

Thelma planned for his rejection. "I'll pack up the extra loaf with hot baked potatoes."

She hurried to the kitchen and Emile called after her, "That is most kind."

"What is kind?" In the hall, her coat unbuttoned, Sari moved her lips awkwardly.

"She made dinner for us to take home. Ready?" Emile walked to the door, put his hand on the knob and said, "Let's go. I have a lot to do."

Sari followed Emile to the car and tried not to feel bitter that he had not asked how she was. The earlier ice had changed to falling snow. Chills went through her as she got into the car. Thelma, who had thrown on an old sweatshirt, was setting their dinner in the back-seat.

She whispered in Sari's ear, "Call me tomorrow. Remember, God's will be done."

Emile wasted not a moment leaving the drive. On the way home, her husband seemed oblivious to her pain. Sari's deformed face hurt. Tiny blisters had formed in her left ear. The hospital doctor never warned her about those.

She imagined he was thinking about things that bothered her, like broken windows and handcuffs. Emile had never told her if he was cuffed, too. They neared the main road to their house.

He surprised her by asking, "Did you find a letter in George's room agreeing with terrorism, then throw it away? Because if you did, they found it. Tomorrow morning, I have to take a polygraph test."

"Uh, uh." A glob of drool spilled down Sari's chin.

Emile glanced at her. At the petrified look on her face, he said, "Look, I'm not blaming you if you did find it. You might have shown it to me, first." His hands gripped the wheel.

"I, I," she stuttered, "I did—," Her lips felt frozen to her face.

"You found it in George's room!" Emile's anger at her was undisguised. "So the government wasn't lying!"

"I—uh—wrote it."

The traffic light turned red. Emile slammed on the brakes, his tires skidding on the wet pavement. "You wrote it?" he roared. "Why on earth didn't you tell me before?"

Huddled against the cold window, Sari shook with uncontrollable sobs. What had she done? How would she ever make him understand she did it to help them?

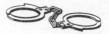

THIRTY THREE

Friday morning, in Harlan's upscale conference room, Emile listened to Darren Fisk, a retired polygraph examiner, show him the workings of the polygraph, a machine that looked like an aluminum briefcase. Fisk seemed capable. But Emile did not understand how the machine measured his heartbeat, blood pressure, and respiration through electrical leads attached to his body. While he heard the details, he wanted to know if the device could tell the truth from a lie.

To ask might imply he would lie, so Emile just listened to Harlan explain that he used Fisk before. The examiner was obliged to keep the day's events confidential. That was fine. But what if Emile failed? The feds would find out and leak it to the media. Harlan said polygraph results were not admissible in federal courts. Even so, agents used them to sort out guilt or innocence in questionable cases. Passing the test could mean his case went away. Which meant, if he didn't, it wouldn't.

Harlan left the room. When Fisk tightened an expandable sensor around Emile's chest, he sensed greater pressure near his heart. Emile's left arm rested on the edge of the table. A thin wire, like black spaghetti, ran from his finger to the polygraph machine, which was out of his eyesight on the table at his left. He did not have to see it to know it was there. His mind and body knew the machine would decide his future. He could not escape the inner voice that taunted him. He was a criminal, going to jail. Just like George.

Fisk was talking to him. "I want you to be comfortable, but sit still during the test. Before I ask the four questions we agreed on, I will first ask five test questions. That's how I monitor your reaction when you lie."

Lie. There it was. Emile felt so uncomfortable at the thought of it, he refused to talk until told to.

Fisk spoke again. "I have the driver's license you gave me. Answer my first three questions truthfully, saying either yes or no. When I ask if this is your date of birth, I want you to lie and say no. Understand?"

Emile barely nodded his head.

Fisk said, "I'll ask the same questions repeatedly and in the same order. Each time I ask if this is your birth date, I want you to lie. That is how I establish a baseline for you."

Once he lied, they would know if he lied again. Incredible. From the corner of his eye, Emile spotted small wands moving across graph paper, recording his body functions on the top of the machine.

"Is your name Emile Jubayl?"

"Yes."

"Are you the CEO of Helpers International?"

"Yes."

Emile saw Fisk make notations on the graph. Beads of perspiration pooled on his forehead and Emile wondered if Fisk noted those on the graph.

Time passed. Several series of baseline questions were asked and Emile lied about his birth date as Fisk requested, "Now I earn my fee. Before I ask you the question about terrorism and banking we agreed upon, I want to make sure you are comfortable."

"I am."

It was quiet for a time. Emile closed his eyes briefly and heard Fisk roll up the fat ribbon of graph paper spitting from the machine.

"Have you ever given financial aid to a known terrorist or terrorist organization?"

"No." Emile opened his eyes but refused to look at Fisk. He heard his scribbling. What did the graph show? Truth or lie?

"Other than the two calls you identified as linked to Hezbollah and your visit to Mr. Wadi, have you had contact with people you knew or suspected were terrorists?"

"No."

After fifteen minutes of repeating the series of four questions, Fisk tore off all the paper and turned off the machine. Emile did not even want to breathe. Not until he knew the results. Fisk disconnected the spaghetti wires and left Emile to wait for Harlan to tell him his future.

Fisk returned with Harlan, who closed the door behind him. He placed his hand on Emile's shoulder and asked the examiner, "Do we take the FBI exam or not?"

Emile held his breath. Fisk wound up the electrical cord, snapped a band around it. "The test did not deviate from the norms of truth-fulness."

Emile looked at Harlan. His heart pounded in his chest. "I failed?"

Harlan smiled at his client, and said with a lilt in his voice, "He means you passed."

The following Tuesday, Trenton looked up in surprise when Ari said without a preamble, "The FBI wants to see your entire file on the Jubayl case." He shrugged, "Routine review, I guess."

An odd request. Trenton shook his head. "Barlow's people combed through it after Emile was taken off the airplane. Is there new evi-dence?"

"Bring it to my office," Ari said and left.

Trenton grew pensive as he walked over to the gray filing cabinet, pulled out the second drawer, and eased out the file against Emile. If it was routine, most likely they had nothing new. On the other hand, if an arrest was near, they might want to scrutinize every fact. The Jubayl file in his arm, Trenton stopped in his office doorway. Maybe his dad could shed light on what the FBI was doing. A strong instinct told him to pick up the phone.

He punched in the numbers to his parent's home. Duke's voice-mail answered. What a disappointment. Trenton told Duke to call, then hung up the phone, reluctant to talk to the FBI about his case. If the guys were anything like Agents Lanning and Quinn, the meeting should be as painless as selecting a DVD.

In Ari's office, Trenton was greeted by cold stares from two sets of hardened eyes. No one shook his hand. Ari was not there.

Trenton held up the bulging file and through tight lips, forced a chuckle. "My evidence against Emile Jubayl."

An African-American agent of medium build opened his cre-dential case and snapped it shut. Trenton saw his gold badge, which trumped Trenton's.

"I am Special Agent Custer. My partner is Special Agent Lee, FBI Internal Affairs."

Internal Affairs! A shudder rippled under Trenton's hairline. He knew from his own experience, and from what his dad had told him, that the only mission of Internal Affairs was to investigate misconduct.

When Lee nodded, her lips were so thin, it looked like she had none. In the fluorescent lights, her silky black hair shone. She shut the door while Custer ticked off Trenton's right to remain silent. His mind froze. What was this, a sick joke? If he needed a Miranda warning, he was in serious trouble.

Agent Custer took out sheets of paper from a folder. "Is this your affidavit for a warrant to search the Jubayl's home? Is that your signature?"

Trenton scanned it carefully. His reply was cautious. "It looks like it. Is there a problem? Do I need an attorney?"

Custer glanced at Lee. "Not if you cooperate and tell us what we want to know."

If he played their game, he might learn something. Trenton set down the folder, but he remained standing, determined not to give them anything.

He asked more casually than he felt, "What do you want to know?"

Custer must have been senior, because he asked the questions. "When the Jubayl home was searched, why did the media show up?"

He smiled and shrugged. "A Fox reporter comes to our office regularly for news tidbits. Probably picked up a reference to it, somehow."

Agent Lee sat on the edge of Ari's desk and wrote down the question and answer.

Her partner continued, "Why was the pen register still working weeks after your former supervisor ordered you to shut it down?"

Trenton eagerly answered, "I filled out the paperwork and shipped it over to Gus Grant. What he did with it was up to him." He pulled a sheet of paper from the top of his file, and waved it in front of Agent Custer. "This is a copy of the form I sent Gus showing that FIG closed the case. Did you talk to him?"

Both agents ignored him. Trenton began to think they were going to be harder to convince than he originally predicted.

"Do you own a Chicago Cubs ballcap?" Custer lobbed this question from out of nowhere.

Trenton stiffened. Why did they want to know about his cap? "Why would I own a Cubs cap? I'm a Yankee fan."

Agent Lee's head snapped toward him. "Answer the question. We know you once lived in Chicago."

Her blistering tone angered Trenton. Her harsh voice was just like that of his aunt when she accused him of killing his sister. Just as he had walked out on her, he would leave these two. They had nothing on him. He'd answer no more of their questions.

He reached down and picked up the file. Before he cleared the door, Agent Lee slid off the desk and pulled a clear plastic envelope from her briefcase.

"The FBI laboratory analyzed this writing tablet and lifted impressions left on the top page. It is a letter purportedly written to a terrorist." She flashed it under Trenton's nose. He recognized the paper. "While you seized half of the letter from a trash pull, this writing pad proves there was more to it. The second half of the letter says the writer has knowledge of someone wearing a ballcap and stealing her garbage. Absent the lower part, it was convincing enough to obtain a search warrant."

Agent Lee's eyes searched Trenton's. "I'll bet you don't know what happened to the bottom half, do you? No wonder you can't remember if you have a Cubs cap." She handed Custer the envelope and turned on the TV.

In a pinched voice, she said, "Watch this, then decide where we go from here."

The black-and-white image on the screen showed a man putting a handset to his ear by the pen register. Trenton stood transfixed as Lee froze the frame on the man's ball cap. The logo screamed out like a fan at a ball game. Cubs!

Where was his cap? In his office? No! It was in his gym bag, in the trunk of his car. They would need a search warrant to get it. He would never consent.

The tape ended and the room grew strangely still.

"I don't know what you think you are doing by showing me that video, but I want to talk to a lawyer. And I don't like you threatening me." Trenton's eyes conveyed what they did in the most heated wrestling match: "Mess with me and you will lose."

Hours passed. Trenton sat in his windowless cubicle. His efforts to reach Duke were futile, which was just as well, as he had no privacy here. He slid on his leather jacket and zipped it to his neck. It was six-thirty and there was no sign of any coworkers. Trenton stalked out, Emile's file under his arm. The office door latched loudly behind him.

Trenton saw no other vehicles in the parking lot. Good. The agents probably left an hour ago. In case someone followed, he drove a circuitous route to his next destination, until he was sure no watchers were behind him. He stopped at a gas station to buy a newspaper. As Trenton drove out of the parking lot, a turquoise car drove in. The driver looked like Hannah!

He stopped by the curb. He had never been to her house. Maybe she lived in the neighborhood. She had not called him back since she missed the appointment with him at GMU, when she went on that errand for Emile. No doubt the FBI had scared her away. Uncomfortable with being the pursued and not the pursuer, Trenton checked his rearview mirror.

A young woman wearing a navy pea coat and gold scarf put a key into her door lock and got back into her car. It looked like Hannah, but was it his imagination? Their long talks filtered through his mind. She drove past his car for the second time. It was Hannah. If only he could talk with her!

He'd follow and see where she went. Turning onto Route 7, Hannah drove past the neighborhood mall, video store, and several gas stations. Trenton ran through a yellow light as it turned red, as did the car behind him. A sickening thought struck him. Maybe Hannah had a date. It would be embarrassing to follow her to another guy's house. His foot stayed on the accelerator, but his mind urged him to back off.

Hannah's left turn signal was on. She suddenly veered into the left lane and turned. Had she seen him? If he turned in behind her, she certainly would spot his car. He drove past that street and into a parking lot. He waited a few seconds for traffic to clear, then aimed his government car, which she had seen at least once, into the right lane. Making an immediate turn, he sped to catch up with her.

Hannah turned into a parking lot at the end of the street. Trenton saw a lighted sign back off the road, "Children's Fun Night. Redeemer Bible Church." He was not going to church, no matter how much he wanted to see Hannah. She got out of her car and removed from her trunk a white board and small artist's case. She'd have no time for him, even if he had the courage to walk inside.

In a split second, Trenton decided to forego his heart and feed his stomach. He'd call her tomorrow. He had something else to take care of. He unzipped his jacket and drove to the first fast food restaurant, the Grilled Onion. He had always wanted to sample their fried onion rings.

The car off, he pressed the trunk release. Before he got out, he checked the mirrors. No one suspicious. A newspaper under his arm, he walked to the trunk. From his athletic bag, Trenton grabbed his Cubs cap, and stuffed it inside his jacket.

He walked straight to the men's room. It was empty. Trenton ditched his cap in the trash container, opened the trash lid and set the newspaper on top. With any luck, it would be hauled to the dump the next day. No one would find it there. He washed and dried his hands, and went to place his order.

His rings and chocolate shake in a paper sack, Trenton stepped hesitantly back to his car. He looked around the parking lot. Everyone seemed to belong. On the way home, he enjoyed eating the rings, but regretted getting rid of his treasured cap. His parents had given him a Yankees ballcap for Christmas. Now might be a good time to start wearing it.

After Trenton drove out of the Grilled Onion parking lot, a man and a woman in an adjacent lot sprang from their car. Dressed in blue jeans and sweatshirts, they were on a mission, but not for food. The woman walked through the restaurant, while the man went to the washroom. Nothing in the empty stall.

Next came the trash can. He pulled out an empty coffee cup, then a wet newspaper, which he scattered on the floor. Reaching back into the trash can his fingers brushed against what felt like the rim of a visor. He tugged out a blue Cubs ball cap. He ran out and signaled the woman with a thumb's up.

Back in the car, the male agent said, "Duke Nash will go crazy. His son hides evidence in the trash at a restaurant connected to terrorists. What must it be like to have such a kid?"

"Custer was right to have us trail him. Seeing him remove something from his trunk, then finding the cap in the trash can, seals his fate. Since you found it, Bob, you write the report."

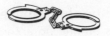

THIRTY FOUR

Several miles off the Socotran coast, Eva pointed to distant mountains. In what she thought sounded like scientific lingo for the benefit of the Omanian crew, she said to Griff and Brewster, "I cannot wait to glimpse the lush Hajhir mountains."

For a brief moment, she thought of Scott and the kids and wondered how they would celebrate Valentine's Day. Another holiday away from home. Eva adjusted the binoculars to see the island. They were still too far out to see much. Minutes later, as they approached Hadibu, Eva scanned the shoreline. The rough outline of a large ship began to emerge.

Griff posed as a novice scientist, but he would secretly board El Samoud's vessel, the *Crescent*. He asked Brewster, "Doctor, will we observe the frankincense trees in the upper regions?"

As the crew scurried to prepare to dock, Brewster explained, "The university arranged for several guides. This afternoon, we will see the trees that the ancients used to cure leprosy, fevers, and as an antidote for hemlock poisoning. We'll photograph the infamous dragon's blood tree, a critical ingredient for violin varnish."

An hour later, the research vessel that they had chartered in Oman was securely docked and their gear unloaded. Eva instructed the charter captain, who spoke broken English, that they would be back for dinner. A few islanders and fishermen lolled about the harbor area. According to plan, as the trio passed by ARC's trawler, they each surveyed a different section of the harbor. Griff slung a leather backpack over his shoulder.

Brewster said loudly in English, "I do not see the guides who were to meet us."

At this cue, Jacques walked to the stern of ARC's trawler and shouted his expected reply, "I speak English. May I help?"

Brewster furthered the ruse by explaining their scientific mission to photograph the island's unique flora, then asked, "Do you know how we can get into town?"

Jacques waved at them, and walked down the gangplank. "Welcome to our island." He lowered his voice. "There is a Jeep over there. Don't look. The driver is one of them."

The Frenchman continued, "Take any other taxi to the Scientific Center where your guides are no doubt enjoying goat's milk. As a gesture of Socotra hospitality, let me invite you to partake some with me when your research is finished. It would be my honor." Jacques tipped his felt cap and walked back to ARC's not-so-secret vessel.

The team avoided the Jeep that Jacques pointed out, and chose instead a driver in a sedan who drove them into the heart of Hadibu. As Jacques predicted, guides were waiting to take them on a walking field trip. Their one donkey was loaded with food and water for the journey.

Binoculars around her neck, Eva marveled. This primitive land contained species of plants and birds not found anywhere on earth. Would this mysterious place be the undoing of El Samoud? Wondering exactly how close she was at that moment to him, Eva wished they could storm the compound Zayed had drawn and take him prisoner. Why wait for another act of terror?

But this was a reconnaissance mission to test and equip Jacques for Operation Thunderbolt, which would not be executed until some unknown point in the future. She would have to be content to wait, but what if they were too late?

Six hours and a hundred photographs later, the American and British research team left the Scientific Center to return to their charter boat. Before getting into the same taxi that had taken them to Hadibu, Eva whispered to her teammates, "Think we'll discover Jacques took El Samoud in the ship and left?"

Brewster's reaction was immediate. "Right. We'd better complete our business without delay." He paid the driver extra to get them to the harbor quickly.

They reached the docks. Eva jumped from the backseat of the taxi, followed by Griff, while Brewster paid the fare. In the growing twilight, she saw the dark outlines of a ship right where they passed it that morning. But there were no lights shining on the *Crescent*. Was Jacques aboard, or was he somewhere else with El Samoud?

By prearranged signal, Brewster removed his pipe, tamped down cherry scented tobacco, and lit it. Eva shifted her backpacks. Griff walked behind her at a slow pace. Shadows fell across the dock and the port side of the ship. Still, they waited for Jacques's signal. As fishermen stowed their nets, Eva turned and saw, back on the street, the Jeep Jacques had warned them about. It was idling on the street at the dock entrance. Was he following them? Probably.

It was now almost dark. A veiled form walked toward them. Eva's eyes narrowed. The shrouded figure grew closer. El Samoud wore a face scarf! Her pulse quickened. She hurried to Brewster and said, "Doc, look behind us."

Brewster turned his head, puffed on his pipe. The darkened form grew closer, carrying a black object that looked suspiciously like an AK-47. Eva hustled toward their charter boat.

Griff's hand moved around to his waist. The veiled figure reached him first. A light came on in a small porthole in the ship. Then, Eva saw the shrouded figure was not a man. She was an old woman, bent over, walking with a stick. The strap over her shoulder was attached to a woven bag. But what was in it?

The woman walked to the gangplank, where she made a guttural sound. Jacques stepped out to the edge and looked around. He replied in Arabic and walked down the plank.

Griff walked over to Eva, "Maybe she's bringing our dinner, direct from her sterile kitchen, or maybe she's talking to Jacques in code."

Jacques took the mesh bag. The woman walked back the way she had come.

Eva and Griff were joined by Brewster. Eva said, "Maybe that bag contains something more potent than dinner."

In their pre-op briefing, they had discussed the possibility that once back on the island, Jacques could easily betray them and his sister. Brewster reached for his hidden knife.

Jacques allayed some of their fears when he held up the bag and said in English, "You doctors are just in time. Our cook brought me fresh goats' milk, cheese, and bread. I am not permitted to invite westerners aboard the ship."

What did he mean by that? They had to get aboard.

Jacques motioned them to follow him to a small shed on the dock that served as the ship's office and store. "Join me for a feast?"

Brewster replied, "We would be honored. I will tell our captain we are delayed."

Eva wasn't going to be denied going home to Scott and her kids by being careless. She stayed just outside the doorway. She could dive into the water if she had to. The ICE agent, posing as research scientist, watched her French informant put bread and cheese on an oilcloth-covered table in the ship's office, then pour goats' milk for his guests, including Brewster who'd returned. She comforted herself with the thought Jacques seemed the type who wanted to live long enough to spend his millions.

In a low voice, Jacques said, "I spend much time down here on the docks. Others from ARC are used to me mixing with visitors. Eat."

They sat on three-legged stools. Eva took a hunk of bread, but kept it in her hand until she could get rid of it. She'd go hungry rather than eat Jacques' food. She still did not completely trust the giant man, who had not been told of their exact plan.

Eva nodded toward Griff and said, "He is one of the FBI's fore-most electronics experts and will outfit your ship with some of the latest equipment."

Jacques looked cautiously down the dock, lit only from the ship's small porthole.

"Come aboard in the middle of the night after everyone is in bed. I will help you."

Griff asked about the ship's engines, electric system, and fuel sup-ply systems. The food remained largely uneaten except by Jacques who consumed a loaf of bread and several chunks of cheese. He wiped off his moustache and beard with his hand and turned to Brewster.

"How is Camille? I assume you're looking after her."

Brewster replied, "Your sister sends word, she is well. She is anx-ious to be released, when you complete your mission for us."

Jacques nodded. "Now, I will tell you. There is a development."

Before Griff snuck into the *Crescent's* engine room, Eva and Brewster had assured him the charter boat crew was asleep. His two team mem-bers watched nearby and would let him know, via miniature two-way radios, of anything suspicious.

In the belly of the ship, a small flashlight held between his teeth, Griff was on his back, wedged between the bulkhead and the engine. In the near total darkness, he felt cold grease and oil seep through his shirt, and something more ominous. In the musty, cramped confines, Griff felt close to panic. When he flew a Cessna Skyhawk, Griff never suffered from claustrophobia in the small plane. Probably because he could see outside, and he was in control of his environment. Tonight, his dread of being closed in gripped him with the force of a mighty storm.

For some minutes, he was powerless to do anything but take short breaths and sweat profusely. Griff squeezed shut his eyes and reminded himself that, as soon as he completed his work, he could escape his temporary prison. If he could fly in small planes and choppers, he could do this. He would do it.

Griff felt the pounding in his ears subside. While sweat dripped from the wire that ran under his shirt up to his earpiece, he was composed enough to begin his task. Static rattled, then Brewster's distinct accent blasted Griff's ear as he said to Eva, "Still quiet by you?"

Griff lowered the volume on the radio mounted on his belt. He heard Eva's reply, "I saw a few varmints. The four-legged kind. Goats wandering around. Griff, everything okay?"

He removed the light from between his teeth and whispered into the microphone clipped near his neck, "Need another hour down here. Keep an eye out for Jacques or his crew."

Eva's voice crackled in his ear. "10-4."

Griff made Jacques draw a sketch of the ship's systems, then go to his quarters to sleep. That way, if Americans and a Brit were discovered on his ship, Jacques could deny knowing about it. As he spliced two wires above his head, Griff blocked from his mind how long it would take to finish.

Brewster's accent and the strong smell of diesel fuel reminded him this was unlike any installation he'd made in the U.S. Griff was used to sneaking into homes, offices, and cars to install court-ordered listening or tracking devices. This was his first secret job in a foreign country, let alone in the inner-sanctum of the world's most wanted killers.

Over the next hour, Griff installed the transponder in the ship's electrical system. Then he used a test device to verify a steady electrical signal was being transmitted by the ship's radio antenna and received by a U.S. Defense satellite above the earth. Griff watched the LED screen of his monitor. Would it display the GPS location of the *Crescent* at the dock in Hadibu, Socotra? Yes. It worked! Now, they could find the ship no matter where it went.

Griff called Eva on the radio, and whispered, "I'm about to install your little surprise."

When done, Griff conducted a final test. He was satisfied. ARC's trawler was now a pawn in the hands of U.S. law enforcement. He packed up his tools, every bit of wire insulation, then checked again. Once, he'd inadvertently left his pliers on the floor next to a Congressman's bedside stand. He never wanted to live through that again, especially on a terrorist-infested island. Nothing hinted of his presence, except for the equipment he had hidden so well he doubted even Jacques could find it.

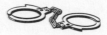

THIRTY FIVE

Emile waited with Harlan in the FBI reception area. Two American flags were displayed in floor stands, and a round FBI seal hung on the wall above their heads. Since he passed the private polygraph with flying colors, Emile was not as nervous. But the constant filtering in and out of federal agents frayed his nerves. Which one was trying to charge him with a crime?

A smiling receptionist wearing enormous glasses sat behind a massive wall of bulletproof glass. She pushed a buzzer for agents to pass through an inner door. Emile watched as one younger man approached the door, but there was no buzz. With a thud, his body folded against the solid wood door.

Emile did not hide his chuckle. Good. He hoped all the agents collided with an impassable barrier, including whoever was hooking up the lie detector machine. He or she deserved to be as stressed as he. The rookie agent stepped back, removed his leather credential holder from his pocket and showed it to the receptionist. "It's my first week here," he admitted sheepishly.

She tapped her temple with her finger, then buzzed him in. She beckoned for Harlan to approach her station. He stooped to get his ear near the small hole. She said, "Mr. Rosen will be right out."

Looking confused, Harlan asked, "I understood Trenton Nash is the investigator."

The receptionist dismissed him with a shrug. Before Harlan returned to his seat, the door with the buzzer opened and a man with thick black hair held it with his foot. He summoned Harlan and Emile inside, shook their hands, and introduced himself "Ari Rosen, supervisor of the Terrorism Task Force. Investigator Nash has been detained. Follow me."

Emile walked down the hallway past several agents wearing suits that no doubt concealed guns. He really felt tense, sure this operator would not be as nice as the one Harlan hired. Ari stopped at a door posted with a "Do Not Disturb" sign.

He said, "Mr. Scribbs and I will agree on the questions to be asked." He turned to Emile with a smile, "Then, we leave you with the examiner."

His heart thumping, Emile followed his attorney into the examining room. He glanced around. It looked bland, but his future would be made or destroyed in this room. Emile's eyes went past the desk to the glittering machine at the end of the table.

The polygraph looked the same. Would he react the same? A woman in a navy pantsuit stood by the examiner's chair. His eyes moved to the other chair. With its elevated concave arms, and wires draped across the back, Emile thought it looked like an electric chair he had seen once in a movie. He let out a long, slow breath he could never take back. This was it.

Ari Rosen introduced the woman as Special Agent Haddad. His examiner was petite, young enough to be his daughter, and reminded Emile of an earlier version of his sister, Reni. He was comforted by her appearance and found himself relaxing, a little.

Harlan negotiated the four crucial questions with Agent Haddad and Ari. After a series of generic preliminary questions, Emile would be asked the same questions as his private test, except for one. It was that one which concerned him.

Now alone with Emile, Agent Haddad hooked up a wire around his chest. He felt her tighten it. Emile was strangely thankful for the test polygraph in Harlan's office. Otherwise, he might pass out from fear. If he failed this one, he might be charged as a terrorist and wind up in prison.

This time he was used to the sounds of the machine and the examiner's pen scratching. Yet his heart beat irregularly. Even though the routine questions were exactly as before, Emile could not get the new question from his mind. *Concentrate on what she is asking you, fool, or you will fail.*

He breathed deeply. As Agent Haddad wrote something down, Emile watched her eyes and recalled Reni chopping spearmint for tabbouleh. Then, Agent Haddad asked her first question about terrorism, and Emile realized that, by taking an FBI polygraph, he had played right into the feds' hands!

Emile dreaded the question about Hezbollah. His palms began to sweat, and his breathing was uneven. The more he tried to control it, the more he dwelt on the test results and the more moist became his hands.

"Have you given financial support to Hezbollah in Lebanon?"

This was the question he felt was structured as a trap. "No."

A blast of air followed. The test continued. Haddad made her scratches. Emile tried to be calm, but he knew that question would be asked again. He was right.

In a moment, she asked, "Have you given financial support to Hezbollah in Lebanon?"

He steeled his body. "No."

Emile thought she overemphasized the word "Lebanon." Why? From the corner of his eye, he saw Agent Haddad close her notebook.

"I want you to relax," she said.

It was over. He passed!

Emile watched her hold the scroll of graph paper protruding from the machine and examine it as it passed through her hands.

At length, she spoke. "I am not able to pass you. You are showing deception."

Emile was crushed. He'd been trapped, and his own lawyer was to blame. Beneath his starched white shirt, rivers of moisture ran down his sides.

Haddad looked at him with sincere brown eyes. "Help me understand why I detect deception."

This was some kind of interrogation technique. Emile said flatly, "I have done none of the things of which I am accused."

Agent Haddad pulled her chair next to his. She looked so much like his sister, he was tempted to ask about her family. Then a sinister thought occurred to him. The FBI probably used Chinese examiners to test Chinese suspects, Japanese for Japanese, and so on. That Haddad was his examiner had to be more than a twisted coincidence. They probably had a photo of his sister, too. When Emile inhaled, the smell of perspiration was overwhelming—and it was not from Ms. Haddad. She had him right where she wanted him.

"When you denied giving financial support to Hezbollah in Lebanon, the reaction of the needles on my machine says otherwise. Is it Hezbollah that troubles you? Or Lebanon, or both?" Her eyes were friendly. "I want to help. If we end the test this way, I have to report you are lying."

Emile feared that question would trip him up, and it did. What could he say? Maybe the truth. With the lie detector turned off, he told of his emotional ties to Lebanon, including the death of his brother. He casually mentioned that Hezbollah was involved in various layers of society.

"I am never sure of the sympathies of people, even those I know well. In fact, my cousin Duma was courted by Hezbollah while in college." His look, the one that swayed many a reluctant donor, was sincere. "My wife Sari and I are sympathetic to the Lebanese, but we remain totally loyal to our adopted country, the United States of America."

Ms. Haddad interrupted his passionate defense. "Tell me about your relationship with Duma. Is his name Jubayl also?"

Emile nodded, then told her he and Duma were as close as brothers and of their contacts prior to his mother's funeral.

As though she were a psychologist, Haddad asked, "And you feel responsible for him?"

"I do. Mainly because so many family members were hurt by the violence in Beirut, and Duma still lives there."

She probed more deeply. "Have you sent money to Duma?"

"Several times he hinted of hardships and I sent a thousand dollars. That's legal."

"Is Duma still involved with Hezbollah?"

How did Haddad know these things? "I wonder about his financial dealings. That is one reason I do not send him more money."

Emile refused to tell her about Duma's $50,000 from his mother, which he had yet to send.

The examiner leaned forward. "When I asked you the question about support for Hezbollah in Lebanon, were you thinking about Duma?"

If this explained possible deception, he would agree to it. "Yes, but I did not how know to give more than a yes or no answer."

Satisfied, Agent Haddad smiled ever so slightly. She placed a hand on Emile's arm that was attached to the electrical wire. "Such thoughts could impact the test. I will rephrase that question and run the test again."

Emile did not know how to react. Was this all part of the FBI's effort to get him to confess something, or was she really interested in arriving at the truth? Did she have any way of knowing how much he sent to Duma or what he did with the money?

Agent Haddad returned to her chair just outside Emile's line of sight, but he could see her open the notebook. "I am going to ask you the same questions, but will change the troublesome question to this, 'Other than funds sent to your cousin, Duma Jubayl, have you given support to Hezbollah in Lebanon?'"

Feeling slightly at ease, Emile replied, "That is much better."

"Relax and breathe normally. The test is about to begin."

Twenty minutes later, Ari Rosen entered the reception area where Harlan was reading a file to make use of his billable time. Ari cleared his throat to get Harlan's attention. "Ms. Haddad is finished. We can join her now."

Harlan bundled up his file and followed Ari to the examining room, which smelled like a gymnasium. Emile was disconnected from the machine and sitting in a different chair.

Agent Haddad wasted no time blurting out, "We had trouble clearing Emile. Once we discovered the issue that bothered him, we completed the test. No deception was detected."

Emile gave Harlan a puzzled look. Harlan briefly shook his head. He would never approach a snarling dog, and he was not about to have her explain the trouble.

Instead he asked, "Will that be the official conclusion in your report?"

Agent Haddad flashed a beautiful smile and nodded. "Yes."

Ari extended his hand to Emile. "I will call Alexia Kyros with the results. You may not have to wait long for this case to be resolved."

In the quiet of the elevator, Emile asked Harlan, "Is it too soon to sue the government?"

His attorney looked incredulous. "We've convinced them not to charge you based on your passing the polygraph, but there is sufficient evidence for a more ambitious prosecutor to indict you. Why do you want to poke a stick in their eye?"

Emile's jaw dropped a fraction. "They could do that? Forget I mentioned it."

Having spent the last six months working with federal agents, Trenton had mixed feelings as he stepped into the Jefferson County Sheriff's Office. The crackle from the radio room, and the dispatcher speaking to the deputies in their cars, reminded him of his first day riding solo. He answered a call for a home invasion and found a boy hiding in a tree in the back yard, his cheek mottled black and blue. The child was afraid to talk at first, but Trenton coaxed him down. He admitted his father struck him because he'd left the door unlocked when he came home from school. Trenton brought the child to Child Welfare. Where was that boy now, six years later?

Duncan called yesterday, asked to see him. Trenton suspected Custer and Lee had paid the seasoned sheriff a visit. Let them try to find his Cubs cap. By now, it was probably buried beneath heaps of garbage at the dump. Tamping down a feeling of despair, he knocked on Duncan's door.

"Come in," the Sheriff said.

Trenton entered Duncan's compact office, where everything was in order, down to one pad and one pen resting on the metal desk. A former Marine, Duncan did not favor frills of any kind and did not waste time on small talk.

He motioned toward a chair across from his desk. "Sit, Nash."

Trenton did as he was told.

Duncan opened his top desk drawer, drew out a typed paper, and handed it to Trenton. "It's your resignation letter. Sign it."

Trenton took the letter and stared at it as though in a trance.

"The FBI paid me a visit. I do not like their allegations that you broke the law, maybe more than one, trying to build a criminal case. It's hard enough to read disparaging news about the Jefferson County Sheriff's Department. I can't tolerate a deputy gone bad. At least the news will read, 'former' deputy is investigated for illegal conduct."

Trenton interrupted, "Nothing is proven against me!" Even to his own ears, he sounded desperate.

"Too late for that." Duncan's cropped gray hair looked like polished steel, just like his voice sounded. "I told you when you were hired, your badge was more than a symbol. It is a badge of honor. I do not allow my deputies to carry even a whiff of scandal."

"Sheriff, let me explain." Trenton unzipped his jacket.

Duncan held up his hand. "Save it for a judge or jury." He pointed to the letter. "After you sign that, I want your badge and credentials. Nash, you are fired."

Trenton yanked the pen off Duncan's desk and signed the resignation letter without reading it. If Duncan could treat him so coldly after Trenton tried for years to make him look good, he had no regrets. Angrily, Trenton took the equipment from his pockets.

"Your gun, too, Nash. Set it down, carefully."

Trenton removed the pistol from his shoulder holster, and laid it on top of Duncan's legal pad. Trenton stood and said, "After all these years, at least you could have heard me out." He was tempted to add, "I won't forget this," but thought better of it. A threat charge on top of everything else would not be good.

Trenton Nash stormed out of the Sheriff's office without looking back. Unemployed and facing criminal charges, Trenton did the only thing he could think of. He walked down the steps toward his government car and called his dad on his cell phone.

While the phone rang, Trenton saw two people leaning against his car. He recognized the long black hair of Agent Lee and the large frame of Agent Custer. Without realizing it, he pulled the cell phone away from his ear, and his anger anything but in check, Trenton challenged the FBI Agents, "What do you think you're doing?"

Agent Custer walked toward him. "Nash, since you are no longer employed, you do not need this nice government car."

"Says who?" Trenton backed up a few steps.

Agent Lee swung around by her partner. "The federal Grand Jury. They indicted you for theft of government property, illegal eavesdropping, obstruction of justice, and lying under oath." She waved a paper. "You're under arrest." From her coat pocket, she withdrew a pair of handcuffs exactly like the ones Trenton used on Farouk.

Trenton shoved the cell phone in his pocket and put his hands behind his back.

How had it come to this? Trenton sat on a scuffed bench in the Alexandria City Jail, where the federal government housed its northern Virginia prisoners. He refused to look at the drunk drivers, thieves and crooks in the large holding cell. At least his dad wouldn't see him in this place. His one phone call was placed to the defense attorney Eva used to kid him about. The guy promised to meet him at his arraignment that afternoon.

Someone nudged his toe. "Think you're better than the rest of us, huh?"

Trenton ignored the barb. Out of the corner of his eye, Trenton stole a glance at a skinny man, whose arm was crawling with a snake tattoo. The blue-and-red snake seemed familiar. Hadn't he once arrested a guy for fighting with his wife who had a tattoo like that?

Trenton flexed his arms, ready to defend himself. The prisoner kicked his foot.

Trenton snapped to his full height, his eyes blazing. "Go bother someone else." He rolled his hands into fists.

The burly prisoner edged closer. "You're the one, all right. You arrested me in Jefferson County. Whad'ya do to get in here?"

"Beat it, buddy." With no legal authority in this place, Trenton still had plenty of the bravado he had used his entire life to succeed. He wouldn't back down now, even if it meant bloodying the guy's lip.

A jail guard stepped to the cell door. "Nash, you have a visitor."

His lawyer must have come early. Taking advantage of the reprieve, Trenton left his adversary without looking back. Minutes later, he was ushered into a small room marked "Professional Visitors."

The guard remarked, "I'll be back."

As the man in the gray suit turned, a bolt of pain caught Trenton off guard. It wasn't his lawyer. It was his dad!

"How did you know?"

Without one word, Duke did the unexpected. He engulfed his only child in a bear hug. Trenton would have been more comfortable with a tongue lashing.

Duke released him. "You called me on your cell phone, remember? I heard Agents Custer and Lee put you under arrest. I heard them criticize you in the transport vehicle. No one turned off your phone!"

Duke Nash's face was so white, the skin under his eyes was blue.

"Dad, I'm sorry." He had no idea what else to say.

"Son, I am glad to hear you say so. Your mother and I want you to know, whatever you have done, we will stand by you, as long as you take responsibility. No excuses, or legal mumbo jumbo. You tell me what you did, we'll face it together, with God's help."

Trenton's shoulders slumped. "I called a lawyer," he managed.

"Who?"

"Bernie Miller."

"That radical? It will send the wrong message to the Judge. You need Harlan Scribbs. All the federal judges respect him."

Trenton shook his head. "I can't. He's representing the guy I was investigating."

Duke was thoughtful. "Harlan's old partner went on his own a couple years ago. I'll give Stan Ritchey a call. He is a former AUSA, too."

If Trenton told Duke everything, could he understand what it was like to be accused of wrongdoing? He doubted it.

"Dad, I can explain."

Duke replied, "There were times in my career, I had to decide whether to cross that imaginary line. Remember the hostage case?"

Of course Trenton did. Hadn't he bragged about it more than once?

"After I fired my gun, I had miles of paperwork to fill out because I killed the hostage taker. Even though I did everything by the book, human rights advocates criticized me and waged protests in the community, claiming I should have taken the terrorist alive. I am no lightweight when it comes to scrutiny."

Trenton needed his dad's support but the two situations were different. His head slumped. "I didn't do everything by the book."

Duke laid a hand on his shoulder. "From what I heard Agent Lee say, I suspected as much. Don't tell me in here. Let me call Stan. Bail will be set, and you'll be released after your arraignment. Son, do not talk to anyone in here about anything."

Trenton was comforted by his father's presence, and for the first time in his life, the urge to compete with him was gone.

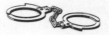

THIRTY SIX

Outside at Dulles Airport, Eva ducked her head and climbed into the back seat of Nathan Barlow's stretch Mercury limo, driven by the agent assigned to guard the Assistant Director. Griff stepped in and sat next to her. In the seat across from them, Barlow said, "What is so urgent to call me from my home at ten o'clock?"

Lights from the Dulles toll road flickered over Barlow's face. He did not look happy.

She said, "You need to know something of vital importance. The plane had no secure phones." From habit, Eva lowered her voice. "Our source told us before we left Socotra that he was ordered to prepare for an extended period at sea."

"What does that mean?" Barlow asked.

"There is no way to sugarcoat it," Eva replied. "El Samoud is preparing to launch the largest ever coordinated attack against Western and Jewish targets during the Jewish holiday of Purim. According to my calendar, that's March 14."

Three weeks away, and the very day she planned to celebrate her parents' fiftieth wedding anniversary! Now she understood the dream urging her to save Queen Esther's people. It had been another premonition. In the backseat of the limo, Eva lifted up a silent prayer for courage.

In her silence, Griff interjected, "Jacques knew only the date, not where."

Eva added, "Mr. Barlow, Jacques did say that El Samoud sees it as one massive attack around the world. My guess is Israel will be a target."

The gravity of the situation touched her deeply. It could be a replay of September 11, or worse.

"Who else knows?" Barlow asked.

"The MI–5 agent landed in London a few hours ago. I'm sure by now, he's elevated it up the chain of British intelligence."

Eva saw they had connected with Route 66. Where were they going?

Barlow finally said, "You were right to call me." He picked up the secure phone, entered a number, then said, "Alexia, I have the agents. Yes," he nodded, "even more so. Meet us in my office in thirty minutes. The guards will let you in."

Barlow also called the Director of the FBI, so he could notify the Director of Homeland Security Director and the Attorney General. Eva glanced at Griff. So, this was what it was like to be in the inner circle during a crisis. The wheels of the U.S. government rolled along to protect its citizens. She kept to herself two burning questions. Did Farouk know of El Samoud's Purim plot, and was he playing another dangerous game?

Two days later, Hannah carried a box of pamphlets when Emile asked her to come to his office. She followed him down the wide hall. Her boss left the door open and asked when she would graduate.

"After this semester, I take two classes over the summer. I have an internship, which I hope will be at the Washington Star." She added, "It's twelve hours a week. I would like to continue my part-time job here, if that's okay."

Emile told her she fit in well. Then he handed her the day's newspaper.

"Speaking of the Washington Star," he said, "Turn to page four."

Hannah set her bundle on his desk and flipped through the pages. A photo jumped out at her. It was Trenton, being led into the courthouse, hands cuffed behind his back! The headline blared, "Former Deputy Sheriff Indicted for Obstruction of Justice." Hannah dropped the paper on his desk with a questioning look. Why did he want her to see it?

"Since journalism is your major, I thought you might like to see the other side of the story. Deputy Nash was the one after us. I hear he is against religion."

Hannah sensed Emile watching her closely. Maybe he knew that she talked with Trenton, and this was a test. He probably brought her in to fire her. She inhaled deeply. Honesty was best. Well, up to a point. Her boss had not actually asked if she knew him.

"Mr. Jubayl, Trenton Nash attends George Mason. We met there a couple of times. I told him about our wonderful mission. He seemed truly interested."

Emile snatched up the paper and scrutinized Trenton's face in the photo. "I have no doubt he was, Hannah."

"What did he do wrong?"

Emile carefully folded the newspaper and set it on the edge of his desk. "He made up the whole thing. We are not associated with terrorists!"

Hannah suddenly felt a wave of guilt. She had been worried about her job, while Trenton, an officer she had come to trust, was in deep trouble. She pointed to the paper and asked softly, "May I read it in the break room?"

Emile waved away the paper and sat behind his desk.

She said, "The Star and the TV stations will have to retract what they said about you."

Emile looked at her sharply. "That is exactly what I will tell my attorney."

She turned and left him to make his call. In her heart, she grieved for Trenton. Hannah found a quiet place to read and pray for him. He needed God's help now, more than ever.

"Happy Birthday, darling, a day early," Eva said.

They were celebrating Scott's March 1 birthday a day early with dinner at Lo's, a Chinese restaurant near their home. For the occasion, Eva wore a long-sleeved lavender dress and the gold heart necklace from Scott. She was overdressed for the neighborhood eatery, yet Scott rarely saw her in anything but sweats or a suit. Eva gave him a square package wrapped in fly fishing paper. Scott shook it, then tore off the wrap. He lifted out a watch with a leather strap.

"It's perfect, Eva Marie. Thanks." He put it on his left wrist. His old one now had a home somewhere in Kazakhstan, where he had lost it.

"See the multiple time zones?"

Eva was glad to have gotten something he needed, but she was beginning to worry about the kids. The sitter was new, and Eva wanted to give Andy his nebulizer treatment before bed.

"Dinner was great, but shouldn't we get back?"

Scott grabbed her hand. "A few more minutes won't hurt. What's happening with your overseas case? Since you got back, we've barely had time to say hello and good night."

Eva rested her hand inside Scott's warm one. "You know the threat level was raised again to orange. The borders are tightened, and no new visas are being issued."

Scott nodded. She looked around. There were only a few diners scattered around the restaurant. Still, she did not want to take chances.

"Let's go. I'll tell you in the car."

Scott paid the bill. On the way, Eva reached over, hugged his neck and whispered, "It's my case!"

Scott turned his head and the little bug swerved. "Why whisper? Only I can hear."

"Scott, remember the meeting you arranged for me with Chief of Naval Operations staff? I have to meet with them again tomorrow. I want you to be there, but it's restricted. Ask Secretary Cabrini if you can join in."

Scott drove into the driveway. As the garage door opened, he said, "My job deals with the media. Maybe it's better if I don't know the details. That way if they ask, I know nothing."

Eva shook her head. "I wish you would come. The Defense Department will need a press release prepared, just in case. This operation is risky. We may have to take the kids to my folks. Pull them out of school." Her voice broke.

Scott asked, "Are you crying?"

As if caught, she quickly wiped her eyes. "Honey," she stopped. She needed to tell him. "I have a terrible sense if I go out there, I may not come back." This was no vision or dream. She had not had any of those since the woman in yellow silk. After that, she'd started praying regularly. This was something different.

Eva choked back a sob. That was all it took for Scott to reach out and hold her tightly. They did not feel the cool night air, nor the time that passed. With that embrace, Eva assured Scott she needed him, which was something she had not done in a long time.

Emile called Sari an hour ago, not to check on how she was doing, but to boast about the arrest of the officer investigating them. She walked by the mirror on her dresser. Most days, she dreaded looking at her face. Today, she studied what she had become. A living wreck. Emile said Deputy Nash was to blame, and he rejoiced in the man's fall.

Her lip drooped on the left side of her face, and she used her finger to close and open her eye lid. That eye could not even blink to moisten itself. The blisters in her ear cleared up after several weeks. Sari brushed her hair, now flecked with gray. Maybe she should color it back to deep brown.

After Emile called to gloat, Sari thought her husband was right. Nash had caused them tremendous pain and insult. She felt glad that justice was finally done. Then she had read Psalm 27. "Be strong and take heart and wait for the Lord." Now she felt uneasy.

She got out the cold cream jar, swiveled off the top and plucked off the cotton balls. Sari stared at the gems and the silver key with squared off teeth. The mystery of them haunted her many nights. She showed them to Thelma, who cautioned against sticking her nose where it did not belong.

"Sari," she had said, "if God means for you to find out, he will make a way."

Sari had replied, "Why did I find this in the first place, then?"

Thelma was silenced, and Sari found a new obsession—finding what the key opened. She tried every suitcase and toolbox. None had locks large enough for the key. The brass box she found it in had no keyhole. Unlike any key for their cars or house, it had no grooves.

Sari fingered the cedar tree on the key ring. Maybe the ring meant the key belonged in Lebanon. If so, she'd never find what it opened. Maybe Thelma's advice was wise. She should throw it away and forget it. But, the gems were not so easily disposed of. Thelma said they looked like diamonds. What if George had stolen them?

Wait for the Lord. That she could do. Sari dropped the key back into the jar, closed it, and shut the drawer. Sari ran the brush once more through her shoulder length hair, then donned a plum wool dress and gold chain Emile brought back from their homeland. She walked down the stairs to start his favorite Lebanese meal, tabbouleh salad and fish fillets with sesame seeds.

In the kitchen, she found her apron. Preparing the Lebanese delicacies brought life to her heart. Perhaps she and Emile would talk at dinner as they used to before George became a teenager. Thoughts of her son deflated her buoyancy. He flatly refused to attend church when Emile asked him to, the day Sari was rushed to the hospital. Maybe that was just as well. Emile tried to talk to him. George stormed out, claiming his dad hated him, and Emile was unaware she heard it all. George had come home once, asking for money. Sari had none in the house that day and told him so. She had not seen him since.

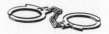

THIRTY SEVEN

The next morning, Eva stood in the rear of the Justice Department press room. In a trim leather jacket and wool slacks, she blended in with reporters and staff. Alexia Kyros walked to the microphones, alone. Nathan Barlow stayed in back, next to Eva, which made it easier for Alexia to avoid answering certain questions.

"I will read a short statement," Alexia began.

At words condemning Trenton's illegal acts, Eva wanted to plug her ears. Alexia announced his guilty plea that morning to obstruction of justice.

"In return for his plea today to that one count, all other charges against him are dropped. He will be sentenced in ten days."

A reporter shouted, "What about the Jubayl family? Are they suing the government?"

Alexia ignored the outburst. Beside Eva, Nathan Barlow squirmed.

Eva's muted cell phone tickled her waist. She had an incoming call. Instinctively, she felt for it, wondering if it was an emergency. Was this the moment she'd drop everything and head for Socotra?

The vibration stopped. Alexia apologized to Emile and Sari Jubayl, neither of whom were there. Eva did not blame them for staying out of the spotlight. They already had a large dose of publicity.

When Alexia gave details about the case that undid Trenton, Eva thought she'd said enough. "The U.S. Government closed its case against Emile Jubayl. We regret the difficulty caused to them as a result of Nash's illegal act. George Jubayl entered a plea of guilty to misdemeanor assault at the State Department and paid a five-hundred-dollar fine. He has not been implicated in any role in the bombing."

Alexia praised the good works of Helpers International while Eva's phone whirled again. It did not ring aloud, but she was distracted by it.

Alexia might be offended if Eva left before the press conference was over. The reporters peppered Alexia with questions, which she fielded herself. Eva decided to stay a few more minutes.

Then, Alexia announced, "Thank you all for coming."

Eva was relieved. Her name had not been mentioned. She slipped out before the swarm of reporters beat her to the door and hurried to the elevator, where she waited.

Someone said in a loud voice, "Mrs. Montanna, you said you were going to give me a heads-up on a new case. Is this the one? Because I don't remember getting a call from you."

That could only be one person. Eva pressed the down button again and looked over her shoulder at Kat, the reporter, pen and pad in hand.

Eva answered, "I said I would call and I will, at the appropriate time. What happened to the Jubayls is exactly why I do not leak information to the media. I want to be sure we have it right."

The elevator arrived and the doors opened. Eva stepped on, said, "Good day, Ms. Kowicki," and pressed the close button. Thankfully, the doors shut and she was alone.

On her cell, she read the numbers. It was Griff who called. She punched in his number.

"Eva where are you? I've been trying to reach you," he exclaimed.

"No kidding. I felt your urgency in front of the world's news media. Alexia's press conference, remember?"

Griff sighed. "I forgot about the groveling before the world because of Trenton."

"Okay, you're sorry. You got me now, in the elevator."

"Eva, I tried to be his partner, but he resisted. I don't know what more I should have done."

Before now, Eva had only considered her own hurt feelings. She had a lot to learn about leading a team. She said, "Griff, there is nothing you could have done. It is my fault for not supervising the shutting down of the pen registers. If only I had—"

Griff cut her off, "Ari was his supervisor, but Trenton did this to himself."

She asked, "What did Jacques say?"

The elevator reached the garage, and her cell connection broke off.

"Griff, can you hear me?"

Nothing but static. Eva got into her car. Once out of the garage, she pushed the send key. Griff's line was busy. Hang up, Griff! She pulled over to the curb on a side street and tried again. This time he answered.

"Eva, meet me at NGA. After hearing from Jacques, I called them. They have some satellite photos from yesterday. I'll tell you the rest there."

"I can be there in twenty minutes," she said, hanging up.

Things were moving fast, beyond her control. Admitting her fears to Scott helped relieve the worst of them. Ever since her promotion, Eva had been pushed to face dangers she never dealt with when working white-collar crime cases. And the fertility specialist was postponed, again.

There must be a better way. She and Scott woke at five and she left for work by six to avoid rush hour. They could move closer to their jobs, take a condo in the District. But, that was no life for kids. Besides, she loved her garden. Her emotions stirred up like a hot stew, Eva realized the things that bothered her were nothing compared to what Trenton faced. His offense did happen on Ari's watch. Still, she failed to notice that Trenton wasn't ready for the independence she gave him.

Signs were there, like what happened in London. He was so eager and likable, she thought of him like herself in younger years. Eva had taken him off Emile's case. It was his choice to transfer to Ari's task force. Like a parent who allowed a teenage son too much freedom, an inner voice told her she failed Trenton. She'd go to his sentencing and tell him so.

Guilty of obstructing justice. It was unbelievable. Trenton sat in his leather recliner, the one his folks gave him so he could watch the Daytona 500 in style. He could care less about the next Bristol race. He was a convicted criminal. The microwave beeped. His steak sandwich was hot, but he had no appetite for food.

A beer sounded better. It was just what he needed after the morning he had before Judge Pendergast. He twisted off the metal cap and took a long swig. The brew burned down his throat, but he liked the taste. Maybe after he finished this one, he'd have another. Trenton took the sandwich from the microwave and put it on a plate. He bit into it. The melted cheese tasted like glue. He threw it in the trash.

Trenton chugged down the beer and went for another. He heard a knock at his apartment door. He grabbed the bottle, twisted off the cap, and took another drink. The knocking became louder. Let them beat in the door. He was in no mood for company.

Trenton glanced out the window. Down front, he recognized his dad's car. Trenton frowned. He'd told him after court that he was busy. Trenton had run down the courthouse steps and roared out of the parking lot in Alexandria, the one he first parked in with Eva, and passed his dad on the sidewalk, trying to wave him down.

Duke never liked the word no. That was probably where Trenton got his stubbornness. Of course, his dad wasn't a criminal, like him. The knocking grew softer.

His dad said through the door, "Son, I saw your car. If you're home, let me in. Let's talk."

Trenton took another swig, then thought, what could it hurt for Duke to say how sorry he was about his son being a convict. Maybe he owed Dad that much. He unlocked and opened the door. Duke was still dressed in his going-to-court suit. A bottle of beer in one hand, Trenton motioned him in with the other.

His dad shut the door. Without commenting on the beer in Trenton's hand, even though Duke never drank, he said, "I came to apologize. You came to me for help on your case."

Trenton felt defensive, but said, "You didn't encourage me to break the law."

"How about we sit."

Trenton went to the couch, gave Duke the leather chair.

"Hear me out, son. I pushed you to get into the FBI, like me and your grandfather. That was part of it, wasn't it?"

Trenton nodded weakly. He guessed it was always in the back of his mind.

"That was wrong of me. Plain wrong. Can you forgive me?"

Trenton said, "Dad, I—"

Words stuck in his throat, tears stung his eyes. Trenton wiped them away with the back of his hand. "It was what I wanted, too. Now you can never be proud of me."

Duke walked over, sat next to him. He put an arm around his shoulders. "If you only knew how much I love you. None of this changes how I feel about you. You made a mistake, and now you're facing your punishment."

He paused, then said, "Your mother and I are facing it with you. Please don't turn to drink. Lean on us. Better yet, lean on the One who created you. I love you as my son, and the Lord loves you so much more."

In between sobs from both men, Trenton asked his Dad, "Can you forgive me, Dad?"

Duke Nash hugged his broken son and said, "I already have."

When he asked Trenton if he could pray for him, his son replied, "Okay."

At NGA, Griff and Eva examined the latest satellite photos of the *Crescent*, docked at Hadibu harbor. When the NGA rep went to get them coffee, Eva said "Quick. Tell me what Jacques said."

"His exact words were, 'Most of ARC's leaders are on Socotra. They plan to depart on the ship in four days. I will call before they leave.' Then, I lost the connection."

"Is El Samoud on the island?"

Griff pointed to a dark shape on the largest photo and said, "The ship's in port. Jacques is there. Where else would El Samoud be?"

Eva narrowed her eyes. "That's what I want to know. We need to see our contacts at the Department of Defense who are monitoring the transponder you planted. I hope your bags are packed."

Trenton got up early and drove to the spot he remembered. After his dad left the night before, he had poured the rest of the six pack down the drain, ate a peanut butter sandwich, and went to bed early. It was the best sleep he had gotten in weeks. When he awoke in his apartment, the fact that he was jobless settled upon him like a fresh blanket of snow, chilling him to the bone.

His life had been a flurry of activity since he started kindergarten, mostly because of Duke's career. When Trenton started college and got hired as a Deputy Sheriff, the long hours satisfied not only his drive to succeed, but a desire to be rarely alone.

He had thrown back the blankets and changed into running gear, not bothering with breakfast. On the long run, each time his feet hit the cold, hard pavement, Hannah's words pounded into his mind like a sharp nail.

Forget what she said, he told himself now. He shut off the car by the tall pine tree, its boughs bright green against the dull sky. Two years since he was here, Trenton hoped he could find what he was looking for. His Yankees ballcap was on the seat next to him. Trenton threw it in the back seat. He would never wear a baseball cap again.

As he stepped from the car, wind battered his face. Why did he think that throwing the Cubs cap in a wastebasket would remove suspicion from him? Instead, it proved the government's case. He wore it on the video. Trenton did not understand why he listened to Emile's call in the wire room.

Well, he could not go back now. Trenton tried to get his bearings. To the right of the splendid pine tree was a hedge of box elders that made a low wall. Trenton walked along the hedge, looking for another landmark. His meeting yesterday with Hannah at the GMU commons was the reason he was here today.

The tears in her eyes, tears for him, had moved him. She had given him information about Emile because she wanted him to see the good that Helpers was doing. Why didn't he? He had no answer then, and sure had none now.

The belief that Emile aided terrorists never left him. Now, Emile was free and Trenton was going to jail. It was not the first time his actions led to tragedy. Thoughts of Tena's death stung him. He kicked the ground with his foot, but his running shoe wasn't sturdy enough to absorb the blow. His toe jammed, sending sharp pains up his leg. If he pounded the ground with his fists, what good would it do?

Trenton did not see what he had come for, but he continued. The memory of Hannah's light touch smothered his heart. It was what she asked him to do that perplexed him. "Tell the Jubayls that you're sorry. As a Christian, Sari will forgive you. She is still sick from the whole mess."

Trenton would not tell Emile that. Or George, either. And hadn't Sari written a letter supporting terror? An inner voice reminded him that the other half of the letter talked about faith as his parents did. He had grown to despise their faith. Maybe that was why he tore off the bottom of the letter and threw it away. Despite their disappointment in him, his parents loved him. Their faith in God must mean something.

As a child, he did feel that love and closeness to Jesus. In Sunday School, he raised his hand along with Tena to show Jesus was his friend. Tena talked often of being a missionary in Papua New Guinea. He now saw that, with her death, that feeling of love had withered within him. In its place he had built a high wall around his heart, until he was certain no one could hurt him again.

Trenton reached the end of the hedgerow. Looking down, he saw it—the gray marble stone, carved with two praying hands. His hand reached down to touch the words, 'Beloved daughter and sister, Tena Nash.'

He cried aloud, "Tena, I should never have made you jump!"

Trenton slumped to his knees, by her grave. Oh, how it hurt to remember. His body convulsed with sobs long suppressed. He should suffer! Tena died because he coaxed her to jump. It was a mistake to come here.

Then, with the tears came a memory of something Tena once said, "You're the best big brother a girl ever had, 'T'." Through her words came the hope that she would forgive him if she was alive. Then the memory of his Dad, the one he looked up to for twenty-five years, asking *him* for forgiveness.

His frozen heart began to thaw. Trying to prove that pastor wrong all these years was in vain. Trenton needed to get his life on track; he had veered far from the upward path he had set for himself after Tena died. There, beside Tena's grave, years of shallowness and lies were unearthed.

Trenton needed forgiveness, first from his sister, whose death he never meant to cause. The words, "Forgive me, Tena," were hard placed, like driving up a mountain path over ruts and rocks and dangling close to the edge. They finally came, and the peace they brought was well worth the trouble to climb that mountain.

Hands rolled into fists, Trenton stayed awhile by Tena's grave, thankful no one else was in the cemetery. He had more business to attend to. With his shame and guilt fully before him, he laid it all before God. He asked him to forgive the wrongs he had committed and to be a part of his life.

Before leaving, he traced his finger over his sister's name on the stone. "Tena, with God's help, I'll do everything I can to live differently and make it up to you."

THIRTY EIGHT

Scott drove Eva and the kids to Richmond that morning to have breakfast with her folks. After blueberry pancakes and sausages, Scott winked at her as they sipped freshly ground coffee.

He asked, "Want to go for a ride"

Her Mom beamed. "Go have fun. Kaley and I will make gingerbread cookies. Andy and Grandpa are setting up the trains."

Laughing like college students about to play a joke, Eva and Scott piled into the van to complete the surprise party next week.

Scott opened the ornate wooden door at the banquet facility.

Eva asked, "Do you think Mom and Dad have a clue about the party?"

The manager ushered them into an office that had silk flower arrangements on every available surface.

Eva's cell phone rang. She had forgotten to turn off the ringer. "Scott, can you go over the menu? I know it's Saturday, but I need to see who it is."

She started to leave, but Scott protested, "I'm the fast food king, remember?"

"My case," she whispered.

Scott shook his heaad, turned to pictures of roast beef and duchess potatoes.

Eva went out to the parking lot and answered her call. Was Griff in the office on Saturday?

"Ma'am, this is Lieutenant Oliver at Naval Intelligence. I called your home and got your answering machine. My orders were to keep searching until I found you."

"You have me now." Eva held her breath.

"Ma'am, I am to give you the following message, 'The red moon is rising.'"

El Samoud's ship had left Hadibu! If Jacques called Griff to warn him, why hadn't Griff called her?

"Lieutenant, are you observing the moon? Is there anything more you can tell me?" On a cell, she was definitely limited in what she could ask, or say.

"Ma'am, you are to be at Andrews at 1600 hours today. Also, arrangements have been made for you to be joined by Mr. Miles in the region."

"Sir, I will be at Andrews on time."

The connection ended. She called Griff on his cell. After five rings, his voice mail came on. She left him a terse message for him to call her. In less than five hours, she had to go to her folks, get the kids, drive home, get her gear, and be at Andrews Air Force Base. And, it was a two-hour drive back home, if traffic cooperated.

Her face set, she hurried to find Scott, panic etched on her fine features.

Without a word, he said, "Fax us the menu we discussed." Scott placed his card on the table, took Eva by the arm, and escorted her outside.

"You look terrible. Are the kids all right?"

She nodded. "I have to fly out of Andrews at four today." Her bottom lip trembled.

Scott held her in his arms, knowing this might be his last chance until they reached Andrews.

"Your Mom and Dad will watch the kids tonight." He opened her door. "Then, you and I can talk all the way home."

Eva climbed in and called Griff at the office. When he did not pick up, she left another message. She did not intend to be the only one risking her life in the Indian Ocean, or wherever El Samoud was heading!

Sari was so glad to see George in the family room watching television, she decided to make him popcorn. On her way to the kitchen, she passed Emile coming down the stairs. Her family was together again, and she relished the togetherness, even if they were in separate rooms, not talking.

"Want some popcorn?" Sari asked Emile, who followed her to the kitchen.

She put a bag in the microwave and set the timer. Emile stopped long enough to tell her, "No," then continued toward the back door.

Sari stepped around the counter. Her heart skipped a beat.

Despite her facial paralysis, she said cheerfully, "If you're going to the office, look into airline tickets for Lebanon. We could all fly, pay respects to your mother," leaving unsaid that due to his being taken off the plane, Emile had not attended his mother's burial.

Emile's hand hovered over the doorknob. He turned to his wife, who lifted sagging lips with a tired smile.

"Do you mean it, Sari? You will go with me and George? You hate to fly."

Sari did not hesitate. This was something she must do. "I want to go soon."

The microwave bell sounded. Her popcorn was done. Emile seemed relaxed, now that the case against them was over and they had been cleared. Even the Washington Star ran the apology from Alexia Kyros. Helpers International had survived the dip in donations.

"I'll tell George."

Emile sounded happy for the first time in months, maybe years. Within moments, father and son returned to the kitchen. George, too, looked different.

"Mom, can we really all go?"

Sari nodded, then realized George's tongue stud was gone. She was ready to do this for her family. Besides, if she could find out about the diamonds and key, she would feel a whole lot better.

"Dad's taking me to buy new stuff for our trip!" George pushed his arms into his jacket. Emile closed the door to the garage.

"Your popcorn!" Sari cried.

Alone again, she plunged her hand into the popcorn bag. Did she have the courage to fly and face Lebanon again? She never told Emile why she refused to return. Tasting the salty treat, Sari scolded herself. Those days were over, and she should put them behind her. But could she?

On the chintz sofa, Sari drank her tea, glad she was giving happiness to those she loved. Of course, Emile was in the dark about her other motive for going. When the doorbell rang, she guessed it was the Palmers, coming to say goodbye. Their house was sold, and the movers were due any day to take away twenty years' worth of belongings. Sari planned to make them a chicken casserole for their last dinner at home.

She set down the Helpers International mug on a coaster and hurried to greet her friends. Sari was startled to see a young man wearing a leather jacket. She took a large step backward, prepared to close and lock the door on the stranger.

He said, "Please wait, Mrs. Jubayl. I am Trenton Nash, the deputy who worked on your case. May we speak a moment? I promise not to stay long."

"The one who rummaged through our trash?"

Trenton swept back his hair with his hand. "That's one of the things I want to talk about."

A flicker of sadness in his face appealed to her motherly instinct. The Palmers' car was in the driveway; she still had time to make them dinner. Sari opened the door and Trenton stepped in the front hall. The fresh scent of popcorn hung in the air.

"I am sorry," he said. "You have guests. I would have called, but thought you might not see me." He unzipped his jacket, but left it on. "What I have to say is best said face to face."

Skeptical, but wanting to know more about the man who worked so hard to arrest them, Sari motioned Trenton to sit. "There is no one else here. Would you like some popcorn and a soda?" Her lips pulled toward her chin as she talked.

Sari returned in a few moments and placed refreshments on a small table next to him.

Trenton sipped the cola, then said, "I was here the day your home was searched. You were handcuffed where you're sitting now. You might not recognize me."

Sari flinched at the memory but simply said, "It hurts to talk about it."

"Mrs. Jubayl, will you—"

She interrupted, "Call me Sari."

He smiled thinly. "All right. I am so sorry for the pain I caused, and I don't mean going through your trash. Many good officers do that to find evidence. I went too far and was wrong. This past week, I pleaded guilty in Court and am out on a bond until I am sentenced."

She could not believe he was apologizing. Was it a ploy for sympathy? "You caused us pain, with the TV news." She pointed to her face.

Trenton asked her to explain. Tears spilled down her cheek, but Sari wiped them away. She did not want to cry in front of this man.

Trenton was moved to say, "Mrs. Jubayl,—Sari—I need to ask. Can you forgive me?"

With the speed of lightning, she flashed to struggling against the handcuffs. Bitter words at Joe's Market: *"We don't shop with terrorists."* She had lain in a hospital bed, thinking she had a heart attack. How could he casually sit here and ask her to wipe it all away? The whispers, the taunts, the brick, the broken window, all told her, *Do not forgive him! He should roast with a conscience seared by a hot iron.*

While Sari struggled against a dark force resembling hate, Trenton drank his soda and waited. Dizziness rushed over her like a wave.

"Excuse me." She dragged herself up the stairs, and went to her room. Her blood pressure medicine was in her top dresser drawer. She took out the bottle of pills from next to the jar of cold cream.

Sari swallowed the pill, and tried to press down a bitterness she knew as a believer of Jesus she must relinquish. He forgave those who crucified him on the cross. She walked down the steps. Trenton was at the bottom looking up at her, his hands on the railing.

"Are you all right? I was afraid something happened."

His eager face broke down her resistance. In those few words, he seemed to care for her more than her family had in all the weeks of her illness. And this young man had been her persecutor!

"I do," Sari reached out her hand, "forgive you."

Trenton shook it. "Knowing you do not hate me will help me deal with prison."

This nice young man was going to prison? George didn't have to.

Trenton walked toward the front door. "Do you mind if I ask a question?"

"Okay." Sari felt a chill. She walked to the hall closet and put on a wool sweater.

"Did you write the letter I found in the stinky fish?"

Oh, that! She briefly nodded, not wanting to discuss it.

"You wrote it in two parts, which confused me. First, you made it sound like you saw the terrorists' side. 'Brothers in the struggle,' you said. Then, at the bottom when you talked about your faith, I thought George wrote that to convince us not to target him. It had the opposite effect. When the FBI said a woman wrote it, I did not know what to think."

Was he saying the letter she wrote made him think they were guilty? The truth weakened her legs. She reached out and steadied herself against the hallway table.

Trenton offered her his arm. With Sari leaning against him, he walked to the living room and helped her sit on the edge of the sofa.

"I was angry at you," she stuttered, her tongue feeling thick and useless. Sari's breathing became rapid. "Our trash ... thawed the fish ... tried to help George ... I was wrong."

Sari's cheeks flamed with red blotches.

Trenton asked, "Can I call someone? A doctor or a pastor?"

She managed to give him Thelma's number, whom Trenton reached. She promised to leave without delay.

Sari touched his arm. "Stay?"

Trenton waited for Thelma to arrive and held Sari's water glass. A glimmer of what Sari had experienced living in that family sprawled before Trenton like a morning dawn. Sari tried to help her son. Instead, she inflamed a case against her husband. Trenton helped her take a sip of water. Sari could be his mom. Now, this poor woman might never recover.

"Is there anything else I can do?"

"My medicine ..."

"Can I get it for you?"

"I took it."

Sari's breathing sounded more regular, for which Trenton was thankful. Still, with her flushed face, he wondered if he should call an ambulance. He lifted up a prayer for the second time that week. And it was the first time in a long time Trenton was concerned for someone besides himself.

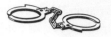

THIRTY NINE

Eva's ponytail slapped her in the nose as a brisk wind whipped across the deck of the aircraft carrier. She should have gotten a haircut, but there'd been no time. Operation Thunderbolt was underway. The Navy briefing over, Eva waited to see Griff depart, to fly over the *Crescent*.

The moment of reckoning was upon them. Purim and ARC's heinous attacks were four days away. Would the system Griff installed and tested on the ship work? If it didn't, the U.S. Navy had contingency plans to board and take the ship by force. But more lives were at risk under that scenario. Griff had seen weapons aboard, but there was no way he could have disabled or removed them without revealing his presence in ARC's inner sanctum.

Dressed in a dark green flight suit Griff joined Eva, and pointed at the E2C Hawkeye aircraft. "That's what I'm flying in! I wanted to get catapulted off in the Viking jet, like the one we arrived on, but the Navy techies insist I fly out with them."

Eva put both hands over her ears. "Flying in that jet is the last thing I want to do."

The Viking's abrupt tailhook landing on the *Constellation* had satisfied Eva's curiosity about Navy jets, for a long time. But perhaps Griff was on to something. The Hawkeye, with its propeller engines and giant mushroom-like radar dome on top, did not look very fast. Could it fly high enough to avoid a missile fired from the *Crescent*?

While Griff inspected the electronic device that would track ARC's trawler, Eva took in a deep breath of sea air. Before arriving on the carrier, they planned and counterplanned for every contingency. Operation Thunderbolt should succeed, yet something nagged at her.

Griff pointed to the LED screen on his control box, slightly larger than a PDA, and said, "The Navy told me their aircraft can find the ship's location without my device."

Eva did not like it. "No tricks. We can't afford to take *any* chances."

Eva was about to say she'd come along, when Brewster walked up, and Griff repeated the E2C pilot's claim.

The MI-5 agent replied, "You mean, the Navy thinks their radar will find ARC's ship if they know just part of the frequency for the transponder you installed?"

"Exactly!"

With a wave of his hand, Brewster dismissed his colleague. "With the Hawkeye, your chances of finding your target are twice as good."

"I'd be happier in the jet."

Eva knew one thing. If Griff's shenanigans blew any part of Operation Thunder Bolt, she'd have him fired. Eva told him so.

Griff's eyebrow shot up as he grinned. "It's under control. Watch and see."

Airmen started to board the E2C. Griff shook hands with his team, donned his flight helmet, and climbed aboard the Hawkeye. Eva wanted to trust that he properly connected all devices when he was aboard ARC's ship weeks ago. If only she could have been in that engine room, to see the test results for herself. Trenton had gone to London without her, and look what happened.

Then she realized what was bothering her. Jacques was supposed to call and let them know when the *Crescent* left Hadibu. He had not called! That meant one of two things: Either he had turned on them or was taken out by El Samoud. She had to get aboard ARC's ship and make sure the targets were arrested and every shred of evidence found.

But could she get there in time? Griff had not yet taken off in the Hawkeye. She had no idea how long it would take to execute his part of the plan. Eva prayed for God's help in capturing El Samoud. It was out of her hands.

Long after liftoff, Griff still scanned the horizon. The sun was beginning to set. They'd better find something soon. Yet Griff saw nothing but swells of the ocean.

Minutes later, his headset crackled and the pilot announced, "The radar operator says we should see the ship soon. Look out your window."

Griff moved closer to the window and looked through binoculars. Nothing. He set down the powerful eyes. He loved to fly and didn't feel claustrophobic. But the longer he was in the Hawkeye without spotting their target, he began to sweat.

He whispered, "You're out there somewhere, sweetheart. Show yourself."

Then an idea hit Griff like a body blow: Jacques had double-crossed them! He must have found the transponder and moved it to another vessel. Eva was right to be wary of the Frenchman, even if he did stand to split thirty million dollars. Admiral Topping's adage was true, "Old loyalties are like a hunting dog. You let them loose, and pure instinct takes over." And Griff had accused Trenton of being played for a fool by Farouk.

The pilot shouted in his ear, "There! Two o'clock position."

Griff's eyes drifted far below the aircraft and saw a dark object in the distance. But was it ARC's ship?

The pilot turned and nodded to Griff in the jump seat. "Your satellite feed should confirm my prediction. Our equipment has delivered us to your target."

Griff checked his monitor, then showed the LED screen to the pilot. He need not have worried. The second phase of Operation Thunderbolt was minutes away. Jacques was down there, and should be anticipating the problem that was about to befall him as captain.

Griff said, "You made me a believer."

Navy pride sprinkled in with his words like salt on steak, the pilot replied, "You should sleep better back home knowing we use nothing but the best to keep our country safe. We got you here, now it's your turn."

They flew high above ARC's trawler. Below, Griff saw the telltale white V of a wake, trailing behind what now appeared to be a toy boat.

Into the microphone on his headset, Griff warned the Navy flight crew, "Be alert. When I sneaked aboard in Socotra, they had crates of surface-to-air missiles."

The ship grew larger through the aircraft window. For the benefit of the techies aboard, Griff said, "When I was on the *Crescent*, I installed a special switch. It's radio controlled. When I push the button on this control box," he snapped his fingers, "the ship's engines will be starved of fuel and stop."

With no fanfare, Griff pressed the red button. Now he had to make sure it worked.

"Can you begin to turn? I want to keep the ship in sight."

The pilot lowered the wing on Griff's side of the aircraft. The ship's wake was beginning to fade! She was dead in the water. The engine shut down, just as Eva said that night in London. She had told him, "If it can work on a mobster's car, it can work on a terrorist's ship."

Griff knew that while Jacques would pretend to search for the problem, his efforts would be in vain. The ship would have to be rescued. By the American Navy, of course.

Griff gave the pilot a thumbs up. "Mission accomplished."

The pilot radioed their position back to the carrier. "Red moon disabled. Phase three of Operation Thunderbolt is a go."

Aboard the nuclear submarine USS Columbia, beneath the surface and just two miles from the *Crescent*, a detachment of fourteen Navy SEALs and two SEAL Lieutenants boarded a SEAL Delivery Vehicle, known as an SDV, which was housed in a Dry Deck Shelter affixed to the Columbia. The SDV launched from the shelter and transported the fourteen SEALs and two officers underwater to the *Crescent*.

Before daylight crept over the horizon, the SEALs popped to the surface. Twelve swam to the trawler in the cover of darkness and found ropes left dangling to the water's edge by the one on board who was in league with the U.S. government. Two SEALs remained in the SDV, beneath the surface. The Navy's special forces silently boarded the *Crescent*, ready to fight. They soon discovered the entire crew was asleep, in various rooms and suites, below deck. In the engine room, the captain and a crew member slept next to disassembled engine parts. The ship had drifted in the water for hours.

By first light, the SEALs had rounded up nineteen members of the Armed Revolutionary Cause, now prisoners confined in the dining area. To a man, they were surly and uncooperative. The SEALs had been told one ARC member was cooperating, but it was not evident by their hostile attitudes. Four SEALs searched for weapons and ensured there were no booby traps or rigged explosives that might threaten the USS *Constellation* when she arrived later that the morning.

Along with Brewster and Griff, who had safely returned, Eva watched from the bridge of the USS *Constellation* as the sun's early rays painted the horizon. The bright sentinel seemed as far away as her quest to take El Samoud in custody before March 14, three days from now. She was uneasy and would be until she had him in cuffs. Captain Wright, the commanding officer, had just briefed them on what happened during the night.

The SEALs successfully boarded the ship and took nineteen supposed ARC members into custody. But they had a problem. They were unable to identify those captured. No one was talking. The SEALs had yet to find out if the prisoners included El Samoud, the Cobra, or any ARC leaders.

Eva was desperate to get off the carrier and onto that ship! Captain Wright refused to helicopter them out. His stalling irked her. He was so military, he could not stand the thought of civilian law enforcement officers running the operation. The Captain dismissed several requests she made for a helicopter to take her, Griff, and Brewster out to ARC's trawler ahead of the *Constellation*. He was confident in the SEALs. They were trained to keep things secure until the carrier arrived. Eva replayed their multiple conversations, and anger worked like too much yeast in a batch of bread; it rose within her until she felt she'd burst.

The tall, seasoned captain entered the bridge and approached Griff. When he spoke, he had one of those gruff voices that sounded like a scratched record.

"Agent Topping, Lieutenant Fitzburgen of the SEALs informed me they have interrogated the prisoners. They are a bunch of low lifes. No one significant is on board."

Eva scowled at Brewster. She'd been afraid Jacques had found a way to warn El Samoud. But she wouldn't know for sure until they got on board. The sooner the better.

Eva tried to keep her temper concealed. "The SEALs are interrogating the crew? Captain, I insist we be taken there immediately."

Turning his weatherbeaten face toward her, he glared at her for a moment, then turned to Griff, "You will get there, in due time. The SEALs will counter any threats of violence."

Captain Wright ignored Brewster completely. That was understandable, since the Brit was a guest, with no authority on the operation. But,to not even look at Eva when he was speaking was rude.

Eva tried reasoning with him one more time. "El Samoud is under a sealed indictment in Virginia. As team leader, I represent the Secretary of Homeland Security and the Attorney General when I tell you he is a criminal defendant, not a prisoner of war. His underlings have been indicted as unnamed co-conspirators. While the SEALs are fantastic at what they do, I am uncomfortable with their collecting and preserving evidence on that ship, or interrogating defendants. Captain, I ask you again, please fly us out to that ship."

The Captain replied, "This is my ship. I decide how to use her assets."

Both of Griff's eyebrows arched. He went over to the coffee pot and topped off his cup.

Captain Wright said loudly, "Mrs. Montanna, we are just over two hours away. The SEALs will control things until we arrive. If we fly you out, it would take forty-five minutes to gear up. It is the extra expense I object to."

Eva recalled the meeting with the Chief of Naval Operations at the Defense Department. His promised support was severely lacking. In her dark blue ICE jacket, her Glock secured in her holster, Eva struck her most confident pose, and asked the Captain, "Will you patch me through to the Pentagon?"

"Mrs. Montanna, we have a chain of command. I will not."

Eva felt she was locked into a new war, an interagency one. She turned to Griff, who drank his coffee and looked out at the ever moving ocean. Eva had a plan to show this surly Captain a thing or two about chain of command, and started to leave the bridge.

Over her shoulder she said, "Griff, I'm going to my quarters to get my satellite phone."

Griff nodded, then sauntered over to Captain Wright. "The Chief of Naval Operations assured Mrs. Montanna and me that the Navy would do everything possible to make this mission a complete success. Your SEALs have control of the *Crescent*, but finding out if we have El Samoud and preserving evidence is what we consider a complete success."

Griff drank some coffee and asked casually, "Do you know the name of the Secretary of Defense's press secretary?"

Captain Wright looked puzzled. "Tall guy on the cable channels, Scott Montanna. Why?"

Before Griff answered, Wright gave a short whistle.

Griff said, "I think my boss, Mrs. Scott Montanna, is about to call her husband's boss, the Secretary of Defense." He disappeared through the hatch, letting his words soak in like spring rain.

Minutes later, Eva returned with her satellite phone, expecting to find Griff. Instead, she found a pleasant Captain Wright.

He held out his hand. "Agent Montanna, I have an SH-60H Seahawk helicopter with sufficient range to go to our captive ship and safely return. Two of my pilots need additional flight hours to maintain their proficiency. Stand ready to depart in eight minutes. Be on the flight deck with your party."

Surprised by his change in attitude, Eva nodded graciously to the Captain, "ICE is thankful for your assistance, sir."

The Seahawk descended, then hovered above ARC's ship. As Eva prepared to be lowered, adrenaline surged through her body. She stood behind Griff near an open door, with Brewster beside her. The Stars and Stripes furling in the breeze on the *Crescent's* mast, caused her to take a second look.

Eva shouted above the noise from the whirling blades, "Look! The SEALs remembered the important things!"

As close as safety permitted, the helicopter lowered near the stern of the ship. Griff dangled from a cable and dropped to the deck below. It was her turn. A crew member helped her into the cable harness and adjusted it for her lack of girth.

"Push off, Eva!" Brewster commanded from where he stood to follow her.

Eva jumped off and swung out at the end of the cable. The trawler's deck bobbed in the building waves, and she hoped she wouldn't have a hard landing. She was almost to the deck. Suddenly, the ship rose or the chopper dipped and she hit with a thud. For a split second, with everything swirling, her feet and ankles took the full punishment. Eva tasted blood, she'd bitten her lip. But at least she could walk!

She stepped out of the harness and walked slowly over to Griff, from where she watched Brewster execute a perfect descent, his years of Royal Service on fine display. The chopper banked and flew away, the cable harness trailing like a spider on a web.

The Commander of the SEALs approached in full tactical gear and extended his hand. "I'm Lieutenant Fitzburgen. You are?"

After introductions, he continued, "The crew is handcuffed and detained below the deck. They've been yelling in Arabic. One guy in particular is a real pain, fighting us all the way."

"Who is he?" Eva rubbed the pain in her ankle as her dad had taught when she was little and fell on her bike.

"No, idea but he's cussing up a storm in French, a language I speak fluently. I will not repeat what he said in front of you, ma'am."

"Does one stand out as their leader?" Brewster removed a small tape recorder from his flak jacket pocket. "We'll interview him first."

Fitzburgen turned to Eva. "My orders are to allow you to obtain evidence and conduct a criminal investigation. So far, we found RPGs, grenades, explosive materials, surface-to-air missiles, communications equipment, and on the Frenchman, a broken satellite phone. He claims it's not his, somebody gave it to him. You might be interested to know I was a JAG lawyer before joining the SEALs. If you want to split up interviewing them, I could help."

Eva asked, "Do you believe the prisoners are lying about El Samoud not being aboard?"

Fitzburgen motioned them away from the hatch so the captives below did not hear. "They pretend not to speak English. I think most do. There doesn't seem to be a leader, but with my Special Ops and Psy Ops training, I sense," he pointed down the hatch, "one of them down there is big."

Eva shot back, "How can you tell?"

"I see it in their eyes. For all their yelling, I see fear. Want to meet your prisoners?"

She ordered, "Brewster, you and I will talk to Frenchie. Griff, you and the Lieutenant talk to one of the others. Don't forget to remove the fuel cutoff switch so this ship runs under its own power."

Fitzburgen guided them below, but Eva pulled Griff aside on the stairs. "I plan to find out if Jacques is still on our side and who's aboard. Then we'll talk to the others. We don't want it to appear we are singling out our French connection."

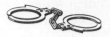

FORTY

In the men's room at the U.S. District Court, Trenton gazed in the mirror. He straightened the red, white, and blue tie he had worn at his Dad's official retirement party. In a navy suit and short haircut, he looked like an attorney ready to begin his case. Trenton closed his eyes to his reflection. He was no attorney. But there was one in the hall, waiting to defend Trenton.

Except for the strength from his newly acquired faith, Trenton would be heaving up breakfast. After telling his parents he had gone to Tena's grave, they hugged him and cried. Their outpouring of love convinced him to share with them something he had intended to keep to himself. Jesus had restored him to a relationship with God.

He washed his hands, then stepped into the corridor. His lawyer, Stan Ritchey, had told him the U.S. Supreme Court had recently ruled that the federal sentencing guidelines were advisory and not mandatory. Which meant that Judge Pendergast could sentence Trenton to anything less than the maximum of five years.

Under the guidelines, Trenton would get less time if the judge agreed he had "accepted responsibility" for his misdeeds. He might do six months in prison. If the judge did not agree, Mr. Ritchey thought he was looking at two years. No matter the time he served, he'd have a felony conviction the rest of his life.

His parents were talking to Sari Jubayl and his lawyer, who waved him over. His mom seemed scared. Trenton couldn't tell from the engaging smile on Stan's lean face that he had a client about to go to prison. Were all defense lawyers this pumped up before court?

Trenton said hello to Sari. Even though part of her face drooped, she looked healthier than she had the day he visited her. Was she here to help or to let the court know how much he hurt her? The tilted

smile on her face told him she would be fair, which was all he could
ask.

The elevator rang, and his insides lurched. Telling himself he could
not avoid Eva or Griff if they came, he was surprised to see Hannah
step through the doors. She looked great, dressed in a black dress and
flats. He moved toward her, then stopped. While he wanted to tell her
what happened to him since they last met, she might not want to talk
to him. Trenton edged back to his parents. Hannah nodded in recog-
nition, then walked past.

Stan pulled Trenton aside. "Who is that young lady? Is she involved in this?"

Trenton sighed. "Hannah works for Helpers International. She
was one of my informants, I guess. Why she's here," he shrugged. His
heart pounded at the sight of her.

"She is lovely. Let's hope she's here to support you. I'll ask Midge
Hopper if Hannah is here to speak on behalf of the government. Remember to say 'Yes, Your Honor,' and stand when Judge Pendergast
comes in. I reviewed your prepared statement. It's fine, but," Stan's
hand clenched Trenton's arm, "don't read from it, sound natural."

Trenton eased his arm from Stan's viselike grip. "I am sorry for
what I did."

His attorney nodded. "I know. We just have to convince Judge
Pendergast." Stan's light brown eyes, the same color as his hair, shone.
"His initial blast will be hot, but don't be afraid. While he is proud of
his legendary lectures to defendants, he aims to serve justice."

Stan disappeared behind heavy wooden doors with small square
windows and into his domain, the courtroom. Trenton peered through
a glass pane and saw his lawyer shake Hannah's hand, smiling the
whole time. He looked away and saw his parents and Sari staring at
him. Trenton held open the door.

With more bravado than he felt, he said, "Mom and Dad, thanks
for coming. We should go in."

His mom was dressed in her Sunday suit and matching coat.
Blonde curls framed her round face. She looked up at him, from her
height of barely five feet two, and whispered, "Dad and I have been
praying."

As his wife walked by, Duke said, "Son, tell the judge the truth.
That's the best way."

"I plan on it, Dad. You can count on me, this time."

When Sari reached him, she said, "I dreamed you planted a vineyard. People came from all around. You grew the best grapes ever grown. I believe all will be well."

Trenton shook his head in amazement. He had no idea what she was talking about. It looked like Griff and Eva were not coming. Trenton did not blame them for staying away. He followed Sari down the aisle, his eyes not wavering from the back of Stan's head.

As he sat next to his attorney, a U.S. Marshal stared at him from the wall next to their table. The AUSA, Midge Hopper, was seated at the table across from them. She wore a stern expression behind red-rimmed glasses. Sitting next to her, FBI Agent Lee looked as dour. They faced the elevated wooden bench, where Judge Pendergast would sit when he came in.

Wondering where the never-friendly Agent Custer had gone, Trenton was relieved he was absent. But what if he was in chambers, talking about him to the judge? Trenton was about to ask Stan, when his lawyer leaned over.

"Hannah wants to talk to you, but she's afraid if she cries, she'd upset you."

Trenton eased his head around. Two rows behind his parents, she looked straight at him, hands clasped under her chin. She blinked a couple times, then smiled. That smile would be a lifeline to hold onto when he lived behind bars.

The gavel banged. Trenton glanced at his parents, then pivoted his head to the front of the courtroom.

"This honorable court is now in session."

Judge Pendergast stepped from behind a mahogany wall. In his black robe, he was as intimidating as his reputation. He settled his six-foot-one-inch frame into a specially made leather chair. Silver spectacles posed on the edge of his nose. He called Midge Hopper to state her case for sentencing.

As part of the plea agreement, she made no recommendation, leaving it to Trenton's lawyer to convince the Judge his client was worthy of a break. The AUSA simply urged the Court to consider the seriousness of Trenton's offense, then gave Trenton a look that suggested he was slime.

"The government does not say much." The judge's eyes seemed to bore a hole right through Trenton. "I recall it gave up that right in the plea agreement. Mr. Ritchey, you may begin. Then, I have a few things to say to this defendant."

Judge Pendergast's voice dripped with ice. Trenton felt his insides shake. Stan walked to the podium where a microphone recorded every word. Trenton took a deep breath.

Stan began his plea for mercy. "Thank you, Your Honor. It is my privilege to represent Trenton Nash today, who fully acknowledges that, in the war against terror, he strove beyond the bounds of the law to make our country safe. While his motives were noble, his methods were not. As proof of his contrition, Sari Jubayl is here to address the court."

The government had no objection. Judge Pendergast called her to the witness stand where his clerk administered the oath. Sari promised to tell the truth, stated her name for the record, then sank into the chair. After Trenton's visit, she had gone back to the hospital.

Stan asked, "May I approach the witness, Your Honor?"

The judge did not look up from his writing. "You may."

Smiling, Trenton's lawyer walked over to Sari in the witness chair. In a gentle tone, like a grandfather speaking to an ill grandchild, he said, "You traveled some distance today, Mrs. Jubayl, and we appreciate your effort. Please tell the court of your meeting with Mr. Nash."

Sari looked puzzled. Trenton swallowed. That dream clinched it. She was taking too much medication.

"Do you mean Mr. Duke Nash, whom I met outside the courtroom, or his son, Trenton?"

"I apologize for the confusion. Please tell the court about Trenton Nash coming to your house and what he said to you."

"Objection, Your Honor. He is leading the witness."

Judge Pendergast gazed at Midge Hopper over his glasses. "This is a sentencing hearing, not a jury trial. I think the government can trust the court to consider what the witness says, and its importance, if any."

The judge said to Sari, "Take your time. What you went through must have been dreadful. Every news channel covered the search of your home and the arrest of your son. When the Department of Justice proclaimed your innocence, only local papers covered it. The court is anxious to hear what you have to say about this defendant."

Sari began to talk slowly. "I was stricken with Bell's palsy, because of ... everything."

The judge nodded profusely. Trenton imagined him thinking, "Nash is to blame for extreme cruelty. Throw the book at him."

"It's hard to speak. At first, I blamed Trenton for my difficulties," she stopped to swallow.

"Let me pour you a glass of water," Stan hurried to the table and returned to her with a glass. Trenton thought it might be better if her throat grew dry. So far, she'd said nothing to help.

Sari pushed the corner of her mouth up to keep the water from dribbling down her chin. "I was wrong. When he found my letter, he was doing his job."

Tears pooled in her eyes. She faced the judge. "I knew someone searched our garbage, and I was angry. What I wrote made it sound like we supported terrorists. I wanted to make fun of him and convince him we didn't. I was mixed up about my son."

Judge Pendergast gaped at her. Sari sniffed and drank more water. The courtroom was deathly quiet. Trenton's pulse throbbed in his ears.

"At the end, I wrote of my faith. By then, Trenton was convinced he found terrorists." Sari was crying now. "He came to see me and ask me to forgive him. I did. Your Honor, please do not send him to jail. It's my fault."

Stan Ritchey brought her a tissue from the table and said, "Thank you, Mrs. Jubayl."

Judge Pendergast asked, "Does the government want to question?"

As Stan sat beside Trenton, Midge Hopper rose at the opposite table.

"Just one, Your Honor. Mrs. Jubayl, are you asking the court to excuse what Trenton Nash did?"

Sari removed the tissue from her face. Her mouth pulled as she said, "But for my letter, he might not have thought we were criminals and been driven to break the law."

Trenton felt sorrow for her, as he was sure she felt for him.

"No further questions," said Midge Hopper, incredulously.

Pendergast adjusted his glasses, but gave no hint of what he thought. "You may step down, Mrs. Jubayl. Thank you for having the courage to come here today. The court has read the defense counsel's brief asking to place the defendant on probation due to his standing in the community. Do you have anything more to add, Mr. Ritchey?"

Stan did an admirable job arguing that Trenton deserved probation because he had no record and volunteered his time with the Boy
Scouts. Trenton loved that organization, having risen to Eagle Scout
by the time he was fifteen. He threw himself into earning his Eagle
rank after Tena died.

"Does the defendant wish to address the court?"

Trenton stood, his back straight, like his dad had taught him.
"Your Honor, Mrs. Jubayl is not to blame for my illegally listening to
her husband's phone call or falsifying my affidavit. It is true, her letter encouraged me to keep investigating, but I am the guilty one, not
Mrs. Jubayl. I am prepared for the court's punishment, whatever it may
be, and to pay for my crime."

He said nothing more, but thought plenty. Could he forgive himself for what he had done?

Judge Pendergast gathered his papers into his arms. "The court
will take a thirty minute recess to consider these developments."

"The defendant will please rise," ordered the court clerk.

Stan stood with him. Trenton's stomach flip-flopped like he was
on a roller coaster. Judge Pendergast's silver half-glasses dangled on
the edge of his nose, and his black eyes pierced Trenton's soul. The
look on the judge's face defeated any hope Trenton had for probation. Pendergast was about to hammer him. He steeled himself as he
had to when stopping a speeding car on the freeway in the dead of
night. No doubt, he'd be bunking with one of his former arrestees,
who could finish him off behind bars. He'd just be another victim of
prison violence.

Trenton told himself that, after the judge pronounced his sentence, he would not face his parents or Hannah. The sight of their
tears would undo him when he needed all his resolve to face prison.
Trenton sneaked a look at Stan, whose eyes stared at the judge's face.
Trenton had heard courtroom gossip that said if the judge meant to
go easy on a defendant, his left brow rose up. Which one was it for
him? He could not see.

The judge spoke. "This case bothers me for several reasons. First,
as a federal judge sworn to uphold our Constitution and laws, I am
grieved when a fellow officer who took the same oath treats it as if it
means nothing more than a movie ticket to be tossed out."

As Judge Pendergast shook his head, Trenton felt the greasy eggs
and bacon he had eaten two hours ago resurge in his stomach.

Stan kept his gaze steady and reached out to touch Trenton, as if to say, "Here comes the blast I warned you about."

The judge picked up a large brown envelope. "Mr. Nash, you entered an early plea to obstruction of justice, which resulted in the other charges being dropped. Under the federal sentencing guidelines, which I am taking under advisement in your case, the offense level is lower than if you were convicted of every crime you committed." He waved the envelope.

"This contains the letter Mrs. Jubayl testified she wrote. While on break, I read the part you so willingly used to frame her and her husband as suspects of terrorism. Throwing out the bottom-half was despicable, Mr. Nash. Such conduct by law enforcement is not to be tolerated. Like a rotten apple, you could infect the whole crate if you are not punished."

Here it comes. Stan said he could get two years in prison. Trenton could only hope he did not get more.

The judge's glare was steady, and Trenton wished the judge would get it over with. His parents must be in agony.

"Your illegal act casts doubt upon the veracity of other agents testifying in my court. You were caught. How many are out there, violating our laws?"

Spots of red appeared on the judge's cheeks. Pendergast took a sip of water from a glass. This judge had touched the depth of Trenton's crime. Someone wept softly behind him. Trenton wondered who it was, yet he did not dare remove his eyes from the judge. Three women sat there, and he had hurt them all in varying degrees. Dad, too, although he doubted he would cry openly in court.

"You brought a false affidavit before the court, and asked the court to believe it was true. We allowed the search of the home of innocent people. Such treachery erodes public trust in our legal institutions. I intended to sentence you to the maximum and not give you the two point reduction for acceptance of responsibility. Still, the court is moved by Mrs. Jubayl's plea for mercy. She has forgiven you, and the court does not take forgiveness lightly."

Judge Pendergast was still for a moment. He looked down to read something. Trenton was too far away to see what it was. The judge returned his penetrating gaze to the Defendant.

"The court read the fine memorandum prepared by your attorney. Mr. Ritchey has represented you well. The court is also mindful of your statement here today accepting the wrong you did, your community service, and your family's contribution to the justice system. Duke Nash served our government faithfully for thirty years and testified credibly before me several times." The judge looked at Duke and nodded.

"I have also read the letter from your former supervisor, Agent Montanna. She spoke highly of your work while under her charge; however, we do not agree with her that lack of guidance from her led to your lapse in judgment."

Judge Pendergast removed his glasses. "Trenton Nash, you are granted the two-point reduction. Therefore, the court sentences you to the custody of the Attorney General for a six-month prison term, to be followed by supervised release for at least one year. Mr. Ritchey, will you obtain the Standard Conditions of Release form for your client to sign?"

Stan took the papers from the clerk. Trenton stood in a stupor behind the table, not knowing whether to be elated at six months' incarceration or grieve at not getting probation. He found the judge was not finished.

"After your release from prison, you will reside with your father and mother for six months of home detention. The court recommends you serve your time at Eglin Air Force Base, away from criminals you might have arrested while a Jefferson County Sheriff's Deputy. The Court imposes the maximum fine of twenty-five thousand dollars and five thousand dollars in restitution to the Jubayls for medical expenses and to fix their door. Does the defendant understand the sentence? Are there any questions?"

Trenton whispered to Stan, "Can my dad take me to Eglin? Do they have to cuff me now?"

"I forgot," Stan replied. He quickly rectified his oversight and asked the judge if Trenton could have time to get his affairs in order.

Judge Pendergast looked at his folks again. "Duke Nash, will you faithfully discharge the courts' instructions and deliver your son to Eglin Air Force Base Correctional Facility, when the U.S. Marshal's office advises a date has been set for his arrival there?"

Trenton turned to look over his shoulder.

His face drawn, Duke stood ramrod straight and said forcefully, "Yes, Your Honor. His mother and I would be most grateful for that opportunity."

Judge Pendergast said, "So ordered." He stood and marched from the courtroom, his black robe the last thing Trenton saw before he felt a hand slap his back. It was Stan's.

"He really had me wondering there for a moment. You heard what he said. Even after reading our brief, he was still going to send you away for a couple of years. You owe a lot to Mrs. Jubayl. Go on and thank her."

His attorney shook his hand, then stuffed several legal manuals into his briefcase.

Trenton had someone else to thank. He would not have gone to see Sari without Hannah.

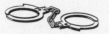

FORTY ONE

Eva stood in the hatch while Brewster grabbed Jacques by his greasy shirt, "Come with us, you big lug."

His hands cuffed, Jacques used strength from years of pounding metal to twist from his grip. Brewster jerked his arms and tightened the plastic cuffs. Jacques spit in the tough Brit's face and kicked with tremendous strength.

The other prisoners' reactions were swift, urging Jacques to resist. Eva was torn. His intense anger bothered her. Either he had second thoughts about taking that final step of turning in El Samoud, or he was acting for the comrades he betrayed. While Jacques allowed them on the *Crescent*, Eva was thankful Griff had the foresight not to permit him to know where the fuel cutoff switch was installed or how it worked.

Well schooled in restraining tactics, Brewster placed his thumb on the pressure point at the base of his prisoner's ear. When Jacques went limp, Brewster hauled him through the hatch. Eva scanned the room. As Griff and Fitzburgen removed a crew member, she noticed a swarthy man edge toward her.

"Griff, I'll get additional SEALs in here. Meanwhile, cuff their feet. I do not want any trying to swim to freedom."

She heard Jacques yelling, "*La, La.*" Eva knew a little Arabic, and that was no nursery rhyme. It was the Arabic word for "no." She asked the two SEALs who were guarding the hatch to the deck to cuff the prisoners' feet.

"Good idea, ma'am," one said.

If Jacques had followed her directives, El Samoud would be on the carrier by midday. She didn't want to even think what awaited them if he refused. Eva reached the galley. Brewster no longer dragged the Frenchman. Jacques sat on a crate, his head down, coughing.

Brewster put his foot up on a stone crock and leaned toward their informant, who was quite sullen. "Cut the act, partner. We don't have much time. This situation could blow apart, and we want you off this rusty bucket."

Jacques shook his head. In a thick French accent, he said, "If I tell you, I am a dead man. El Samoud's henchmen will track me down and do a permanent job on my throat." Jacques looked at Eva. With pleading eyes, he moaned, "Have mercy."

Eva squatted so she could peer into those eyes. "Like the terrorists showed mercy to the three thousand innocent people killed at New York and those in the Pentagon? My sister died at the hands of your 'Brotherhood of the Blood.' I know El Samoud is not the head of Al Qaeda, but you are one and the same. ARC murders women and children. I do not like you, but if you keep your bargain, our government has agreed you will not be charged."

Her knees ached, and Eva stood, disgusted with having to give one terrorist his freedom. "If you fail us, you and Camille will face trial in American courts, maybe even a military tribunal."

Brewster jumped at the thought. "Which is why I involved the Americans. It may be, you all want to be martyrs anyway, so your life means nothing to you."

Jacques coughed again.

Eva wondered aloud. "Maybe Griff already found El Samoud among the crew."

Brewster agreed. "If he has, we can avenge your sister's death."

Jacques' throat miraculously healed. "What about my reward?"

Eva replied, "If we capture El Samoud, you and Camille split thirty-three million. Other informants divide the rest."

Jacques spewed, "If you have another, you don't need me."

Eva paced away from the mercenary. Farouk and Jacques were alike in many ways, both out for blood but willing to suspend their ideology for the proper price. "And you don't need even one million. When we get the prisoners moved, we'll get another informant to identify El Samoud and save a lot of money." Eva began to leave.

Brewster raised Jacques to his feet and pushed him toward the hatch. He said to Eva, "It's good you're leaving. Jacques might resist and die while trying to escape."

Jacques refused to walk and stumbled forward. "Wait," he cried. As he fell, he banged his chin on a barrel. Blood spurted from the wound. Eva retraced her steps. Their ruse had worked.

In a mangled heap, Jacques was almost crying. "If I point you to El Samoud, you must assure me you will proceed with our original plan. I don't want to be confined with him, because he'll know for certain it was me."

Eva agreed. "You must go back down there or he'll be suspicious. Trust me."

Jacques sat on the crate and said, "El Samoud removed his *isharb* and blends in with the rest of the crew."

"What does he look like without the veil?" she asked.

Brewster helped Jacques to his feet.

Sweat glistened off his thick beard. The Frenchman sighed in resignation. "He took the black scarf from his face and tied it around his waist. Before he wiped black grease over his face, I saw many scars on his face. It is rumored he had smallpox in his youth. If you can get off the grease, you'll know."

Jacques looked down at Brewster. "Another scar runs down his whole left side of his face. As a child, El Samoud was told to stop his donkey cart but did not. A British officer christened him with his sword. He vowed revenge and has lived his whole life getting it."

Eva considered what Jacques had just said about El Samoud. Neither Camille nor Zayed had mentioned what moved ARC's leader to commit such evil acts, and she had never formed any picture of him as a child. With all the people he had killed and hurt, that was impossible. After meeting Camille, Eva had a better idea of what drove her.

What would it be like to come face-to-face with the leader of the world's most vicious terrorist organization? She would soon find out.

A thought struck Eva. "What about the Cobra, El Samoud's second in command? Which one is he?"

The big man shook his head. "He was not on Socotra when we left. I have no idea where he is."

Eva preceded Brewster and Jacques from the galley, down a narrow passageway, to where the SEALs guarded the ARC prisoners in the dining area. Besides being damp, the hold reeked of dirt, mildew, and remnants of cargoes past. A generator produced faint light, and she strained to see which one had grease marks on his face. Many men did. How clever!

Jacques still bled from his fall. For the benefit of his fellow terrorists, he disgorged a stream of hatred and profanity. With feigned outrage, Brewster dragged him to a support column and instructed a Navy SEAL, "Secure this one around this post. He will kill you if given the chance."

Eva went up the narrow stairway to the deck to find out if Griff had made any progress. The brightness of the sun, reflecting on the blue sea, hurt her eyes. In the distance, she saw the USS *Constellation*. The time to arrest El Samoud and find out what happened to Cobra was fast disappearing. Even if they arrested those on board, including ARC's leader, the Cobra would be free, an active culture to begin a new organization. The thought frightened her.

On the fantail of the ship, Eva spotted Griff and Fitzburgen questioning an Asian man. She motioned Griff to join her.

When he did, she asked, "Any success?"

"Most claim to speak no English. We're ready to return him below. And Jacques?"

"Resisted at first, but his mercenary self won out," Eva said, then added softly, "El Samoud is down there."

Eva gave him a rapid-fire explanation how the terrorist concealed his identity when the SEALs boarded. She nodded toward the Asian. "Let's take him below. Bring the one with a black scarf around his waist up here, so the four of us can pay him our respects."

Griff turned. She caught his arm. "It's important El Samoud doesn't find out Jacques fingered him."

"I'll handle it."

Griff and Fitzburgen escorted their prisoner down the steps to the dining area below. Eva followed at a discreet distance. After all the weeks of planning, El Samoud was within their grasp. Her eyes adjusted once more to the dimly lit area. Griff pushed the Asian prisoner toward the group.

Griff smiled broadly, placed an arm around that man's shoulder and said loudly, "Thank you. Thank you."

Eva stifled a laugh. He was placing the blame on him. Brilliant!

The Asian struggled to get away. As Eva moved closer, she saw his eyes grow wide, no doubt scared at being wrongfully credited for helping the Americans. Griff held fast onto his shoulder until a SEAL stepped forward and led the prisoner toward a support column to secure him.

To drive another wedge between the decoy and El Samoud, Griff said to the SEAL, "That's not necessary. He's helpful."

The SEAL cuffed him anyway. Griff scanned the other prisoners. He pointed to an older man with protruding ears and black scarf around the waist, and instructed Brewster, "Bring that woman here."

Eva stood inside the hatch so as to be invisible to their target. She wondered at Griff's strategy. Intentionally humiliating a terrorist would get him so angry he'd refuse to talk. But then, Brewster had bluffed with Jacques and won. She would let things play out a little while.

The MI-5 agent dragged El Samoud toward the door. His eyes flashed daggers at the Asian prisoner returned by Griff. Eva saw a look spill over El Samoud's face that reminded her of Camille and then some. It was a visage of pure hatred.

She ducked into the passageway to get away from El Samoud, whose face revealed more to her than streaks of grease. She'd been so busy convincing Captain Wright to fly them to the *Crescent*, she neglected the source of her strength. Eva remedied that now. She uttered a silent prayer. *Father, this man is evil. He means to kill us all if he can. Protect and guide us. Amen.*

Eva heard loud voices. She hurried around the corner. El Samoud was yelling in Arabic and she didn't understand what he was saying. She motioned for Fitzburgen's attention. El Samoud repeated his rant. Fitzburgen quickly translated, "He's shouting, 'Get your dirty hands off me, you demon!'"

Eva lunged into the room. "Get him out, now!"

Griff took hold of the flex cuffs securing his wrists, grabbed his prisoner's long hair and hauled him up the steps. Brewster followed. Eva and Lieutenant Fitzburgen stayed well behind El Samoud's bound feet which missed every other step. His chin banged against the stairs as he was hauled up.

Griff lugged El Samoud toward the fantail and taunted, "You may think this is ARC's cook, but I was just told this one is actually El Samoud." Griff used the flat of his hand and struck him on the shoulder, "Stand up straight! Look like the leader you think you are!"

Wishing Griff would give the jabs a rest, Eva sized up El Samoud. With his hands and feet cuffed, she found him lacking. It had happened to her before. After months locked in a struggle to capture a criminal foe, her mind created an impression of a more deserving adversary. No taller than she, he continued to struggle with the ties that bound him.

Eva looked in the terrorist's eyes. "I am told you are El Samoud. Is this correct?"

He stared at her blankly. In a thick accent, he said, "No English."

Brewster stepped betwen Griff and El Samoud and said in his striking British accent, "Maybe you need to hear it spoken as you learned it."

El Samoud's eyes flickered once to Eva's before he glared at Brewster. It was time for Eva to remove El Samoud's mask. She unbuttoned the left pocket of her cargo pants and removed a small bottle of hand sanitizer. She dripped some on her finger tips, stepped toward El Samoud and said, "Brewster, hold him still."

She reached toward his face. He struggled backwards and tipped his head away from her reach. Brewster tightened his grip and stood the murderer upright. "Easy fellow, you've forgotten that you are a prisoner. Stand here like a man, and this agent, who planned your capture, is going to examine you."

Brewster held his other arm as Eva rubbed the cleanser on the corner of his forehead and down the side of his face. Dirt and grease melted away. The man's pockmarks and scars became visible like the sun after a storm. He was El Samoud. Eva's two witnesses, Jacques and Zayed, could identify him.

Brewster leaned toward El Samoud's face and remarked, "No wonder you hide your face behind a veil. That British officer, whoever he was, really sliced you."

Whether Brewster meant to show empathy or derision, Eva was not sure. Later, when she thought about what happened next, she was certain his remarks were the match that lit El Samoud's fuse.

El Samoud started shouting as loudly as he could, "Destroy the satans of the world! Destroy the satans of the world!"

Those were the words Zayed said would trigger the massive attacks! Purim was only two days away. Maybe El Samoud had the power to transmit his instructions to Cobra at some other location. Just as Griff had installed the transponder, did ARC's leader have a secret way to communicate with his followers?

Before Eva could react, a chorus of shouts erupted from below deck. The other prisoners must have heard the rants. She hissed at Griff, "Get down there."

Griff and Lieutenant Fitzburgen had just gone through the hatch, when El Samoud wrenched away from Brewster. He lunged his small body toward a crate, and struck his hands and wrists against the edge. Eva was shocked by the strength El Samoud showed. In the next second, the flex cuffs burst apart, freeing his hands. Eva had heard of this happening only once before.

El Samoud spun around, still restrained at his feet. She reached for his arm just as Brewster's body enveloped the terrorist and they fell to the deck. El Samoud rolled over and was on top of Brewster. With the speed of a welter-weight, ARC's leader smashed his fists on Brewster's neck and chest. As if there were no nerve endings in his skull, El Samoud repeatedly slammed his head against Brewster's, screaming in Arabic. Brewster seemed dazed by the suddenness of the attack. He tried to reach his hands around El Samoud's neck, but was repelled by the ferocious blows.

Eva went for her gun. But if she shot El Samoud, she risked hitting Brewster. With one swift move, she removed a leather-covered leaded blackjack from the slot pocket of the side of her cargo pants and bashed him on the right side of his head, just above his ear. He fell over, on top of Brewster. The skin above his ear was folded back and bleeding, but he was suddenly still.

Bleeding from a cut on his chin, Brewster pushed El Samoud's limp body off of him. He panted to get his breath as Eva helped him ratchet steel cuffs around the prisoner's wrists.

After El Samoud regained consciousness, a SEAL medic wrapped a bandage around his head. Now came the rewarding moment Eva waited for, one she had rehearsed on the USS *Constellation*.

As the long-sought prisoner sat on the deck, Eva intoned, "El Samoud, leader of the Armed Revolutionary Cause, also known as the Scorpion, and killer of innocent men and women, you are under arrest for violating the laws of the United States, including acts of terrorism. You have the right to remain silent. Anything you say can be used against you in a court of law. You have the right to an attorney, and to have an attorney present when answering questions. If you cannot afford an attorney, one will be appointed for you by the court."

While he was entitled to the same rights as any other defendant, she knew he was thousands of times worse. She had to ask, "Do you understand your rights?"

She was not surprised when El Samoud answered in perfect English, "I do, and I want an attorney."

Out of the corner of her eye, Eva saw a launch from the USS *Constellation* bringing sailors and engineers. Griff and Fitzburgen had quieted the other prisoners and were back on deck.

Brewster whispered in her ear, "The Lieutenant and I can take care of El Samoud."

She nodded. "Griff, come with me. Brewster will get him ready."

Eva walked with Griff safely out of range from El Samoud. She said, "Disconnect the fuel kill switch, so the *Crescent* can follow the *Constellation* if Captain Wright designates someone to start her engines and pilot her."

Her tone turned even more serious. "We have another problem. Jacques claims the Cobra is not on board. You heard El Samoud shout the code words for massive attacks. Is there any way he could transmit those words to the Cobra and his followers not on the ship? Lives of thousands of people are at stake."

Griff's eyes narrowed. He glanced at El Samoud, handcuffed and sitting on the deck. "I think he originally intended to make a speech on some media outlet, but we arrested him first. He was probably shouting that command to those on board, hoping some might escape."

Eva shook her head, "Do you think he has a transmitter here on board that could have broadcast his command?"

Griff looked over his shoulder toward the *Constellation*, "While you start moving prisoners, I'll check the ship for transmitters."

Eva approached the SEAL guarding their ride back to the carrier and said, "Ready the launch for us to transport the prisoners. Get some other SEALs to help. That one," she pointed to El Samoud, "is cuffed hands and feet. He needs to be carried on and then closely guarded. "

The SEAL consulted the launch driver, then beckoned them. "Ma'am, you can leave now."

El Samoud thrashed like a fish out of water as two SEALs carried him into the launch. Besides the cuffs holding his hands and feet, he was cuffed to his seat. Several other ARC soldiers whose feet were uncuffed were loaded aboard and secured to their seats with flex cuffs. Jacques was led aboard by Lieutenant Fitzburgen, who struggled to cuff him to the seat. Secured only at his hands, Jacques jumped onto the seat, yelled a profanity in French, and dove into the water.

"Prisoner overboard," Fitzburgen shouted.

He and the other crew tried in vain to grab him. In moments, there was no sign of the Frenchman. Even the bubbles had disappeared.

Having heard via radio that the transport vessel was returning, Captain Wright waited for two SEALs to haul a prisoner, bound by his hands and feet, up the gangplank. Eva and Brewster followed their first prisoner aboard. The Captain greeted them with a practiced smile. "Welcome back aboard. Whom do we have here?"

The man lifted his head, and scowled at Brewster. His voice edged with hate, he said, "You will pay for what you have done to me."

Eva grabbed him by both arms so he faced the Captain. "Sir, this is El Samoud, the most wanted terrorist in the world. He needs a ride to a court appearance in the United States. We've told him you would be happy to provide the first leg of his trip."

Several nearby sailors murmured among themselves.

Captain Wright showed no emotion in front of the sailors and directed a lieutenant, "Take this man to the ship's brig."

His arms held by the Lieutenant and two MPs, El Samoud was dragged away.

Eva said to the captain, "Sir, Agent Topping and the engineers are determining if ARC's trawler can follow your carrier to port. Meanwhile, we have a problem. El Samoud's second in command is missing. Can you patch me through to the Pentagon?"

This time, Captain Wright did not hesitate. "Follow me."

As they walked away, the captain leaned toward Eva and whispered, "I just received word from the captain of the submarine *Columbia*. As arranged, the SEALs were bringing your Frenchman safely aboard. He swallowed a lot of salt water, but now has a little scuba diving experience."

Captain Wright winked at Eva as they headed to the command center.

Scott toggled through several highlighted words that were not misspelled. Spellchecker did not recognize them. Scott added those words to his computer's dictionary and printed the press release. It was a standard piece for Secretary Cabrini to update the nation on the war against terror. Nothing dramatic had happened lately. Yet Scott believed in keeping the public informed, even if it meant retelling which world leaders were cooperating with American military and law enforcement.

Scott placed his initials by his name, rolled the chair from his desk and walked toward his door. He did not hear the phone ring. Something made him glance at his desk and, when he did, he saw a blinking red light on the phone. *Eva!*

He had not heard from her since she first arrived on the *Constellation*. Scott scooted to his desk and grabbed the receiver, hoping to hear his wife's light voice.

"Hello Scott, it's Celia Cooper, from the *Washington Star*. I had a tip about the USS *Constellation*. Is it true an Arab man, believed to be El Samoud, was captured in the Indian Ocean?"

Scott drew in his breath, then blurted, "No comment."

A reporter with thirty years experience, Celia ignored his terse reply. "My source hinted there is concern whether it is El Samoud. What about ARCs' key leaders? Did we get them?"

Finding his composure, Scott responded truthfully, "I have no knowledge of El Samoud being seized anywhere."

"What about the claim your wife is the federal agent responsible for tracking El Samoud?"

Scott was willing to play the game if he could dissuade Celia from digging any deeper. "Ms. Cooper, surely you know spouses are not part of the Defense Department. We do not comment on private matters involving their lives."

Undeterred, she said, "Since you are employed by the Defense Department, have you seen your wife in the last two days?"

Scott nearly bit her head off. "Ms. Cooper, you keep asking questions about my family, and I will keep saying that you know the drill here. I was on the way out my door. I must sign off. Good bye."

Eva a hero? It would not surprise him, but he wished he could have heard it from her own lips and not from the biggest gadfly in Washington. Scott tore up the stale press release, then fed it to his triple shredder. This was incredible! Pride mixed with worry swelled his heart.

Scott rushed down the hall to find Secretary Cabrini. He was expecting to sign the press release, but surely he'd know if Eva had indeed made the world a safer place for them all.

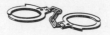

FORTY TWO

I t was cold for mid–March. Trenton rang the bell and waited for
it to be answered. He looked around and saw, for the first time it
seemed, enormous white clouds shaped like giant bears float by
with the steady breeze. Trenton absorbed every sight, every smell of
freedom. Next to the multicolored stone walk, tiny purple and yellow flowers had been coaxed by the sun from their sleep beneath the
earth.

The door opened. He turned. Hannah's freckled cheeks and vibrant green eyes shone on him more brightly than the sun ever could.
Her fresh beauty warmed his heart, but he had no right to tell her so.
Outside the courtroom, she asked him to call. That took courage. He
did call and now he was here, at her house.

She smiled a kind of half-smile, tinged with sadness and regret.
"Come in." Hannah shivered and quickly closed the door. "Can I take
your jacket?"

Trenton shook his head. "I won't stay long. Thanks for letting me
stop by."

Without a word, Hannah walked him to a porch with tall windows. She took a seat on a cushioned wicker sofa, and Trenton was
struck by golden light falling on her auburn hair. *Stop torturing yourself,
man. She can never be more than a friend to you, now.*

"I made flavored coffee, just how you like it."

She filled a cup from a carafe and handed it to him. He blew on
it and watched steam rise. She poured herself a cup.

Trenton drank the coffee in silence as if the sound of words would
cut like ice. At length, an urge to explain overpowered his fear of
hurting her. He put down his cup and leaned toward her, but not too
close.

"It meant so much seeing you at court. When I saw you cry, I doubted you would speak to me ever again. I regret—"

Hannah held up her free hand. "Let's not speak of the past."

Trenton closed, then opened his eyes. He saw glistening tears on her lashes.

He said, "Hear me out, just once."

Hannah flashed that half-smile again and said nothing.

He wished he knew her thoughts. Did she want him to leave?

In his mind, Trenton looked beyond her, to the tall pine tree in the still cemetery. "An amazing thing happened after you urged me to tell Sari Jubayl I was sorry. I was so annoyed at you." Trenton's laughter came easy as he told Hannah of his drive to Tena's grave and what he found there.

"My past is behind me, but in a different way than you think. I am a changed man, because of someone you know, too." Trenton could not keep the smile from his face, despite his circumstances. "Jesus has already made a difference in my life."

Hannah drew her hands together. "Thanks for telling me. It won't be so hard picturing you in a cell, knowing you are not alone."

This time, her smile radiated happiness. He had so much to ask her. Like, when he got out of prison, would she mind if he went with her to that little church? But, doubt assailed him. If he confessed his true feelings, she'd be outraged. Yet her glowing smile kept him sitting in the wicker chair drinking coffee that had grown lukewarm.

"Don't think of me in a cell. Remember, the judge recommended I go to a correctional facility at Eglin Air Force Base. My dad said that white-collar prisoners and those cooperating with the government go there. I'll be in a dormitory and can read, walk, work out."

Hannah smoothed the hair behind her ears. She said, "I'm glad to know that."

They looked at each other a moment and Trenton saw a pink blush climb up her cheeks.

She broke the awkward silence. "I have news. Helpers' donations went down since this whole thing began. Several of us lost our jobs and—"

He felt wretched. Was there no end to the havoc he had caused?

Trenton reached to touch her forearm. "My fault."

Hannah touched his hand with hers. "It's all right. I found a new job, one that's closer to what I want to do as a career."

She trilled a laugh that sounded forced, but when she explained, he thought maybe she was glad to be gone from Helpers.

"The Washington Star is starting me out as a copy clerk until I graduate." She said softly, "Mr. Jubayl was hard to get to know. He was kind one moment, aloof the next."

Trenton ignored the reference to Emile and shook her hand. "Congratulations!"

Was this a good time to mention his plan? Inviting him for coffee in her home was one thing. Being seen in public with him might offend her.

Instead, he asked something different. "What about your mother's job?" Trenton had not seen Penny Strobel since she was excused from the grand jury. That seemed a lifetime ago.

"I'll be back." Hannah went to replenish their coffee. When she returned, she explained, "She's visiting my grandmother in the nursing home."

Hannah had not spoken much about her family, and Trenton wondered about her father or siblings. Maybe one day he'd find out.

She drank some coffee, then added, "She's getting a new job, too. Jefferson Community Hospital hired her to coordinate hundreds of volunteers. Trenton, there is something else I want to tell you. About Helpers International."

The last thing he wanted was to hear about new evidence, but that turned out not to be Hannah's purpose.

"The Central Asian Director for Helpers spent time in prison. When he was young, he got drunk and killed a little girl riding her bike with his car. He served time for manslaughter, I think they call it. While there, he found Jesus and serves him in Kazakhstan. Maybe after you get out—"

Realizing she might find it difficult to use the word "prison," Trenton interjected, "I should like to meet him, one day."

That day seemed as distant as the planet Pluto. Still, she had brought up the subject of the future. Perhaps she was not entirely opposed to him.

"Hannah, will you go to dinner with me in Annapolis to celebrate your new job? We could see my folks for dessert. They saw you at court and want to meet you."

He left unsaid he would be free only a few more days. Hannah glanced his way, her green eyes searched his hazel ones. Trenton held his breath. When she stayed silent, he decided to make it easy on her.

And himself. Before she turned him down, he'd leave. Trenton stood, but Hannah reached for his hand.

"Can I let you know later? I should talk it over with my mom."

Trenton's face fell. No way her mother would let Hannah go out with him. He was a dope to think a guy going off to prison for violating the nation's trust had a chance with a woman like Hannah. It was time to end his misery.

Dull pain squeezed his heart. "Just remember, I'll always consider you one of the most important people I have ever met."

She refused to let go of his hand. "I wanted to ask my mom if it is okay to have you here for dinner. Some friends are coming from my church college group. Most are studying to go into missions and serve overseas, in places like Papua New Guinea. Can I call you later, after my mom gets home?"

That was weird. Papua New Guinea was where Tena had hoped to go. Two months ago, he would have laughed at her for having friends interested in church.

He replied, "If your mother is not okay with it, remember what I said."

Trenton smiled at her, then released her hand. He had to sometime. It may as well be now. He walked outside. Breathing in the cold air, he thought to himself that Hannah probably just thought he needed friends.

He opened his car door, turned, and looked toward the front door. He saw Hannah in the window, her hand up to the glass, waving at him.

Sari wished she had not agreed to fly to Lebanon. Their plane left at eight o'clock that night. Emile had gone upstairs carrying a flashlight and stick. What he was doing, she had no idea. George called an hour ago and said he'd be home for dinner. The problem was, she had not made any. She was too tired to cook.

"Sari, come up here!" Emile yelled down the stairs.

She stood slowly and climbed the stairs one at a time. Pain shot down her leg. Her Bell's palsy was not healed, but her lip did not droop as much. Thoughts of going to Lebanon, to face what she had done as a teen, made her sick. She had not kept down food all day. The ginger ale she drank tasted like soap and felt like hot sauce in her stomach.

The militants had warned her, "Carry our messages, or we kill your father and mother." So, Sari ran across the Green Line, that line separating Christian militia on the East from the PLO and Muslims on the West. With her own small fingers, she passed a message to Hezbollah forces.

Later that day, a bomb exploded on the East side, killing twelve children, one of them her friend. She had only told Thelma what she had done. It was always in her prayers, decades later. Emile had horrors from his own family. He never asked for details. Neither had Thelma.

"Sari!" Emile called again.

She leaned against the wall for support and walked into their bedroom. Suitcases were strewn about the bed and floor. No Emile. Sari poked her head into the master bathroom. Where was he? It had been so many years since she had visited her homeland, she did not know what to expect. After years of violence, it had taken a lifetime for Beirut to provide even the basics. She would never know if the message she carried killed those children. Yet these many years later, it haunted her.

She followed the sound of banging to George's room. Was he home already? It was not George, but Emile. He was crouched on his knees, and his head hovered over the heat duct. The metal register she had so carefully replaced weeks ago lay at his feet, along with a wad of duct tape and the ornate box she found. It was open.

"Emile, what is going on?" She felt an insane urge to laugh, with his arm shoved down the duct, a flashlight wobbling in his other hand.

"Stick your arm down here and see if you feel anything," he ordered.

Sari sunk to her knees, willing herself not to feel nauseous when she put her head down. "Tell me what I am looking for," she pretended.

Emile rolled out of the way. His voice shook. "George tampered with something important of mine. I hid it in here so it would not be found. Now it is gone!"

Sari pushed her arm in the dark hole, her mind reeling. The box and mysterious contents belonged to Emile! Did she dare admit she had what he searched for? All along, she had been afraid the gems and key meant George was involved in something illegal.

She found nothing in the duct and told Emile so. Sitting back on her heels, she admitted, "Emile, I must lie down for a few minutes."

Emile pounded the floor. "You are worried about sickness when our whole retirement is down the drain! I should have secured it at the bank. Sari, don't you understand George made off with thousands of dollars of assets intended for our retirement?"

Sari tried to calm him. "I think I can help, but I want to know exactly what you have been up to. After all that happened to us, I deserve that."

She coaxed Emile to sit with her on George's bed, which she had made that morning.

He ran his hands through his well-groomed hair. "It's simple. On my trips to the Middle East, I bought precious stones at bargain prices. You know how it is over there. I kept them in a small box I got in Lebanon. That box," he pointed to the one on the floor, "was taped in the register. Now, the diamonds are gone! The last time I checked, when you first went to the hospital, after the police searched our house, they were there."

Sari looked closely at Emile. Were those tears in his eyes? "Is that all you had in that box, Emile? I want to know."

Emile creased his brows. "Since you ask, Duma sent me a key. When my uncle died last year, he left me some money, which is in a safe deposit box in Beirut. I wanted to get it out and bring it home."

Sari squeezed his hand. "Why didn't you tell me this before? How much money, Emile?" She waited for his answer, which seemed ages in coming.

Emile stood up and walked over to the window. Some moments passed before he came and sat by her on the bed.

He took her hand. "I have not always treated you fairly. You were so caught up with George and Thelma and your prayer circle, there was little time for me. I began telling you less. I thought you were not interested in my work. He left me fifty-thousand dollars. I kept it in Lebanon as a nest egg. If it was nearby, I would be tempted to spend it. We need it to pay Harlan Scribbs and the polygraph examiner."

Sari was hurt by his words. He was saying his failure to talk was her fault, because she showed no interest in his work! Her memory was completely the opposite. She stopped asking, because he had stopped telling. How could she convince him she cared without sounding like one of those women on the afternoon talk shows? *Lord, help me with Emile. He has not talked with me so openly for years.*

A nudge in her spirit grew to a push. She edged closer to her husband and hugged him. No words, just a complete touch. When she felt his arms encircle her, love rekindled in her heart. She only hoped Emile felt it, too, and that they could build a future upon this moment. Her sickness vanished like fog in the warming sun.

She said, "I have something to show you. I found your box in George's room after the search and kept the key and gems safe all this time."

She thought a moment and offered him a suggestion. "Emile, you told me after your mother died she wanted you to send Duma fifty-thousand dollars. You should keep his money and he can take yours out of your safe deposit box in Lebanon."

Emile pulled his hand away. "That's not a good idea."

Sari laughed. "Oh, never mind. Everything is going to be all right, you'll see."

Since Scott received that cryptic phone call from Ms. Cooper, he managed to speak with Eva. She called on her satellite phone to say she was back from the *Constellation*. That was six hours ago. She said nothing about Operation Thunderbolt. Their connection was lost after thirty seconds.

Now he sat in the third row in the White House Rose Garden, behind the President's cabinet and members of Congress for this hastily called press conference. He was oblivious to the important leaders of the nation. His chief concern was his wife. Had she and her team made it back to the U.S.?

Because he suspected the conference was prompted by Eva's case, he warned the White House press secretary that Celia Cooper called about El Samoud's possible arrest. Wishing he knew what was happening with Eva, he crossed his long legs. Scott had shed a couple pounds since she flew out of Andrews Air Force Base five days ago. Even his mother-in-law's cooking failed to tempt him to eat.

Cold air gnawed at his face and ears. Scott pulled up the wool collar of his overcoat. It was too raw for an outdoor press conference. Secretary Cabrini explicitly said, during the ride over in the limo from the Pentagon, the President had great news for the nation and wanted the maximum coverage, which the Rose Garden inevitably garnered.

The President's personal assistant stepped to the microphones and gave the obligatory two-minute warning. Scott's cell phone pulsed against his waist band. With a split second to decide, he pressed the key to receive the call.

"Honey, it's me. We're on our way to meet with the President at the White House. After that, I'll come to see you. I miss you!"

At the sound of Eva's voice, relief and tenderness passed through Scott. He wanted to hold her in his arms. Instead, surrounded by politicians and diplomats, he hoped only she could hear, "I'm in the Rose Garden. The President is about to address the nation. Eva, it's not a regular briefing, but a live newscast. You may be the star attraction."

"You're kidding, right?"

Scott chuckled. Eva loathed publicity. She'd head for the office if she was driving. "Call it an educated hunch. Eva, I miss—oops, the President is on. Got to go."

Scott ended the call. Would Eva be asked to speak to the nation? The President approached the podium. Scott glanced across the aisle and recognized several reporters assigned to the White House. The Vice President, entire Cabinet, and Alexia Kyros, left their seats to stand behind the Commander in Chief, who stood in the cold dressed only in a suit.

The President, proud of his Scottish Highlander ancestors who had immigrated to America and fought in the Revolutionary War, spoke earnestly, "Courageous FBI and ICE agents and Navy SEALs captured one of the most ruthless terrorists of our time. Six months ago, we raised to fifty million dollars the reward for anyone who helped us capture El Samoud. That money will be paid to several who will never be identified."

The audience applauded. The President's smile and his sound bite were certain to be broadcast that night on the evening news. This was a major victory not only for the Administration but for the civilized world.

"This team of men and women seized twenty million dollars in ARC's hidden bank accounts. Most of ARC's hierarchy is in custody, along with their vile leader. El Samoud, also known as the Scorpion, will soon feel the sting of our courts of justice."

Applause again erupted. Alexia Kyros beamed, no doubt itching for him to be facing the justice he deserved. Secretary Cabrini vigorously nodded his head.

The President held up his right hand. "I wish I could assure all Americans these arrests mean our fight against terror is over. It is not. Even though El Samoud is in custody, we raise our security level to red, the highest level."

Strong murmurs rippled through the group. Scott was certain Eva's identity should never become known. The enemy lurked out there. She was a sure target if it was ever revealed she arrested ARC's leader. Scott looked all around. No Eva. No Griff. What had become of them? He could not see everyone who was seated. Maybe she was in the back.

The President concluded, "El Samoud's chief, also known as the Cobra, is still at large, and poised to strike American and Israeli targets throughout the world on Purim, one day from now. If you want to know more about the hideous nature of these terrorists, get a Bible and read the Book of Esther, where more than two thousand years ago, a man named Haman plotted to kill every Jew. El Samoud sees himself as a modern day Haman. Our intelligence has learned that he planned massive, simultaneous attacks in two known locations, the Eiffel Tower in Paris and the Western Wall in Jerusalem. There could be many others."

With both hands, the President gestured from one side of the audience to the other. "Every American, in the United States and around the world, must be vigilant. Purim begins in twelve hours. Our embassies are closed in Indonesia, Turkey, and in the Middle East. I am told our loyal team responsible for capturing El Samoud—"

Scott looked behind him, expecting to see Eva. He did not.

"—has not arrived. I had hoped to honor them today, but we will do so another time, for each one will receive the Presidential Medal of Freedom. I am not taking questions. We have work to do to secure our nation. May God continue to bless America."

The Cabinet dispersed. Scott's boss caught up with him. "The President sent a Secret Service detail to pick up your wife and team. I'm heading back to the Pentagon. You might want to wait. They called five minutes ago and were turning onto Pennsylvania Avenue. My wife and I want to have the two of you over for dinner."

Scott was surprised at how talkative the Secretary of Defense had become. Curious where this speech was heading, he quickly found out.

"Did you know your Congressman is retiring?"

Scott shook his head. What difference did that make?

"And the current Senator from Virginia who took my old seat may not run for another term. The President wants to back new, fresh candidates for those seats. With your military record as an Air Force captain and your wife's success today," he slapped Scott's arm, "imagine, a husband and wife team on the hill. First time it will have been done. You and Eva have time to think it over. Elections are twenty months away."

With that bombshell, the Secretary walked away, leaving Scott standing among all the reporters eager to get on the air El Samoud was in custody. But no one was more shocked than Scott. Cold air dried his open mouth. He swallowed. What would Eva say to the Secretary's audacious proposal? Is that why they had worked so hard, to give back to their country in an even bigger way? Running for office would definitely change the lives of their children.

He wandered to the seats being stacked by the ground crew and sat in one until a worker tapped him on the shoulder, "Sir, do you mind?"

"Sure."

Scott got up and walked out toward the security perimeter. Eva must not be coming. As Scott reached the gate, a large black SUV with smoky black windows approached the guard station. He cleared through the guard post and prepared to hail a cab when a car door slammed. He heard Eva's squeal, "Scott!"

She ran behind the large vehicle and fell into his arms. Kissing her, he held her tightly.

Eva looked up into his eyes. "We had a flat tire. Can you picture two Secret Service agents changing it in traffic? I missed you so much. I cannot wait to get back to our lives."

Scott smiled, and he wondered what their lives would hold a year from now. No matter what direction God purposed for them, they were together again.

Eva grabbed his hand. "One thing is certain. I'm through working hundreds of hours a month to catch these guys. You put one away and another springs up to take his place. I want to spend time with you and the kids." She squeezed his hand and wound his arm around her.

"Come on," she said. "I have so much to tell you."

Me too, Scott thought, as he hailed a cab.

"Excuse me, Mrs. Montanna. It's me, Kat, from Channel 14. Were you involved in the capture of El Samoud? Why weren't you at the press conference? You promised me a sto—"

Their cab pulled up, and Scott pushed Eva inside, leaving that Kat woman standing alone on the curb. He told the driver to take them back to the Pentagon, the place where they first met.

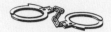

FORTY THREE

Four days later, Eva, sat at a table laid with tea and scones with Griff and Brewster at the Willard Hotel. They had spent most of the day in post-operational meetings at Homeland Security. Eva glanced at Brewster's chin and smothered a smile. Aside from his sutures that stuck out like little whiskers, he was recovered from his tangle with El Samoud. She was still very tired. Her energy tank was empty. Since El Samoud's arrest, Eva tried to catch up on her sleep. She had spent a tense Purim with the rest of her team knowing Cobra was an evil menace out there, waiting to kill.

Eva had done more than wait. She and Scott prayed together these last three nights. While no disaster occurred on Purim, Eva had a hard time accepting that Cobra had not been found. While she believed he would face God's justice one day, if *she* could find a way to stop him in this lifetime, she would. When Brewster summoned their server, her mind returned to the pleasant surroundings.

He asked, "Miss, please bring another pot of tea, and a refill for his coffee." He nodded toward Griff.

As the waitress walked away, Brewster mused, "Jacques will never forgive us for his near drowning. He told me he drank liters of salt water before the two SEALs were able to get an air tank on him and drag him into the SEAL Delivery Vehicle."

Eva chuckled, "Pity."

His voice tinged with pride, Griff replied, "Just think of the genius. If each of our informants keep their mouths shut, they will probably live to a ripe old age. It's possible none will be needed to testify against ARC. At this point, El Samoud is convinced each is dead."

Eva commended Brewster for his earlier idea. "The story you planted to the London papers about a couple drowning in the Thames

was brilliant. Do you think ARC believes that it was Farouk and Camille?"

Brewster hesitated. When the server left, he said, "Our intelligence
sources have filed reports that ARC sympathizers think the woman
was Camille, and the man was her lover from America."

Eva nodded. "Zayed, Jacques, and Camille will get their equal
shares of the fifty-million-dollar reward soon."

Griff laughed. "You finally got revenge on Farouk for spitting on
your shoe."

"That had nothing to do with it."

He replied, "If I remember right, it was *you* who said in our meeting this morning that, because of his attempted diamond smuggling
when he was supposed to be cooperating, he should not receive any
reward."

Her blue eyes shone. "Okay. But I was also the one who said
because he gave us information about Camille and Jacques, his cases
should be dismissed with prejudice—and Alexia agreed."

Brewster joined in with a question. "Nathan Barlow explained
that the witness protection program would change identities for the
four of them. Does that really work?"

Eva traded a glance with Griff. Usually it did, although in the past
government witnesses had gone on to commit other crimes. It was
not foolproof. The Canadian government had agreed Camille could
be relocated in the Quebec province. Zayed and Farouk would end
up wherever the witness program placed them. Jacques was leaning
toward Quebec to be near his sister.

"I know one thing. I would not want to be any of them, looking
over my shoulder every day, wondering if the Cobra was about to end
my life."

As Eva said that, she wished she'd left the words unsaid. The same
could be true for her. She had to trust God to protect her and her
family.

In Thelma's cozy kitchen, Sari smiled as her friend opened her gift.
Thelma slid a large knuckled finger under the lavender paper and
pulled out a beautiful green and yellow scarf.

As she wrapped the square around her shoulders, Thelma cooed,
"Honey, it's simply beautiful. I'm gonna wear it Sunday over my black
dress."

Sari's eyes grew wet as she replied, "For all your help, you deserve
so much more. I found it in a little shop in Beirut. Can you believe it
was made by women in a village in Africa for Helpers International?"

Thelma poured them more hot tea from a pot shaped like a roost-
er. "How was your trip? You look tired from the flight back, but your
lips seem to work better."

Sari stirred honey in her cup, then a bit of lemon. "They do. That
is only one of the wonderful things that has happened. My Bell's palsy
seems to be disappearing. I thought I'd be afraid. But once I landed, I
had such peace."

She touched the top of Thelma's hand. "Thanks for your prayers.
I felt them."

Silence descended as Sari gathered the words to explain what
happened. "Emile's cousin Duma was so kind. Emile and I stayed in a
suite in his large stone house. George was in an apartment room on
the top floor. Duma had guards and a security system. I felt safe. Everything was first class. His cook fixed Lebanese food like my mother."

Thelma passed Sari a platter heaped with banana walnut bread. "I
made it special after you called."

Sari picked up a thick slice and set it on a small plate.

"I prayed for God's help in healin' your past," Thelma said.

A slow smile lit Sari's face. "I visited my friend's grave, the one
who died after I—" Sari stopped. Thelma's eyes, warm and friendly,
urged her to continue. "She died in the bombing after I delivered that
message. I put spring flowers in a vase by her stone."

Sari wiped her eyes with a tissue.

"What about those gems and key?"

"Emile explained all that before we left." Sari quickly explained
how Emile was building them a retirement fund.

"Thelma, the funny thing is, I thought Emile would take me to
the bank when he withdrew the money from the safety deposit box.
But he didn't. He said we needed that money to pay his lawyer. I don't
think he even went to the bank."

Thelma bit into her banana bread, and chewed it carefully, before
saying, "Everything will be all right. Just leave it with the Lord."

Sari nodded. She had told Emile that very thing before they left
for Lebanon. She hoped Thelma was right.

It was May Day. The town of Bemidji, Minnesota still had gritty piles
of snow in shady places. Only a few locals had met their newest citi-

zen, Al Farris, who sat in his recently purchased 1987 Honda Civic. He stared at the towering statue of Paul Bunyan and his Ox, Babe, hating all that he saw. Al felt more than betrayed by the Marshals' Service. He felt alone, abandoned.

During the two meetings with the Marshals in Virginia, they had promised him a new identity, money to buy a car, and help in finding a job. Here he was in the far north. His car barely ran and needed a new muffler, but it was all he could afford. His efficiency apartment was dinky, one giant room with a separate bathroom, where the water in the shower never got hotter than lukewarm. Because Farouk had no work history in the name of Al Farris, his new identity, he could not find a job. He was reduced to living on a stipend of one thousand dollars a month.

Among the other promises the Marshals had yet to fulfill, Al waited for a response to the letter they had agreed to deliver to Camille. She lived elsewhere under a new identity. It was impossible to find her without help from a deputy marshal. His only hope now was that she would respond to his continued expressions of his great love for her. It was within her power to send him some funds, through the Marshal Service, so he could join her. But Al Farris had no way of knowing if the deputy marshal assigned to his case had, or ever would, deliver the letter to Camille.

Al started his car. At the rattle and roar of the old engine, a group of tourists gathered around Paul Bunyan turned to look at him. A large man, with a full head of black hair, scowled at him. Al jammed the shifter into drive. That man looked to Al like Drury Baptiste, his former source in the mailroom at Homeland Security. Even though he was in the Witness Protection Program, he wondered if he would *ever* feel safe from ARC. He sped away, then slowed the car as he turned a corner. He couldn't afford to be caught speeding.

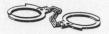

EPILOGUE

The cat in gloves catches no mice.

Benjamin Franklin

It was July, four months since El Samoud's capture. Like a snake with no head, ARC had been quiet. The Cobra had not been seen or heard from.

At the edge of a Kenyan village, near the Indian Ocean, Scott sat around a campfire. Eva was stretched out in a hammock, a green and yellow scarf wrapped over her shoulders. It was wonderful to see her relax after working so hard for months to dismantle ARC's terror network.

To surprise her, Scott contacted Helpers International about traveling to Kenya. Eva agreed and they were here, in Africa. Her hand dangled over the edge of the hammock. Scott wanted to hold it. Instead, he sat on the log, enjoying the sight of his wife swaying in the gentle breeze. His heart was glad.

"Scott, look." Eva pointed.

He popped up the flash on his camera and snapped a picture of Andy and Kaley stringing beads with the African girl Kaley had met at church last fall. Scott was strangely content, with no desire to think about the Pentagon, or the Secretary of Defense's strange proposal that he and Eva should run for Congress. She simply laughed when he told her.

Their host, the Kenyan Director for Helpers, hoisted a log on the fire. Orange embers floated in the air. Mombuto moved closer to Scott and said, "Mr. Jubayl asked me to give you a special welcome. Are you comfortable?"

"Certainly." Scott smiled.

From her resting place, Eva added, "The rice and chicken dish your wife made was good. I want to try to make it when we go home. What do you think of our marshmallows?"

It had been Kaley's idea to bring marshmallows to share with their hosts.

"The cooked outside fooled me about the melted inside." Mombuto clasped his hands, almost as if he was in prayer. "Mr. Jubayl is concerned your experience is a good one. He wants you to know about our work here."

"Please tell us more about what you do." Eva added, "We might return for an extended mission trip."

Scott chuckled. "You have a lot of leave saved up, but could you survive being away from work that long?"

Eva simply laid back her head and swung in the hammock.

Mr. Mombuto tossed another log on the fire, the ideal setting for his tale about building a school and children learning how to use computers. Scott stifled a yawn, but Mombuto was not finished.

His bony hands gestured to prove his point. "You should have seen me before I met Mr. Jubayl. I was a simple farmer and pastor of the village church. He has given me everything I have."

Scott waved his hands around the small village. "Your chapel and cement block houses?"

Mombuto picked up a stick and stirred the fire. "Mr. Jubayl donated fabric and sewing machines. He organized hundreds of women to sew thousands of scarves every year. They made the colorful one your wife wears. Mr. Jubayl arranges for them to be sold throughout the world. Our ministry keeps half of the proceeds."

Scott asked Mombuto what Emile did with the remaining half.

Expansive white teeth glistening against chocolate-colored skin, Mombuto said, "Mr. Jubayl told us to send the other half to aid the Brothers in the Struggle in Lebanon, Syria, and Sudan. But," Mombuto lowered his voice to a near whisper, "he is so humble. It is his way of helping them without others knowing."

Scott's head swiveled away from the flames. He stared at Mombuto. Hezbollah was in Lebanon. Sudan and Syria were terrorist nations, and U.S. citizens could not give them aid. Had Emile found a creative way to use others to fund terrorists? What did Eva think Emile was up to? She was so quiet.

He looked over at her lying in the hammock, heard her deep breathing. His wife, the ever ready federal agent, was fast asleep. It was the end of her first trimester, and she and the baby needed the rest. He did not have the heart to wake her.

ABOUT THE AUTHORS

Diane Munson has been an attorney for more than twenty years. She served the U.S. Department of Justice as an Assistant U.S. Attorney in Washington, D.C., where as a Federal Prosecutor she brought indictments, tried criminal cases, and argued appeals. Earlier, she served the Reagan Administration, appointed by Attorney General Edwin Meese, as Deputy Administrator of the Office of Juvenile Justice and Delinquency Prevention. She worked with the Justice Department, the U.S. Congress, and the White House on major policy and legal issues.

More recently she has been in a solo general practice specializing in helping families and representing children and parents in cases of neglect and abuse.

David Munson served as a Special Agent with the Naval Investigative Service, U.S. Customs, and U.S. Drug Enforcement Administration over a 27-year career. During his career he conducted many investigations and often assumed undercover roles. He infiltrated international drug smuggling organizations. In this role he traveled with drug dealers, met their suppliers in foreign countries, helped fly their drugs to the U.S., then feigned surprise when shipments were seized by law enforcement. Later his true identity was revealed when he testified against the group members in court.

While assigned to DEA headquarters in Washington, D.C., David served two years as a Congressional Fellow on the Senate Permanent Subcommittee on Investigations and as a staff investigator.

Prior to writing this novel, Diane and David were trained as Christian mediators and created a mediation firm where they helped many people seek forgiveness and restoration in their relationships by applying Scripture to their lives. They have seen that justice and forgiveness are possible, no matter the circumstances.

As they travel to research and cloister to write, they thank the Lord for the blessings of faith and family. David and Diane Munson live in western Michigan and are collaborating on their next novel.

www.DianeAndDavidMunson.com